Social Issues for Carers
A Community Care Perspective

Richard Webb, BSc (Soc.), MA, CQSW, PGCE
Lecturer in social care/social work
Parkwood College
Sheffield

and

David Tossell, BSc (Soc.), MSc, CQSW, PGCE
Lecturer in social care/social work
Kilburn College
London

Edward Arnold
A member of the Hodder Headline Group
LONDON   MELBOURNE   AUCKLAND

To my mother and father with love
Richard Webb

Edward Arnold is a division of Hodder Headline PLC
338 Euston Road, London NW1 3BH

First published in the United Kingdom 1991

9 8 7 6 5 4
99 98 97 96 95 94

British Library Cataloguing in Publication Data
Webb, Richard
Social issues for carers: A community care perspective.
I. Title   II. Tossell, David
361.3

ISBN 0-340-53598-9

Whilst the advice and information in this book is believed to be true and
accurate at the date of going to press, neither the authors nor the publisher
can accept any legal responsibility or liability for any errors or omissions
that may be made. All names of clients have been changed to protect
their identity.

Illustrations by David Tossell except where otherwise credited.

Typeset in Linotron Times by
Rowland Phototypesetting Limited, Bury St Edmunds, Suffolk
Printed and bound in the United Kingdom by
J W Arrowsmith Ltd, Bristol

Social Issues for Carers
A Community Care Perspective

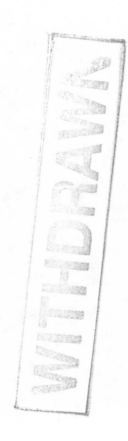

Contents

Preface   vii

Acknowledgements   viii

Introduction   ix

1   An unequal society   1

2   Social class and the creation of an 'underclass'   12

3   Women, gender, inequality and sexism   34

4   Racism, black people and discrimination   64

5   Other marginilized groups   95

    5.1 Introduction   95
    5.2 People with learning difficulties (mental handicap)   97
    5.3 People with HIV/AIDS   105
    5.4 Elders   109
    5.5 Single parent families   113
    5.6 Gypsies and travellers   119
    5.7 Gays and lesbians   124
    5.8 People with mental illness   131
    5.9 People with physical disabilities   139

6   Crime, policing and the penal system   151

7   The media in a democratic society   174

8   Social change, welfare and community care   191

9   Towards positive practice   217

Appendix: Useful addresses   235

References   239

Index   243

Preface

This book is aimed at a wide range of people who are involved in the care of others, whether professionally or on an informal basis in their own homes. It draws on a number of study areas including social care and social work practice, social policy, sociology and criminology.

We could not claim that this book provides a comprehensive academic analysis of society. Instead we have sought to focus on a range of social issues related to inequality, prejudice, discrimination and marginalization. Our aim has been to raise these issues for consideration, to stimulate discussion and to increase awareness of the effect of 'structural' disadvantage on individuals.

The issues dealt with in this book are often complex and controversial and invariably generate strong feelings and reactions whenever they are discussed. In a book of this size it would be impossible to fully explore all aspects of the issues raised. We have not sought to blame or accuse individuals for prejudiced views and behaviour; rather we have tried to shed some light on why discrimination has developed and why it occurs, and we have focused on the harmful effect of this process.

We are mindful of some of our own prejudices and limitations, which stem in part from the fact that we are two white, middle class men who have been brought up and exposed to the conditioning of British society. In order to present a fuller discussion of social issues, we have sought the assistance of a number of different people including women, people from ethnic minorities and people with different lifestyles and sexual orientation. Along with others we are engaged in the lengthy process of discovering and challenging our own behaviour. We hope that this book makes a contribution to a fuller appreciation of social issues and their significance for positive social care and social work practice.

Richard Webb
David Tossell
1991

Acknowledgements

We should like to thank the following people for their advice, assistance and time:

Hakim Adi, Jill Bendelow, Vaun Cutts, Ken Douglas, Bill Downie, Roy Fletcher, Wendy Foulger, Sarah Godley, Richard Grover, Rupert Hensser, Richard Johnston, Peter Latham, Elizabeth Leng, Marion Mathura, Aileen McDermott, Sue McIntosh, Alison Millerman, Howard Millerman, Robin Parker, Bob Prentice, Laura Timms, Phil Timms and Umut Ugur.

We are also indebted to Joyce Tossell for her grammatical insight. In addition, we should like to thank staff and students of both Parkwood College, Sheffield, and Kilburn College, London, for their ideas and support.

Introduction

Aims of this book

This book aims to consider some of the central issues concerned with social care. Caring takes place within a social setting and it is important that the significance of this social context is understood, in order that we as carers are able to appreciate the impact of the wider society on the individual. In this way it is possible to gain a more rounded perspective. It is otherwise far too easy to observe an individual, for example, a person with alcohol-related problems or someone who is physically abusive to members of her or his family, and blame that person, and say that she or he is entirely responsible for her or his situation. Categorizing individuals in this way may make the person making the judgements feel better, even superior, but it does not lead to a helpful understanding of the situation, nor point towards a resolution of the difficulties. Whilst it is fair to say that we are all in some way responsible for what we do, we are not always able to control our circumstances. An appreciation of the effect of external factors enables us to develop a more balanced and less judgemental view of the person we care for.

The focus and related themes

At the root of many clients' experience is a powerlessness which often results in their isolation. Whether working professionally in the field, residential or day care settings, or as carers looking after the needs of dependent adults or young children, social carers and social workers are automatically in a position of power, since those we care for are in some way reliant on us for help in various forms. This help may range from providing counselling advice to giving assistance with practical tasks, which are often those of a highly personal nature. As carers, it is important that we acknowledge the power we have and understand its contribution to the relationship with the client or person for whom we are caring.

In addition to examining the influence of power which exists in the inter-action between individual people, we need also to look at the general distribution of power within society to establish which groups of people hold power and which groups of people are excluded from positions of influence and privilege, and are consequently unable to take a full part in the social, economic and political life of this country. These latter groups, comprising people with similar situations, can be seen to be relatively powerless because they are denied access to many of society's resources. Because of their gender, race, age, religion, sexuality, health, lifestyle, low income, or as a result of a

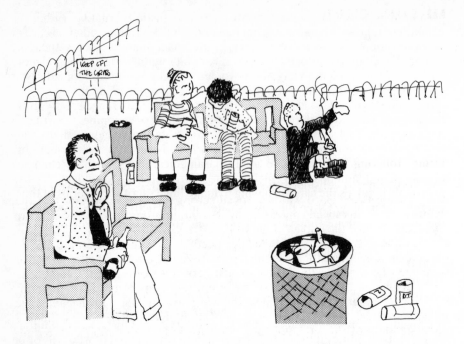

To what extent is society responsible?

combination of any of these factors, people are seen to be experiencing what is known as marginalization – they are said to be marginalized. This process is a central theme of the book.

Social issues are important to carers for two reasons. First, as carers, we need to be aware of the social influences on our clients. Second, as members of society we need to recognize its impact on our own lives. In both circumstances we need to acknowledge the interactional relationship between the individual and society as they are both shaped by and help to shape each other.

Who are the carers?

Most care takes place in the home. Only a relatively small number of people are permanently cared for in institutional or residential accommodation. All children are nurtured and reared in a variety of different home settings. In addition, there are many people who owing to disability, fragility, learning difficulties and behavioural patterns, require continued care. It is currently estimated that one adult in seven in Great Britain is looking after an elderly or disabled person, a figure which represents six million carers overall (OPCS, 1988b).

'Informal' carers
It would be wrong to assume that 'informal' carers who care in our society from the home have always freely chosen to undertake this role. Many have little or

no option because of the lack of a satisfactory, realistic alternative. Either the dependent relative's condition is not bad enough to warrant residential care or hospitalization, or community services are inadequate or not sufficiently developed. Consequently, the burden of care falls mainly on families and more particularly on women. In fact, more women stay at home to care for elderly or disabled relatives than stay at home to look after young children.

The time involved in caring for a dependent relative can range greatly, from a few hours a day to prepare a meal, or to do washing or shopping, to virtual 24 hour support. Tasks undertaken will also vary from simple help with dressing and feeding to more complex or arduous ones. These may include bathing, lifting, toileting and having to apply paramedical skills, such as changing dressings and administering medication. Caring for a dependent relative invariably involves the carer in having to make huge sacrifices in terms of time, energy and money. Often they are isolated in their activity since essentially it ties them to the home, and carers forsake their own involvement in the outside world. Opportunities for paid work and career progression may be sacrificed and their social and leisure time is severely curtailed.

Volunteers

Many organizations in our society depend for their successful functioning on the unpaid efforts and dedication of volunteers. Some voluntary and self-help organizations rely almost exclusively on voluntary help. Other larger voluntary and statutory bodies depend to a lesser extent on volunteers who will often complement the work of paid employees. The motivation to volunteer is varied: for example, some people may not have satisfactory human contact in their daily lives, and have a need to help others; unemployed people may find voluntary work provides a source of fulfilment; others may use the opportunity to gain experience and knowledge in the field of social care or social work. Some people, of course, have a committed spiritual or humanitarian motivation, and others simply have a strong moral conscience.

Social carers

So far we have discussed people who are not paid for their caring. We now turn to those who are paid to care for others. There has traditionally been in this country a somewhat artificial distinction between that which is considered to be *social care* and that which is regarded as *social work*.

Social care has come to be understood to mean only the direct physical care of clients, i.e. washing, dressing, feeding and toileting of the client. Social work on the other hand still stands for purposeful enabling intervention on behalf of the whole person. This has arisen mainly as a result of historical factors. Although there have been social workers and social work training since the beginning of the century, social work practice as it is known today did not become established until the late 1950s when it began to incorporate the prevalent psychoanalytical theories of the time. Since then there has been the establishment in 1971 of the Social Services Departments in England and Wales and the Social Work Departments in Scotland which were created following the Social Work (Scotland) Act 1968. Training has become established within Higher Education for both social workers and probation officers and social work has used such developments to press its claim for professional status. Partly as a consequence, social work has been at pains to distance itself from the more pragmatic, routine element of its function which has in turn been seen to be the province of social care.

A difference in status developed between field social workers and their contemporaries who worked in residential, domiciliary and day care settings. This was compounded by the tendency for field workers to be provided with Certificate of Qualification in Social Work (CQSW) training which was full-time and offered almost exclusively in institutions of Higher Education, while residential and other workers were mainly expected to undertake Certificate in Social Services (CSS) training which was provided on a day release basis and required the student to remain at work. When CSS was first introduced in 1975, it was not regarded as a professional qualification. It was only after it became recognized that the work carried out on the CSS was as thorough and comprehensive as that undertaken on CQSW courses, that they were, in November 1987, officially deemed to be equivalent by the Central Council for Education and Training in Social Work (CCETSW) and social work trade unions and professional organizations. Whereas the majority of field social workers have received professional training, only a minority of residential social workers have had the opportunity to qualify.

The distinction between social care and social work is misleading for two main reasons. First, because physical care is not carried out in isolation. It is an integral part of what has been traditionally regarded as social work. When, for example, a care plan is designed for an elderly person, the person's physical needs such as the planned visit to the chiropodist, the required changing of dressings, dietary needs and toileting arrangements are taken into considera-tion – so too are the client's social needs, such as the need to maintain links with loved ones and to attend gatherings wherever possible. Similarly, the client's intellectual need to be stimulated and to be engaged as much as possible in the surroundings is taken into account, together with the emotional and psycholog-ical need to be able to take risks and make decisions, to express oneself and to feel valued. The client's cultural requirements are also acknowledged and arrangements made to accommodate them. Physical care, essential as it is, is neither more nor less important than any of the other elements of the social work task.

Second, in order to be carried out properly, physical care cannot be performed without an understanding of the whole person; the need for privacy, the need for time and space, and a person's right to have her or his cultural expectations met. In other words what is commonly regarded as social care still needs to be directed by social work principles.

Although in practice those people who are employed primarily as social care workers are predominatly concerned with the immediate, practical caring tasks of clients, their actions form part of a process of social work intervention. In this way social care can be seen to be part of social work.

Social work and social care are part of the same continuum; they overlap in practice. The field social worker may well be called upon to attend to the personal needs of her or his physically disabled clients; medical social workers may well have cause to deal with their clients' incontinence on home visits in the community. In the same way, residential social workers, particularly key workers, are in a position to offer sustained emotional support and case work intervention equivalent to that provided by their field work colleagues. Care assistants or care officers and other residential staff, by nature of their situation are often well placed to form meaningful relationships with clients and so contribute to the social work process. As Joan Beck, President of the Social Care Association, says, 'Living with your clients day in and day out provides the ideal situation to carry out social work. Even doing something like washing up together provides a natural environment in which to talk, unlike the artificial "home visit" situation' (*Social Work Today*, 19 October 1989, p. 12).

Among practitioners and academics alike there is no universal agreement about what constitutes social care and what constitutes social work. Consider the following definition. In your opinion does it relate to social care or social work?

'The *term* used to describe the activities and processes undertaken by all sectors/ agencies (statutory, voluntary and independent) which seek to enable individuals, families and groups who are disadvantaged, or deprived in some way, to achieve a higher, self-determined level of functioning and quality of life. It is about the planned meeting of client's needs. It concerns the physical, intellectual, emotional, cultural and social aspects of the client's development and well-being. It involves mutual trust and respect; it involves a sense of purpose and change; it recognizes the interaction between people and their environments.'

(Mallinson, I., 1988)

In fact the author was defining social care. However, it can be seen from the content that this definition is very similar to a description of conventional social work.

One way of clarifying the confusion that exists between social care and social work is not to focus on the separate tasks carried out by different workers or on the authority and responsibility invested in particular roles. Instead we need to consider the whole activity which is defined either as social care or social work.

As we have already stated social care and social work can be seen to be part of the same continuum, which the diagram overleaf illustrates. It shows the range of personal needs which can be met by the activity of social care and social work. As we move from social care on the left along the continuum towards social work on the right, we pass from more basic, physiological needs, through emotional and cultural needs, to less tangible and more general psychological and social needs. Social care informs social work, just as social work informs social care.

The undervaluing of caring

There can be no doubt that caring, whether informal, voluntary or paid, is seriously undervalued in our society. It is chiefly carried out by women and is largely taken for granted; furthermore, it is usually unpaid. This undervaluing results in a general low status for all those involved in caring. It is manifested in the absence of resources and support available for 'informal' carers and it is reflected in the relatively low salaries of qualified nurses and social workers compared to other professions, and the poor remuneration that residential domiciliary and day care workers and health care workers receive.

Social carers, domicilliary workers and health care workers are predomi-

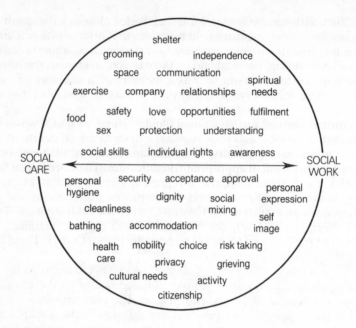

shelter
grooming   independence
space   communication
                              spiritual
exercise   company   relationships   needs
        safety   love   opportunities   fulfilment
food
    sex   protection   understanding
        social skills   individual rights   awareness

SOCIAL   SOCIAL
CARE ──────────────────────────────────▶ WORK

personal   security   acceptance approval
hygiene   personal
        dignity   social   expression
cleanliness   mixing
                                              self
bathing   accommodation   image
    health   mobility   choice   risk taking
    care   privacy   grieving
        cultural needs   activity
            citizenship

Fig. (i)   The continuum of social care and social work.

nantly female and they are also disproportionately from working class backgrounds and many of them are black. This contrasts sharply with the make-up of senior and managerial personnel, who are predominantly white and male. The very name 'care assistant' trivializes the work that is done by social carers and fails to convey accurately the responsibilities they undertake. This is now recognized by some authorities who are rejecting the title of 'care assistants' in favour of 'care officers'. Similarly the range of work and responsibilities carried out by 'home helps' has now been acknowledged and they are now being increasingly referred to more broadly as 'home carers'.

There are other encouraging signs of the revaluing of both social care and health care. The aims of National Vocational Qualifications (NVQ) in England, Wales and Northern Ireland (or Scottish Vocational Qualifications – SVQ) to achieve a better qualified work force will hopefully enhance status and financial rewards. At the same time, the general public's perception of care may become more positive and a fuller understanding of its importance may result.

National Vocational Qualifications (NVQ) and Scottish Vocational Qualifications (SVQ)

Many of you reading this book may be involved in preparation for assessment in the workplace under the newly created NVQ or SVQ arrangements. It is important that those who care for others are acknowledged for the competence and efficiency with which they perform their tasks, although there will always be some immeasurable qualities held by carers that no assessor will discover. However, it is vital that carers recognize fully the needs of others; needs which extend well beyond the hospital bed or the day centre lounge: the need to be understood as a whole person, not as a member of a client group, defined perhaps by their disability, but firstly as a person who also has certain difficulties.

The National Council for Vocational Qualifications (NCVQ) was set up by the Government in 1986 as a response to the acknowledged dearth of trained personnel throughout all industry. Less than ten per cent of all those working in social care had any form of appropriate qualification. The Care Sector Consortium (CSC) was formed comprising representatives from employers in the statutory, voluntary and private sectors, employee trade unions and professional training bodies, such as the Central Council for Education and Training in Social Work (CCETSW), the National Health Service Training Agency (NHSTA) and the City and Guilds of London Institute (CGLI). There is also a care sector liaison group in Scotland.

The CSC has made an analysis of all the tasks involved in caring for people and as a result has drawn up a complete breakdown of all the competences necessary for effective social and health care. The new scheme is 'employer-led' and as far as possible competences are assessed in the workplace, using mainly 'naturalistic observation'. In other words people employed as social carers or health care support workers can now be tested on their performance in the work-place for their practical competence and knowledge. This represents a departure from traditional training where educational establishments and professional awarding bodies have determined the criteria for training. Now employers themselves have made clear the requirements they want social and health carers to possess. In theory at least, it is now possible for an employee to receive no outside training and be tested for job competence within the work setting based on her or his ability to perform certain prescribed tasks. (For further details of NVQ and SVQ see Chapter 8).

How to use this book

This book is designed to be read sequentially or to be dipped into selectively according to the reader's interests. Whichever way you decide to use the book we would stress the importance of you initially familiarizing yourself with the material contained in Chapter 1.

This chapter, entitled 'An Unequal Society', outlines the main themes of the book and clarifies all the key concepts used. It describes how inequality is structured mainly along the lines of class, gender and race. The next three chapters are devoted to each of these elements separately, in order that they may be considered independently. Chapter 2 focuses on class, Chapter 3 looks at women and sexism and Chapter 4 examines issues of race. Chapter 5 outlines how a number of minority groups in society are similarly affected, and denied full social participation. Chapter 6 'Crime, Policing and the Penal System' examines how members of the working class, women, black people and some minority groups have a different experience of crime and social control agencies compared to others in society. Chapter 7 considers the influence of the media in forming public opinion and in shaping prejudiced attitudes to the social groups discussed throughout this book. Chapter 8 reflects on how economic, political and social policies affect structural inequality and comments on future developments in the field of nursing and social care as well as in the wider society. Finally, Chapter 9 examines strategies for change which involve positive practice that can be adopted by individual carers and incorporated into their daily work.

In addition to the text the book contains a number of diagrams, illustrations and quotations from literary sources, and at the end of each chapter there are exercises, questions for essays or discussion and suggestions for further reading. The further reading is made up of both academic references and literary sources. In some instances, we have recommended one specific work by an author, although several of her or his publications could equally have been recommended, as they cover similar or closely related themes.

Exercises
These are designed to broaden the reader's understanding of the issues and to help them to think through the practical implications, particularly in relation to caring. Directions are given on how these exercises may be carried out, although these may be modified to suit the needs of particular groups or settings. All case study material is based on real situations, but the names are fictitious for reasons of confidentiality.

Questions for essays or discussion
Again these are designed to broaden the reader's understanding of the issues. Most build on the text while others introduce new material.

Further reading
Academic sources
In this section we have recommended academic texts which we consider accessible and up-to-date.
Other literary sources
We have selected works of fiction and poetry which comment on or allude to the material in the text. Social care and social work are as much an expression of art as they are theoretical and practical disciplines. They draw amongst other things on intuition, feelings, spontaneity, insight, imagination, compassion and spirituality.

Films or plays
We have selected a small number of films or plays which in some way explore ideas and viewpoints contained in the text (except in Chapters 8 and 9). The name given before the title of a film is that of the Director.

1 An unequal society

We live in an unequal society and this is apparent from an observation of everyday living. Not everybody has the same life chances. Some people, owing to differences of social class, gender, skin colour, physical and mental health, are more likely to enjoy and participate in a fuller range of society's benefits than others. Inequality in society manifests itself in different ways and we might usefully break equality down into three different forms: *formal* equality, equality of *opportunity* and equality of *outcomes*.

Formal equality is the principle that everyone in society is equal. They are born equal and will receive equal treatment at the hands of society's political, administrative and legal institutions. Examples of this are that all adult citizens have the right to vote in democratic elections; they have a number of common civil rights and liberties, and they are all entitled to the same treatment under the law.

Equality of *opportunity* refers to the principle of everybody having an equal chance to achieve their potential in society. Under this principle society provides equal access to health, education and job opportunities. In other words, society endeavours to mitigate against any disadvantages individuals may have with regard to their social class, gender, race, age, culture, disability, sexual orientation, life-style or religion.

Equality of *outcomes* refers to the principle which ensures that, as far as possible, all individuals obtain an equal share of society's benefits. Outcomes would include income, wealth, life-style, influence, power and status, as well as equal health treatment and quality of education, housing and employment.

It is important to stress that these forms of equality are principles, and that in reality no society has, or could, translate them entirely into practice. For example, in our society formal equality under the law is adversely affected by power, wealth, prejudice and discrimination. Statistics indicate that black people have a greater chance of being arrested, charged, remanded in custody and imprisoned than white people. Similarly, most men who apply for care and control of their children in divorce proceedings are unsuccessful.

True equality of opportunity would mean that society would have to control all political, economic and social influences on all individuals from birth. This is clearly impossible to achieve. For example, in our society a child born into a wealthy family that can afford to provide greater stimulation can have an enormous advantage over other children even before the child attends school. According to statistics, the child is already likely to be healthier and more educationally advanced than a child from the working class. Thus, although it is declared that we have a free and open education system, in reality it is not so because some children start with socially bestowed advantages.

Likewise, equality of *outcome* is impossible to implement absolutely since so many variables would require controlling. Intervention would constantly be required to restore imbalances which would continually develop. Income is linked to status and power, and as individuals will always use it differently, so inequalities will always be arising. In addition to individual differences there are also social structures which prevent the achievement of full equality.

There have been attempts within our society to create various equal opportunities policies, for example, those aimed at enabling more black and Asian people to enter social care and social work. It has been recognized that black and Asian people are under represented within the profession, and that this is caused in part by the existence of structural racism within our society. Equal opportunities policies have aimed at redressing this imbalance. However, equality of opportunity can only really be effective if equality of outcome is also established. The two principles are inextricably linked.

For example, the policy of providing access to the Diploma in Social Work courses to black and Asian students can only be successful as an equal opportunities policy if those students go on to complete the course successfully and obtain appropriate jobs within social work. If black access students still face discrimination during training, at the job recruitment stage or later, then equality of outcome will not be achieved.

Similarly, equal opportunities policies aimed at attracting women back into employment will only be ultimately successful if they are accompanied by other social changes. Employers' expectations would need to change, and hours of attendance, leave arrangements, working conditions and facilities would have to be altered to accommodate women's specific needs. Obviously outcomes would ultimately determine the effectiveness of equal opportunities.

Individual and structural inequalities

'During the depression years of the 1930s, cookery classes were organized for women in poor communities in an attempt to help them to provide nutritious meals for their families despite their low incomes. One particular evening, a group of women were being taught how to make cod's head soup – a cheap and nourishing dish. At the end of the lesson the women were asked if they had any questions. "Just one," said a member of the group. "Whilst we're eating the cod's head soup, who's eating the cod?"

(From Langan, M., Lee, P. (eds), *Radical Social Work Today*,
Unwin Hyman, 1989, p. 140)

Inequalities exist both among individuals and within the structure of our society. There are differences between people at birth, including differences in physical and mental capacity. Whether or not these potential abilities develop will depend to a large extent on the person's social circumstances. No social structure can eliminate essential innate differences between people. However, it can help to determine the distribution of power, influence and life-chances.

There is plenty of evidence of structural inequality in our society. Take for example the composition of the House of Commons. In this democratically elected chamber of the 651 members only a small proportion are from working class backgrounds, 46 are women, four are from ethnic minorities and only two are registered as disabled. This is a reflection of the structural imbalance of power, influence and prestige within society. Similar observations could be made of many of society's major institutions, for example, the Civil Service, legal and professional organizations, the media and social and welfare services.

Society can be said to be divided in three major ways. These are social class, gender and race. It is also structured according to factors such as age, disability and sexual orientation. In our society able-bodied, white, middle class, heterosexual males are more likely to achieve social success, obtain power and derive more of society's benefits and rewards. All other groups will experience a corresponding lack of power and influence to a certain extent. In this way they can be said to be *marginalized* within society. A contributing factor towards the process of marginalization is the extent to which people experience *prejudice*.

Prejudice is not easy to define and it can take many different forms. It is usually a strongly held attitude towards individuals, or more commonly groups, which is to a greater or lesser extent unreasonable or irrational. It is irrational because it is *not* based on reasonable, factual evidence. To some extent prejudice is expressed in a person's behaviour, but much of it may remain secret or unconscious and may, as a result, be very hard to recognize or admit to. Usually, it is very deep-seated and powerful, and can affect what a person thinks, feels and does.

Prejudice is either based on fear or on a lack of knowledge, or on both. It is most often applied by the more powerful, those with authority and influence, to the less powerful. When used in education or in work, its application can profoundly hurt the prospects of those to whom it is directed. Again, it tends to be working class people, women and black people who most often suffer from its bad effects. Those in authority who can affect our lives and life chances may express prejudice through fear, because they feel threatened in some way, or because they feel they will lose out. Whatever its cause, an ignorance of those to whom it is directed is nearly always present.

The expression of prejudice leads to *discrimination*, to a situation where people are treated unequally, some favoured and others not. Discrimination may appear to be arbitrary as it will be subject to the whims of those expressing it.

Prejudice is commonly based on or justified by a *stereotype*. The two are closely related. A stereotype 'lumps together' all members of a particular group as if they *all* possessed the *same* characteristics. Examples of negative stereotypes used in our society might be that 'all Scotsmen are mean' or that 'all Jewish people are wealthy' or that 'all men are uncaring'. So a person might say 'I do not mix with a certain kind of person, because they are . . .'. Thus, her or his action has been governed by a stereotype.

Most stereotypes are negative. They may describe a group as 'lazy' or 'dirty', 'mean' or 'criminal'. Whatever the epithet used, they fail to see a person as a whole individual; particular traits or characteristics are isolated, and from this a generalization is made which denies a person's uniqueness.

The actual process of stereotyping is simple and follows this pattern:

> This person is an 'X'
> All 'Xs' are selfish
> Therefore, this person is selfish!

It is difficult to say where stereotypes originate from. It is almost certainly a range of sources, for example, parents, our socialization, our friends or peers, teachers, literature, the mass media and advertising. They are certainly contained in the very language we use and many of them take the form of 'clichés' in that language. There are, for example, more derogatory terms for marginalized groups, including minorities and women, than there are for more established members of society. It is because stereotypes are so deep-seated that they are so extremely difficult to modify, let alone remove completely.

It is important to point out at this stage that we also use stereotypes in a good and positive way. We do this in order to make 'short-cuts', so that living is made easier and more manageable. Huge amounts of information continually bombard our senses and we have to continually select or 'stereotype' in order to make sense of the world. For example, the 400 plus recognized shades of green become a single 'green' for the purpose of conversation and making sense quickly to one another. Again, we refer to a 'drug', whereas in reality there are thousands of different drugs doing very different things to different people. Using stereotypes as a form of 'short-hand' helps us to be definite and to reduce ambiguity which we may feel threatens us.

If we use a different phraseology, stereotyping may be described as labelling or stigmatizing. When a person is said to have been 'labelled', then frequently a stereotype with negative associations is being used. It is common for those in a powerful position to employ a label in order to 'put people down'. Thus, someone in work might 'label' an unemployed person as 'work-shy'.

It is extremely hard for people who are labelled to attempt to modify the label and its associated stigma, let alone rid themselves of its taint completely. They act from an inferior position and lack the power and influence with which to do so.

Marginalization

The overall effect of these interrelated processes of stereotyping, prejudice and stigmatizing is to *marginalize* the victims. This means that they are prevented from taking a full part in the life of our society; they live as it were 'on the edge' or 'margin' of society. They do not share full citizenship with regard to the social, economic and political life of the community.

Many will be unemployed and will be dependent on state benefits, as will many elders and people with disabilities. Others may be among the one million single parent families in the UK, or be among those suffering from mental illness or those who have a learning difficulty. Many of them lack the satisfactory income which enables them to take a full part in economic life. Such groups are likely to be over represented in the so-called 'underclass'.

Poverty is directly related to marginalization in that those people who are poor do not have the same extent of choice or control over their lives as other members of society. For example they have a greater reliance on public utilities and services and are less able to afford to buy labour and time saving appliances for the home. The goods within their purchasing range are often of inferior quality and not cost effective and may need to be replaced sooner than more expensive items.

Poor people undergo a great deal of inconvenience since they are forced to

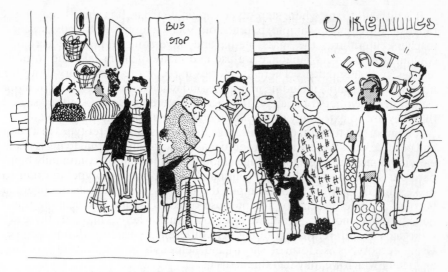

Poor people are affected by 'time poverty' – they do not have the facilties and conveniences in their own homes and are dependent on public utilities and transport.

depend on public transport which is often unreliable. This makes tasks such as shopping more difficult and means that many poor people have to shop in more expensive and smaller local stores. They are not able to take advantage of a monthly trip to the hypermarket in order to stock up their food cupboards and freezers with lower priced goods.

Reliance on public telephones and the nearest launderette add to their inconvenience. More affluent families will not only have all the required appliances within their homes, they will also often buy in domestic help for cleaning, decorating and gardening.

The consequences of poverty are felt just as deeply in rural areas as they are in an urban environment. A recent report *Faith in the Countryside* – Report of the Archbishops' Commission on Rural Areas (1990), highlighted the significance of rural poverty, '. . . the weak, the poor and vulnerable and the elderly have their choices further curtailed, since without readily available personal transport, access to basic facilities is restricted' (p. 311).

The extent to which money buys time in our society is often overlooked. As Sue Ward (1986) has pointed out 'being poor takes up an enormous amount of time and energy' (p. 37). She adds, 'Money also buys better housing and working conditions. These also affect the amount of time you have. Keeping clean, warm and fed – even just keeping going – in a damp council flat on the 14th floor, where the lifts don't work and the nearest supermarket is a mile away, is going to be a struggle anyway' (ibid., p. 38).

As a reaction to their deprivation many people turn inwards to their homes and families and rely exclusively on the privatized entertainment of television and video. Lack of money effectively prohibits poor people from having the chance to fully engage in local activities. Thus the possibility of corporate, communal life becomes ever more remote.

It is not surprising that many marginalized people, families and groups feel 'trapped' in their situation. It is extremely hard to work one's way out of this predicament. For those who have committed offences, the existence of a criminal record will make it even harder still. We may feel it a small wonder that in the early 1980s many large cities saw extensive unrest. Such unrest had many complex interrelated causes, and it would appear that anger and frustration were certainly amongst them.

In addition to those who experience marginalization owing to their material deprivation and the associated prejudice of the more privileged sections in society, there are others who suffer similarly as a result of their so-called 'unconventional' life-styles, or involvement in grass roots political activity. These include groups that are sometimes referred to as 'alternative' such as the Peace Movement, some feminist groups and other alternative life-style groups such as the so-called 'Peace Convoy'. To a large extent such people choose to be unconventional and therefore anticipate a marginalized identity. Whether passive victims because of class, gender or race, or victims who have made a more conscious decision to live 'marginalized' life styles, the result is the same – a substantial proportion of the population do not play a full part in the life of our community.

Carers

It would be accurate to describe the position of informal carers as being marginalized. Less than 10 per cent receive any outside help and many are trapped in a long term, full-time caring relationship. Whether carers undertake this role because of the lack of a suitable alternative care arrangement or because they feel obligated or they harbour strong feelings of love and want to care for their relative, few would have received any training or preparation for the task. Any difficulties which accompany the practice of providing personal care are likely to be intensified when the person being provided for is related to the carer, so that these relationships are sometimes characterized by either physical or mental violence, resentment, stubborness and non co-operation.

> "It is often harder than a paid job, involving longer hours and heavier work (for instance, lifting a handicapped person); statistics on physical injury and mental illness among carers testify to its danger and stressfulness. Yet it arises as an extension of such roles as spouse, daughter or daughter-in-law, and is seen as part of kinship. Carers often disown the name, saying things like 'I'm just being a wife'."
>
> (From Jordan, B., *The Common Good*, Basil Blackwell, 1989, p. 149)

Some people find it difficult to adjust to the role reversal required when a daughter or son provides intimate care to her or his mother, father, aunt, uncle or grandparent, who formerly had provided care to them. The carers themselves are often in need of support yet continue their role in isolation and have

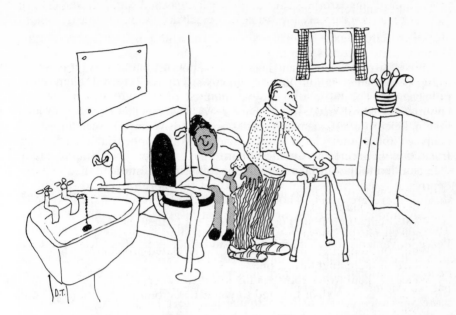

Social care is generally undervalued by society and is mainly undertaken by women. Care is seen as an extension of the traditional woman's role.

to make personal sacrifices. They are marginalized in the sense that the care commitment they undertake often prevents them from living a full life within the community.

Similarly, social care can also be seen to be marginalized within the activity of social work and basic or auxilliary nurse care within the Health Service. The work is regarded as having a low status, it is poorly paid and is mainly undertaken by working class women, many of whom are from ethnic minorities. Until recently very few social care workers or health care workers have been offered any training whatsoever; fewer still have the chance of professional training. As a consequence they are separated from the policy and decision making processes and have little control over their work situation.

Exercises

1. Obtain from your local DSS office information concerning the exact financial benefits to which any of the following people are entitled:

 i) A family of two unemployed parents and two children under the age of ten.
 ii) An unemployed single parent with one child under ten.
 iii) A single unemployed person.
 iv) An elderly male, post retirement age, living on his own.

Find out the average rent and community charge contribution typical of your area. Then make an estimate of essential everyday expenses including a proportion of standard bills such as electricity, gas and water. In the light of this, calculate as accurately as possible how much disposable income remains to meet the cost of other essentials.

2. Either individually or in pairs, make a list of twenty derogatory terms/swear words and consider at which group of people they are targeted. Share these with the whole group. Now, in discussion as a whole group, consider the following question: What does this say about general social attitudes towards those groups which you have identified?

3. *Examining prejudice*   On the opposite page are ten photographs. Study each face carefully whilst considering the following questions:

   i) Who would you be most likely to share a personal problem with? (Rank order the remainder).
  ii) What occupation (if any) do you think each of them has?
 iii) What social class grouping do each of them belong to?
  iv) Which of them might have a drink or drug-related problem?
   v) Which of them might live alone?
  vi) Which of them would most readily resort to violence?
NB: This list is not exhaustive and so you can add other suggestions of your own.

As a whole group discuss your answers to the following questions:

   i) Are you aware of the roots of your own prejudice?
  ii) What steps can you take to eradicate your own prejudice?
NB: This exercise is designed to elicit personal prejudice in a spontaneous way. It should be undertaken in a spirit of trust and no criticisms or blame should be levelled at, or attached to, any individual contribution.

4. *The effects of labelling*   The trainer needs to produce a different label for each member of the group, for example, aggressive, friendly, depressive, assertive, withdrawn etc. These labels should be randomly allocated to each group member and fixed to her or his forehead so that other participants can immediately see the label. Participants will react towards others in accordance to the label they are displaying.

The setting is a social services day centre (for any client group) in which a group of service users are planning a range of future social events. This task should take about 20 minutes. The purpose of the exercise is to focus on the labelling process. It is important for participants to refrain from using the specific word or words which make up the label. The discussion following the exercise should explore the varied responses to the label as well as the different feelings evoked as a result of being labelled.

5. *How we think others see us*   In pairs each takes it in turn to explain to their partner how others will see them in terms of the following criteria:

   i) *Class*: Having established her or his own class position, the participant proceeds to describe in detail how someone from a different social class will see them.

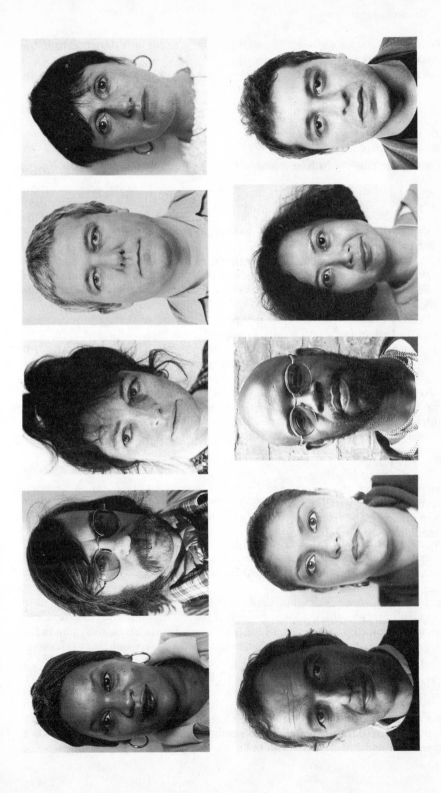

ii) *Gender*: The participant relates to her or his partner how someone from the opposite sex will see them.
iii) *Race*: Similarly, the participants imagine how they are perceived by someone of a different race or culture and relates this to their partner.

When this process is complete, the whole group should examine what they have learned from the experience.

Questions for essays or discussion

1. A.H. Halsey has said 'Society means a shared life. If some and not others are poor then the principles on which life is shared are at issue; society itself is in question'. In what ways does poverty put shared or corporate social life in jeopardy?
2. Which of the following do you consider to be the most significant structural disadvantages – social class, gender or race? Explain your reasons.
3. Often in our society the rich are made richer and the poor are made poorer as a way of encouraging their respective efforts and initiatives. Why should society's approach to the two groups differ in this way?
4. 'Poverty is at the root of powerlessness'. How are poverty and powerlessness linked and what forms does powerlessness take?
5. Explore the ways in which Equal Opportunities Policies can work towards eliminating discrimination and inequality in our society.
6. In regard to a group of your own choosing e.g. women, black people, working class people, homeless people, unemployed people, gay people and people with physical disabilities or learning difficulties, describe what form their marginalization takes.

Further reading

Academic sources

Archbishop of Canterbury's Commission on Urban Priority Areas, *Faith in the City*, Church House Publishing, 1985.
Archbishops' Commission on Rural Areas, *Faith in the Countryside*, Churchman Publishing Ltd., 1990. Produced as companion studies by the Church of England, amongst other things they highlighted poverty, inequality and social division, and the economic and social factors which had contributed to them.
Goffman, E., *Stigma*, Penguin, 1968. Subtitled 'Notes on the Management of Spoiled Identity', this classic sociological study examined the close relationship between stigma and stereotypes and looked at the strategies open to the stigmatized with which they could minimalize what we would now refer to as their 'marginalization'.
Golding, P., (ed.), *Excluding the Poor*, Child Poverty Action Group – CPAG, 1986. This very readable book outlines the many ways in which poor people are excluded in our society and depicts the barriers which exist that prevent people in poverty taking a full part in the life of their community.
Lister, R., *The Exclusive Society – Citizenship and the Poor*, CPAG, 1990. A short text which examines both the responsibilities and rights of citizenship

in Britain. The author goes on to study how poverty threatens full citizenship, especially in relation to black people, women and children. Along the way she attacks the concept of an 'underclass'.

Taking Liberties Collective, *Learning the Hard Way*, Macmillan, 1989. This book is made up of working class and black womens' experiences of oppression and discrimination and their struggles in everyday living.

Walker, A., Walker, C., (eds.), *The Growing Divide – A Social Audit 1979– 1987*, CPAG, 1987. Published just before the 1987 General Election, this book examines inequality in Britain from a number of themes including poverty, unemployment and health.

Other literary sources
Crisp, Q., *The Naked Civil Servant*, Flamingo, 1977.
Dickens, C., *Little Dorrit*, Penguin, 1967.
Greenwood, W., *Love on the Dole*, Penguin, 1969.
Hesse, H., *Steppenwolf*, Penguin, 1965.
Orwell, G., *Animal Farm*, Penguin, 1989.
Steinbeck, J., *The Grapes of Wrath*, Pan, 1987.

Films or plays
Huston, J., *Fat City*, US, 1972.
Lynch, D., *The Elephant Man*, US, 1980.
Pollack, S., *They Shoot Horses Don't They?* US, 1969.
Schlesinger, J., *Midnight Cowboy*, US, 1969.

2 Social class and the creation of an 'underclass'

Think of what our nation stands for,
. . . free speech, free passes, *class distinction*,
democracy and proper drains.

(John Betjeman, In Westminster Abbey,
from *Collected Poems*, John Murray Publishers, Ltd.)

Introduction

In 1934 in the Cutteslowe area of north Oxford, it was proposed to re-house some 28 'slum clearance' families in public housing adjacent to a new private housing development. In December of that year, the company that had erected the private housing responded by building large brick walls topped by metal spikes across the two roads which connected the separate developments. An outcry from many sections of the local community followed, but it was not until March 1959 (following protests, court injunctions, partial demolition and re-building of the walls) that the walls were finally removed.

For 25 years the 'Cutteslowe walls', or 'snob walls' as they became known locally, had remained *in situ*. Edmund Gibbs, a city councillor, whose father had campaigned vigorously to have the walls removed, ceremoniously knocked out the first bricks with a pickaxe in 1959. He said later, 'I was delighted to be there when those dreadful walls came down at last, but it is depressing that class prejudice is still around, and even getting stronger' (*Limited Edition*, October 1988, p. 12). This was an extreme and unique example of class prejudice and indicates the depth of feeling that can sometimes occur around the issue of social class. Most of us have some concept of class, and of our own place within a 'class system'. We might rank ourselves or others as 'working class', 'middle class' or 'upper class'. We will do this according to various factors: the way we speak or dress; what we or members of our family do for a living; where we live; what kind of car we drive; what we spend our leisure time doing, and so on.

Some people think of social class hierarchically, implying that being 'upper class' is somehow better than being 'middle class', which in turn is better than being 'working class'. Many object to the generalized use of the term 'social class' on the grounds that it emphasizes differences and inequalities between people who are essentially the same, and creates an unfounded snobbery.

Social class is an extremely complex concept which in common usage has almost as many meanings as there are people prepared to make generalizations about it! However, a refined and generally accepted use of the term 'social class' is extremely important for people who study society. Above all, it is a useful *analytical tool*. It enables researchers to make observations about social need and the effectiveness of social policy. Most importantly, it can highlight the plight of particular groups of people, defined by their social class, and consider whether their needs are being met. In this way the effects of policies concerning education, housing, health, social care or income maintenance can be examined.

Some possible misconceptions about class

We need to remember that there is nothing 'natural' about social class. Rather it is an artificial concept designed for the benefit of social analysis. Social class is not *fixed* – there is movement between classes, both within generations and between generations. If we perceive class as a hierarchy, this movement can be either up or down the social scale. A child born into a particular social class may change her or his position as she or he grows older and enters the worlds of education and work. We refer to this movement as 'social mobility'. It takes place usually between adjacent groupings, rather than extremes of 'top' and 'bottom'.

As we shall see later, the concept of social class alters over time. It has to be updated in response to changes in society, particularly those concerning the people who make up the work-force.

The concept of social class applied in Britain will not necessarily be transferable to other countries or cultures. It has evolved from the analysis of our own particular society. All nations are unique, having a different history, culture and traditions. The work-force will be organized in different ways and patterns of income and wealth will not be the same. We must treat each nation state in ways which are sensitive to its own particular qualities. One of these qualities will be its own unique pattern of social class.

Social class is an objective analytical tool and no moral judgements are implied or intended when using class analysis. For example, if we discover that working class children do less well at school, the implication is that the education system is failing to deliver effectively to such children, not that they are less able or intelligent than children from other social classes.

What is social class?

Outside of an ideal society, it is hard to imagine a society which is not divided in some way between those less well off and those better off. In reality, all societies past and present have been divided into a range of groups of varying material resources (wealth, income, property, land etc.). All societies are said to have been stratified, i.e. divided into different *strata*, a concept which social scientists borrow from geology which refers to the various layers found in the structure of the earth.

Social stratification is a neutral term which simply refers to the different divisions or groups within society. *Social class* is simply *one* of the ways in which societies can be divided.

Not all previous societies have been divided along *class lines*. For example, they may have been divided (or 'stratified') by *age* – in which older people occupy the most powerful authority positions and have more status than others. Societies can also be stratified by *gender* – they can be *patriarchal* or *matriarchal*, where those in powerful positions are either male or female, respectively.

Race or *ethnicity* (or colour) may be the crucial stratifying factor, for example the present *apartheid* system in South Africa. This is based on the supposed superiority of a minority white group who, by dominating the major economic and political institutions of society, are able to treat the black majority as subservient and keep them under repressive control.

Some societies have been divided on *status* lines. This has taken many forms. *Slavery* was one example where masters literally *owned* their slaves and treated them as their property.

In some countries, e.g. India the *caste* system is another example. This fixes a person's social position at birth and strict rules govern what relations there will be between castes. At the lowest end of the caste system, the 'untouchables' are barred from social interaction with all higher groups and lack the civil rights enjoyed by others. This system has of late undergone change and a 'loosening up' of rigid divisions has occurred.

It is important to point out that such stratification systems are not mutually exclusive, i.e. more than one system can operate in a society at any one time. For example, gender and age could be the prevalent factors, with older women in positions of authority; gender and slavery could be prevalent, with male masters holding power.

To sum up, social stratification refers to the structural inequalities in society: that is, inequalities between different groupings of people which are determined by the way society is organized. Ruling groups may have a vested interest in preserving inequalities in order to continue deriving benefits and privileges.

Most modern societies are today stratified by what we call *social class*. Unfortunately there is no absolute agreement about the definition of class and there are a large number of competing definitions, theories and explanations. Broadly speaking class refers to *socio-economic* differences between groups of people. These differences will affect peoples' life-styles, life chances and future prospects.

Explanations of social class tend to include both *objective* factors (e.g. those tangible, material factors that can be more easily measured, such as *income*, or *wealth*) and *subjective* factors (e.g. a person's *attitudes* and *values*, including perhaps how they view their own class position). Whereas it is reasonably straightforward to assess the former, it is far more difficult to assess the latter.

We will now turn to three of the most prominent explanations of social class which have been applied to the British class system, in order to consider their usefulness in helping us to understand our present society.

Karl Marx (1818–83)

Marx, a German economist and political scientist who lived and wrote for most of his life in London, has to be included in any discussion of social class. His work is still extremely important for social scientists today, despite being over one hundred years old. Marx was the first to make social class central to an analysis of society.

For Marx, 'the history of all hitherto existing society is the history of class struggles' (Marx and Engels, 1975, p. 32). In other words he felt social class characterized all previous forms of society. In ancient societies the division was between masters and slaves and in feudal times society was fundamentally divided between landlord and serf (although there were intermediary group-ings). In each case the former group dominated the numerically larger latter group. The social class system changed once more when society was trans-formed from being basically agrarian to a society based on industry and commerce.

In Marx's theory, a person's social class is determined by her or his relationship to what he called the '*means of production*' – the means by which material goods are actually produced; the technology, situated in workshops and factories. Within this system, *capitalists* (or industrialists) *own* the means of production, while *workers* (or the *working class*) earn their living by selling their labour to capitalists.

Capitalists derive their wealth by exploiting workers, who are never paid a wage which reflects the true value of their labour. This wealth, 'creamed off' by the capitalist class, was referred to by Marx as 'surplus value'. In this way profits were made by the capitalist class, while workers had to continue working day after day, week after week, simply in order to survive.

As the capitalist class gained in wealth, they also gained in power and influence, although a small, landed aristocracy remained. They were therefore able to control and dominate all the institutions in society; the law, the education system, religion, politics and the media. Their ideas, attitudes and values (or *ideology*) became dominant, and contrary views had to struggle to find a voice and be heard.

Thus, Marx viewed social classes as real, objective entities. The class system required inequalities to exist in society. We could describe these inequalities as *structural*.

Criticisms of Marx's concept of class

We must not be unfairly critical of Marx, and should appreciate that our society has changed a great deal since his death in 1883. Society today is far more complex. It has become less easy to place certain groups of people in one or other of Marx's two great opposing classes: the working class or *proletariat* and the middle class or *bourgeoisie*.

With the development of our modern, industrial society, a large state apparatus has grown, including the Civil Service and other large bureaucratic organizations operating at both national and local levels. These include, for example, the Department of Social Security (DSS), the National Health Service (NHS) and the local authority Housing Departments, and Social Services Departments (or Social Work Departments in Scotland). Marx did not foresee these developments in the public sector and so his class analysis is unable to accommodate the personnel working for such government organiza-tions. They are clearly not capitalists in Marx's sense of the word, and neither are they working directly for the capitalist class. They perform their duties for the good of the community, or society as a whole. Such people we would now refer to as 'middle class', because in a sense they fit between Marx's two classes, but they cannot be accepted into his scheme of things on his terms.

Another fundamental criticism of Marx is that by focusing exclusively on class he ignored other ways in which society is stratified, e.g. race, gender and age. In his day, most waged workers working outside the home were male. Consequently women appear to be largely *invisible* in his work. Yet today women form over 40 per cent of the work-force and this is increasing rapidly. Despite this, however, most top jobs are held by men. We might conclude from this that in terms of employment *gender* is as much an important factor as *class*.

Third, some of Marx's historical predictions have not been borne out. He believed that the two major classes would become more clearly demarcated but in fact they have become more fragmented and, as we have seen, divisions between them have become blurred. The working class has shrunk in size (not grown as he predicted) and its revolutionary potential has not been realized in this country. So much then for Marx's referring to the working class as the 'gravediggers of capitalism' (Giddens, 1982, p. 63).

The Registrar-General's Classification of Occupations

This classification, first published in 1911, was produced by an official government body – the Office of Population Censuses and Surveys (OPCS). The first use of the data by the government of the time was the analysis of infant mortality statistics. Since then the classification system has been revised a great deal. It recognized five basic social classes, and occupations were placed in these classes according to their 'standing within the community'. It was therefore a classification based on *status*. A major change took place in 1980 when 'social standing' was replaced by 'occupational skill' as the basis of categorization.

The way in which classification is made is under further review. At present, however, the five classes are listed in Table 2.1. Note that social class III is divided into two sub-divisions.

Below are some examples of actual occupations in the various class categories used at present:
Social Class I Accountant, architect, chemist, doctor, judge, lawyer, optician, solicitor, university lecturer.
Social Class II Aircraft pilot, chiropodist, farmer, manager, publican, Member of Parliament, nurse, police officer, school teacher, social worker.

Table 2.1   The Registrar-General's classification of occupations.

Class	Category of Occupation
I	Professional and higher administrative occupations
II	Intermediate occupations
IIIN	Skilled occupations (non-manual)
IIIM	Skilled occupations (manual)
IV	Partly skilled occupations
V	Unskilled occupations

NB The Armed Forces are included as a separate sixth class, but this is a relatively small number of people.

Social Class III N   Clerical worker, estate agent, sales representative, secretary, shop assistant, typist.

Social Class III M   Bus driver, bricklayer, carpenter, cook, hairdresser, miner, police constable, train driver.

Social Class IV   Agricultural worker, bar person, bus conductor, hospital orderly, postman, street vendor.

Social Class V   Chimney sweep, kitchen hand, labourer, office cleaner, railway porter, window cleaner.

In all, there are over, 20,000 different occupational titles used by the Registrar-General.

This classification is used in the analysis of a vast amount of data the government produces by way of surveys, such as the National Census which is carried out every ten years. Much of the data and subsequent analysis will concern social policy and welfare services. Through analysis, the effectiveness of such policy and services can be assessed.

Criticisms of the Registrar-General's Classification of Occupations

Firstly, the many revisions to the classification which have taken place (and which continue today) create confusion. In particular, they mean that comparisons in class changes made over time may have little validity.

Secondly, data which is based on occupation leaves out of its reckoning all those not in paid work. This is a majority (57 per cent) of the British population. Seventy seven per cent of males and 56 per cent of females of *working age* do some kind of paid work – that is, work of all types, full time, part-time, self-employed. However, these figures do not include 23 per cent of all men and 44 per cent of women of working age who include students, housewives and unemployed people (*Sociology Update*, 1990, p. 33). Consequently, far less women than men are included in the classification. This may be seen as an example of how women are marginalized and how their contribution to society is unacknowledged.

Thirdly, the very rich who have great existing wealth, private incomes, and who may deal in land and property are also left out of the classification. They do not have an occupational title and so are excluded. Such people might be called 'upper class' or even (but less commonly) the 'aristocracy'.

Finally, the British census, which places people in classes according to the class of the 'head of household', makes the *patriarchal* assumption that there is only one such 'head' and that that person is male. This notion of one single male 'breadwinner' is now outmoded.

To sum up, a classification which relies solely on occupation, is far from satisfactory. It should be related more to a systematic theory of social stratification.

The third explanation of social class may be more complex than the previous two, but it is more comprehensive, and therefore of more use.

John Goldthorpe's class model

In the course of many years work on class and social mobility (how people move up and down the class system), John Goldthorpe (working largely from the 1960s onwards) has devised a sophisticated model of class in Britain. His work is highly respected by other social scientists who have also studied class. For example, a major recent study of class in this country, which is part of a larger, world-wide study involving some nineteen countries, found Goldthorpe's analysis the most useful. This study, based at the University of Essex, involved a national sample survey of men and women aged 18–65. Almost 2,000 responses were received and the survey included a 1½ hour interview with each respondent (Marshall *et al.*, 1988).

At its most elaborate, the Goldthorpe model of class identifies eleven social classes. These can be reduced to seven, five and even three major classes depending on their use. These are entitled *service, intermediate* and *working* classes (1980).

The *service* class includes all professionals, administrators and managers, along with the supervisors of non-manual employees. (*NB*. Goldthorpe's term 'service' should not be confused with terms like 'service industry' or 'service sector'.) The *intermediate* class is made up of routine non-manual workers, such as clerical and sales personnel, lower-grade technicians, the supervisors of manual workers and the self-employed. The *working* class constitutes all skilled, semi-skilled and unskilled manual labourers, including agricultural workers.

Goldthorpe has reviewed his class categories at times in order to stay up to date with changes in the workforce and other social developments. His classes are determined by two major factors fused together – a person's occupational title (including their source and level of income, financial security and financial prospects) and their employment status (how much autonomy they have, or what control they exercise over their roles and tasks at work).

Criticisms of Goldthorpe's class model

Although Goldthorpe's class analysis is an improvement on the Registrar-General's classification because it involves employment *status* as well as occupation and occupational skills, there are still inadequacies in it.

First, social class positions are still too much determined by a person's occupation – the kind of job they do. Therefore, (as with the Registrar-General's classification) those who are very rich, those with other sources of income and those who do not need to work are not included. Again, those not classified as working, such as the unemployed, pensioners, housewives and students, are also 'invisible' to the analysis.

Second, women generally tend to have many more part-time, less well paid and less secure jobs than men. The relationship between women and work and men and work is thus very different. Goldthorpe's class analysis does not do full justice to this situation, because the nature of much of women's paid work leads to their being over represented in the 'working class'. This is a distortion since it ignores other social class determinants, such as life-style, leisure pursuits and cultural interests. In fact, this particular issue has led some writers on class to suggest that we should seek to devise a completely different class analysis for women as opposed to men. This may therefore be a future development.

Summary

So far, by focusing on three important contributions to an understanding of social class we have seen that the concept remains far from simple. So many different variables need to be taken into account depending on our definition of social class – occupation, income, wealth, status, skill, autonomy in work, values, attitudes, life style, leisure interests – the task is a daunting one! A major problem is that these complex variables frequently contradict each other making classification difficult. Consider for example, where a high earning manual worker living in a leafy middle class suburb and whose friends and leisure activities are middle class should be placed? Further, where would you place his wife, who does not have paid employment?

Each explanation of class which social scientists have put forward appears to be incomplete or inadequate in some way. In particular, two issues of key importance – *gender* and *race*, appear to be largely ignored in class analyses.

The class analyses are very *male* oriented and still use outdated concepts like 'head of household'. Many households in Britain today do not comprise the traditional 'nuclear family' i.e. two parents and the average number of children – now somewhere between two and three. There are now over one million single-parent families and many of these parents will not be able to take any kind of work because of their child-care responsibilities. Most are women. They are not represented in our 'gender-blind' class theories and analyses.

Analyses of class also ignore the fact that there are racial issues of importance. For example, a large proportion of black people are to be found in poorer-paid, less secure, and in the case of black women, part-time jobs. Black people, along with people with disabilities and those with learning difficulties, are not evenly represented in all occupations and a social class analysis fails to portray this. British society is stratified by gender and race in ways too important to be ignored, or rendered 'invisible'.

'Class gets so complicated with working class, lower middle, middle, upper middle and aristocracy – I suppose I'm working-middle class and rather proud of it.'
(Richard Briers, Actor, *Options*, March 1990, p. 82.)

Why use the concept of social class at all?

For all its inadequacies, inconsistencies and incompleteness, for all that it is a crude measure involving generalizations and the grouping of individuals into wide categories, social class *does* continue to have some value. It can still inform us about the quality of life for some groups of people. Let us look at its application, when examining important areas of social policy.

Social class and health

Social scientists are able to demonstrate that people from class positions higher in the social scale tend to be on average healthier, taller and to live longer than those in lower class positions. Class differences are greatest in infant mortality and the death of children. Additionally people from lower class positions are more likely to die at all ages in life than people from higher class positions. There are a number of reasons for this, but the main one is the lack of financial resources of those in lower class positions. This leads to a poorer diet. A recent report from the Health Education Authority written by a National Health Service dietician, Issy Cole-Hamilton, stated that people on low incomes could not afford to eat healthily. Lack of money, rather than lack of knowledge as to what healthy foods to eat, led to this situation (*Observer*, 15 October 1989).

The report estimated that in 1986 the weekly cost of a healthy diet for each adult in a family of four was £14. However, the average adult in a family of four on a low income only had £9.82 to spend per week on food. The report's research showed that the cost of healthier food, e.g. green vegetables, fish, wholemeal bread and citrus fruit, has risen in recent years faster than the cost of less healthy food items, e.g. biscuits, white bread, sausages and butter. Compared to the low-income average £9.82 per adult per week spent on food in 1986, wealthy people at the top of the class scale spent £18.72. This represented a quarter of the average income compared to about one-sixth of a wealthy person's income. In order for people receiving state benefits, in the form of 'income support', to obtain a healthy diet they would have to spend from between 40 to 50 per cent of their disposable income on food per week.

In addition to diet, there are a number of other factors involved in the relationship between health and class. Those lower down the class scale tend to live in poorer housing and environmental conditions. Those with jobs tend to suffer from poorer working conditions (dirtier, noisier and more dangerous) and those lower in the class structure generally are less able to afford holidays or breaks, which are an important part of a healthier life-style.

Such findings were aired in a major report called *Inequalities in Health*, written by a working group set up in 1977 and chaired by Sir Douglas Black (the Black Report). The report was published by the DHSS (as it then was) in 1980. It created a good deal of controversy because of its disturbing findings. Its most important conclusion was clear – that *material deprivation* played the most important part in poor health for those in lower social classes. Other contributory factors were biological, cultural and those centred around life-style.

The report indicated that those in higher social classes tend also to benefit more from medical care. They have more access to such care, being able to draw on private as well as public (NHS) services. Such people are more likely statistically to self-refer to such services. They also spend longer on average in sessions with their General Practitioner.

In 1986, the Health Education Council commissioned research which would update the evidence of the Black Report. The report, *The Health Divide: Inequalities in Health in the 1980s* (1987), stated:

> 'In some respects the health of the lower occupational classes [Registrar-General's] has actually deteriorated against the background of a general improvement in the population as a whole. While death rates have been declining, rates of chronic illness seem to have been increasing, and the gap in the illness rates between manual and non-manual groups has been widening too, particularly in the over-65 age-group.'
>
> (p. 266)

One of its conclusions was that 'the weight of evidence continues to point to explanations which suggest that socio-economic circumstances play the major part in subsequent health differences' (p. 304). Another conclusion indicated that, 'disappointingly, in the intervening eight years [since publication of the Black Report] there seems to have been little progress on the basic problems underlying inequality in health' (p. 350). Amongst these underlying problems are mentioned 'poverty', 'poor nutrition' and poor 'housing and working conditions' (ibid).

'A new health warning deserves to be publicized on every hoarding, in every newspaper and on every TV programme. Poverty damages health; poverty kills.'
(Town, P., in *The Growing Divide*, 1987, p. 87)

Social class and education

The education which our society provides for our children and young adults tends to re-affirm class inequalities rather than change them. The tripartite system of state (or public) education introduced by the Butler Education Act 1944, i.e. Grammar, Technical and Secondary Modern schools, enshrined the principal of 'equality of opportunity'. It aimed to offer children of all classes the chance of winning a grammar school place. Grammar schools were committed more to academic achievements than the other two types of school, and young people leaving them tended to have gained better qualifications and thus were more likely to go on to Higher Edcuation (Polytechnics and Universities) and better paid jobs with better prospects.

The 1944 Act also introduced the 11 plus examination and success in this secured a grammar school place. What has been discovered since is that home environment was the dominant feature in a child's educational success or failure. Those children from higher social classes whose homes were more comfortable and conducive to study did better. It was also felt that the 11 plus examination contained an inbuilt cultural bias which favoured children from higher social classes (the style of language used is a key feature here – it being more 'foreign' to children from lower social classes). There also tended to be too few grammar schools in working class areas of our towns and cities, so there was a dearth of places for less privileged children.

An Oxford University social mobility study (Goldthorpe, 1980) surveyed 10,000 *men* asking them what their own occupation was and what their fathers' had been. Using John Goldthorpe's three major class divisions – service, intermediate and working class, the movement between them over a generation was studied. What was discovered was a 1:2:4 rule. This means that whatever chance a working class boy had of moving into the service class, a boy from the intermediate class had twice the chance, and a service class boy had four times the chance.

Working class children are far more likely to drop out of education earlier than others. In the Oxford survey, the service class child was four times more likely to be still at school at sixteen, eight times more likely at seventeen and eleven times more likely to enter university. Less than one in forty boys from working class families gained 'O' levels, compared with one in four service class boys.

Of course, not being so successful in educational terms has a 'knock-on' affect for lower class children. It means their prospects of higher education and of better paid jobs and promising careers are severely curtailed. Add to this the fact that more privileged people in top social classes can also afford to take advantage of the growing sector of private education, and the result is considerable inequality.

'I suppose I am middle class. I would define it as being slightly boring and sending your children to private school!'

(Sue Arnold, Journalist, *Options*, March 1990, p. 78)

Social class and the clients of the personal social services

'The majority of social workers are white middle class and the majority of clients are working class.'

(Jones, C., *State Social Work and the Working Class*, 1983, p. 9)

No substantial research has been carried out into the social class position of the clients of the personal social services. From our own working experience and the testimony of others in social welfare, we know that the majority of clients are working class and poor. We know that material deprivation (as experienced by lower class people and families) will be the root cause of many problems which people, as clients, will take to a social worker.

In 1969, Frederick Seebohm (chair of the 'Seebohm Committee' which reported in 1968), considered that poverty and bad housing 'probably caused something like 60 per cent of the work that is now carried on by social workers'. We know that poverty and poor quality housing (the two of them are closely linked) will be suffered disproportionately by members of lower social classes.

The class position of the clients of the personal social services will, of course, vary depending on the need. For example, residential care for elders and day care for disabled people, or for those with learning difficulties, will tend to be provided to a wider cross-section of social classes in Britain. We *all* get old, and disability or learning difficulties occur in all kinds of families from all kinds of social class background. However, those individuals or families who approach a social worker and whose problem has its root in deprivation will be more exclusively drawn from a lower social class.

It is also important to look at the other side of this question, i.e. why are members of the higher social classes able to *avoid* becoming the clients of the personal social services? There are three possible answers. First, their general level of affluence means they do not suffer, either directly or at second hand, from poverty, poor housing or a poor environment with few facilities. Second, they are able to purchase what is often (but not always) a higher standard of care from the private sector and to employ carers in their own home for themselves or their children. Third, research such as the Black Report and *The Health Divide* shows clear signs that the better off actually derive more benefit from public services such as education or the National Health Service than do lower class members. Middle class people tend to be more assertive and better able to seek out what is available to them.

Also to be taken into consideration is the social class background of professional workers within the personal social services. This is dealt with at the end of this chapter. What this section has illustrated is the contribution which material deprivation makes (poverty, low-incomes and poor housing) to a client's difficulties. These are often inextricably linked with emotional, relationship, or psychological problems that clients may experience. For carers and clients it is frequently unclear precisely where the origins of difficulties lie.

Changes in the British class structure

Society is never static – change is constant. In particular, the nature of work and the constituency of the work force has changed dramatically in the last few years. Although the work people perform is only one of several factors which influence which social class they belong to, it is extremely important. Changes in work and the nature of the work-force must be considered, therefore, in any discussion of social class. Some of the important changes in the work-force are indicated below.

A decline has taken place throughout Britain, but particularly in South Wales, Scotland and northern areas of England, in the traditional 'heavy' industries such as ship-building, steel and coal mining. These industries had always employed a large number of people belonging to the working class – workers (virtually all men) of a skilled, semi-skilled and unskilled *manual* nature. This has led to a corresponding decline in the communities in which they lived in large numbers. Particular areas hit by unemployment in these types of work were: the shipbuilding industry in the north-east of England, and on the River Clyde in Scotland; steel manufacture was hit in the 'steel-city' of Sheffield and in surrounding districts in the English north-midlands; and coal mining was severely run-down in the valleys of South Wales and in Yorkshire and Lancashire.

The decline in other types of work affected different parts of the country, For example, the complete closure of the London docks in the east of the City and the Isle of Dogs occurred in only a few years. Many thousands of dockers lost their employment in these areas. Recently, the last remaining colliery in Kent closed down, and all the work-force was made redundant.

Whilst the 'heavy' industries have seen dramatic decline, the service sector and white-collar work has seen a tremendous growth. As old technologies are phased out, so new technologies have gained rapid growth. Automation, computerization and the massive growth in the use of micro-chip technology has brought about what might be referred to as a 'revolution' in working practice. New areas of work have blossomed, such as information systems, whilst more established areas of work have completely changed their working practices. The newspaper industry is one such example. The move of all major national newspapers out of Fleet Street has been accompanied by investment in new plant and new technological ways of communicating news and producing the finished article.

Many young people have entered these new types of work – information systems, computers, specialists in the new technologies, and some have received very high financial rewards for their work. Those who work in certain areas, such as the City area of London, in banking and the financial markets, have even earned themselves a new name – 'yuppies'. The term is short for 'young, upwardly-mobile, professional people'. It highlights the belief that such people are increasing their affluence and improving their position in the class structure.

Following the end of the demographic post-war 'baby boom', the numbers of young people leaving school and going into the job market has declined. As a result the government and employers have had to think of ways of encouraging other people, who may well have left the work-force, back into it. Two groups in particular – older people and women, have been targeted. In order to do this successfully, however, certain means of encouragement have needed to be used, such as better child-care facilities for women with children or 'career breaks' for those looking after a dependent person.

All of these changes have had two important effects: first, they have led to an expanded middle (or 'intermediate') class and second, they have increasingly fragmented this class into new divisions as the nature of work has changed.

A good example of the last point is that of *clerical work*. New technologies, such as the computer and word processor, have made the work physically easier, but more routine and monotonous. People in such work increasingly have only a single task, for example, switchboard operator, filing clerk, or keyboard operator. For this reason, some writers believe the clerical worker has suffered downward social mobility or 'proletarianization' and some writers have even placed such workers in the working class. In the 1800s such clerical workers had a high social status and their work, within which they did not 'dirty their hands', was much respected!

Those members of the working class who have remained in work have, from the 1960s onwards, enjoyed an increasing level of affluence. From that time, some have been able to own their own car, buy a range of labour saving gadgets for their homes and to enjoy holidays abroad. In the 1980s, a growing number of this 'affluent working class' have been able to buy their own homes. Home ownership for all households in Britain now stands at 63 per cent and is still increasing (*Social Trends*, 1990: **20**; 138). (The proportion of home ownership is significantly lower in Northern Ireland and Scotland.) Many households in Britain have been able to buy their 'council' (or public sector) house at a reduced rate in accordance with recent 'Right to Buy' legislation.

This increase in working class affluence has led some social scientists to believe that all workers may be becoming middle class. A French writer, André Gorz (1982), published a book entitled *Farewell to the Working Class*. For Gorz, new technology means that we will not in the future have to employ people to carry out the manual tasks that we have hitherto. He foresees a future in which full-time, paid employment as we know it today will disappear, and people will merely have to spend a much reduced length of time devoted to 'socially useful' work. All the signs are that, in fact, he may have heralded the end of the working class a little prematurely!

> 'We can state that middle-class people in comparison with the working classes, enjoy better health; live longer; live in superior homes with more amenities; have more money to spend; work shorter hours; receive different and longer education, and are educationally more successful; marry later in life; rear fewer children; attend church more frequently; belong to clubs more often; have different tastes in the mass media and the arts; are politically more involved – to mention only a few examples.'
> (Reid, I., *Social Class Differences in Britain*, Grant McIntyre, 1981, p. 297.)

The emergence of an 'underclass' in Britain

In the past few years some commentators on social class have begun to talk of a new phenomenon in Britain, particularly in our class structure. This is the emergence of a so-called 'underclass'. For many social scientists and those concerned with the future of our welfare services, this new development should deeply concern us all.

Debate on the concept of the 'underclass' itself has intensified. The term has been used both by those on the 'right' and on the 'left' of the political continuum. When used by those on the right it tends to have a morally judgemental element in that members of the underclass are depicted negatively as 'fickle' or 'immoral', 'criminal' or 'work-shy'. For those writers the concept appears to be a resurrection of the Victorian idea of the 'undeserving' as compared to the 'deserving' poor who they would now refer to merely as 'the poor'.

For those on the left, there has been disagreement as to the use of the concept and it is recognized that the very word itself has negative connotations. Ruth Lister believes it is imprecise, emotive and value-laden. Bob Holman agrees, rejects the term completely and prefers to simply refer to those who experience 'social deprivation' (*Social Work Today*, 16 August 1990). Both authors believe that the very use of the term is likely to worsen the plight of those to whom it refers and to increase the social stigma they face.

Others, such as Frank Field, whose definition of the term is discussed more fully below, and Bill Jordan, use the concept, but in doing so they concentrate on the economic, political and social *forces* or *structures* which exclude certain poor people from full citizenship. They focus on what Miller has referred to as 'the insufficiences of current economic and social policies to bring a subsection of the poor out of poverty conditions' (cited in Bulmer *et al.* 1989). Bill Jordan (1989) considers that we have 'a social structure in which the most important division in society is between the relatively comfortable majority and an underclass' (p. 18).

Despite the disagreement surrounding the use of the term 'underclass' it still has its usefulness. We use the concept throughout this book in a non-judgemental way as a means of drawing attention to the economic, political and social elements which have conspired together to exclude a section of our society from full citizenship. Perhaps a more satisfactory term will soon be discovered. For now we have placed the word in inverted commas in order to emphasize its imprecise nature.

The concept of an 'underclass'

There have been a number of varying concepts of an 'underclass' used in the past. In fact Marx himself referred to a capitalist society, such as Britain, as having a 'surplus population' or 'reserve army of labour'. Within this were five different groups of people:

1) Older workers who lose their jobs.
2) Agricultural workers who wish to move into industry.
3) A number of people who are employed on an irregular basis, in a casual way.
4) Paupers and others who are unable to work – they are not physically capable of doing so. This might include those with mental or physical disabilities.
5) To use his own word – the '*lumpenproletariat*'. These were, for example,

criminals, vagrants and prostitutes. Marx was very condemning of such people on moral grounds.

Some of these five groups of people would be able to find work when the economy is in 'boom times', but would speedily lose their jobs in a time of 'slump'. Hence the term *'reserve* army of labour'. They are used by capitalist employers for their own convenience. However, this is not the sense in which we are currently using the term 'underclass'.

Neither is it the same as that concept used in the 1970s by the sociologist Anthony Giddens. In a key text on social class (Giddens, 1973), he refers to a 'massive urban-based underclass' which he says is 'in a variety of ways, a specifically American phenomenon' (p. 217). In the same work he uses the concept in a different way. After saying that 'female workers are largely peripheral to the class system', he describes women workers in the service sector and clerical work as 'in a sense the 'underclass' of the white-collar sector' (ibid., p. 288).

In 1979, Rex and Tomlinson, writing about the British class system, referred to 'colonial immigrants' (we would now say 'ethnic minorities') as a distinct underclass. We should make clear that in no way was this a negative comment about the 'underclass'. Rather, Rex and Tomlinson were at pains to point out that their inferior position in the class structure of Britain was actually compounded by white racism.

What do we mean by an 'underclass' in Britain today?

For a more accurate account of what constitutes the 'underclass' in Britain today, we can turn to the sociologist Ralf Dahrendorf. In 1987 he noted that in this country (as in all Western societies) more goods could be produced by a shrinking labour force, because workers have become increasingly skilled and can draw on new technologies. This means that those people without such skills or educational qualifications are increasingly finding it more difficult to obtain work. They are no longer needed by society or more particularly by its economy. Many will face a future with no prospect of paid employment at all (*New Statesman*, 12 June 1987).

Dahrendorf notes that in America an 'underclass' has been spoken of for some time, but it is a much more recent development in Britain. Members suffer from a number of interlocking social problems, e.g. a low level of education attainment, family breakdown, miserable housing and environmental conditions and few public facilities in the areas in which they live, frequently the 'inner-city' areas. He also believes that members of ethnic minorities are over represented in the 'underclass'.

Perhaps the description of the 'underclass' which appears to be the most appropriate is that recently spelt out by Frank Field (1989), a Member of Parliament and former Director of the Child Poverty Action Group (CPAG). He believes the modern 'underclass' has been recruited from three groups of people. First, the long-term unemployed. Second, single-parent families and third, elderly pensioners. All are on *fixed incomes*, i.e. they receive state benefits of one kind or another.

It is important not to think of these groups as being homogenous; their situations, ages, gender and race are various. For example, the long-term

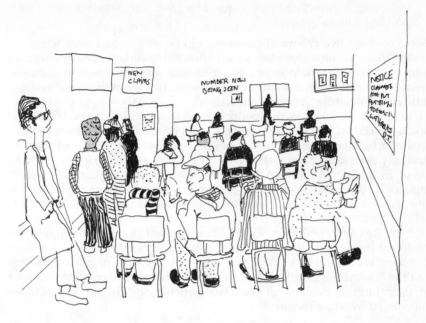

A common characteristic of the 'underclass' is their reliance on welfare benefits. The process of obtaining benefits often incurrs delay, frustration and sometimes humiliation.

unemployed will include young people who have not had paid work since leaving school, and older workers who have lost their jobs and owing to the ageism in society they find it difficult to obtain new employment. A large proportion of the unemployed are to be found in or near inner-city areas due to the earlier mentioned decline in heavy manufacturing industries. There is also a higher than average proportion of ethnic minority members among them, (given their numbers in society) whose families had originally moved to inner-city areas for the available work in traditional industries. Again, because of racism, people from ethnic minorities have found it extremely hard to obtain work. There are now over one million single-parent families in Britain and the vast majority of parents in these families are women. Child-care responsibilities are most frequently taken on by mothers and the plight of those who have been on welfare benefit for a long time is particularly harsh. Their child-care responsibilties mean they cannot work, especially in full-time jobs.

Those elderly pensioners who are completely dependent on their old-age pension and income support are also particularly deprived. They do not have an additional occupational pension, they often live in very poor housing, and they also have to contend with the increasing ill-health and disability which growing older can bring.

A final group that we should include are people who suffer from disabilities. An official report from the Office of Population Censuses and Surveys (1988c) estimated that there are six million disabled people in this country i.e. about one in ten of the total population. Another report from the same source published soon afterwards noted that two thirds of disabled people were living at, or below, the poverty line.

Around the same time, a report from the Disability Alliance (1988), (which represents about 100 voluntary organizations who champion the interests of the disabled) showed that disabled people of working age are twice as likely to be living on or below the poverty line, than are their able-bodied counterparts. Those particularly hard hit were disabled people who had never been able to work and who had therefore never made any national insurance contributions. Such people only receive basic state benefit for disabled people. The elderly disabled are particularly badly affected because of this.

The 'underclass' – permanently marginalized

The most depressing and distressing aspect of the social position of members of the 'underclass' is the *fixedness* of their situation. They are *trapped* and their situation is almost certainly permanent. If they earn a little money on a part-time or casual job their benefit is cut. It would appear that their only escape is well paid, secure employment, and this is extremely unlikely given their multiple deprivation.

Blaming the victim

As they are not needed any longer by our economy as workers, it is easy for our society to ignore and lose interest in them. It is possible to make the mistake of treating the deprivation from which members of the 'underclass' suffer (poverty, poor housing, etc.) as being the 'cause' of their plight. If this mistake is made, it becomes dangerously easy to unfairly 'blame the victim', for her or his predicament.

Bob Holman has pointed out that the behaviour of the rich carries less public censure. "Cabinet Ministers who beget children outside marriage, Oxbridge students who use drugs, Stockbrokers who commit fraud, the London Docklands' affluent who . . . build security fences to make themselves a separate group, do not lead [commentators] to write an attack on the 'overclass'. By just blaming the poor [they make] them victims" (*Social Work Today*, 16 August 1990).

How large is the 'underclass'

It is probably impossible to come up with an accurate figure for the number of people in the 'underclass'. We must be clear that this is not equal to the number of people living in poverty, of whom there are far more.

In 1987, Dahrendorf estimated that the 'underclass' he defined was around 5 per cent of the British population – that is nearly three million people. John Vincent as a supporter of Church Action on Poverty (an organization representing a number of different church denominations) calculated the size of the 'underclass' at the close of 1989 to be between one and two million people (Radio 4, *Today*, 11 December 1989). Not only is it extremely difficult to measure the number with any accuracy, but the situation is of course changing all the time, as social and economic factors and conditions alter.

Deprived of full citizenship

'Society means a shared life. If some and not others are poor then the principles on which life is shared are at issue; society itself is in question'.
(Halsey, A.H., Foreword to Mack, J., Lansley, S., *Poor Britain*, 1985, p. xxiii)

The material deprivation which members of the 'underclass' suffer also deprives them of a number of other things. Their children's education, which will be impoverished by poor living conditions, and diet – the direct result of poverty, will be further harmed by a lack of financial resources. Parents are not able to send or take their children on educational visits, trips or 'exchange holidays'.

The same families' mobility is severely restricted because they will not have access to a car and they have to rely on an often limited public transport (especially in rural areas). This also means they will have to rely on local shops, where prices are often higher than in larger stores in city or town centres, or in super-stores on the edge of urban areas.

Entertainment, hobbies, leisure pursuits and sport all cost money to some extent, and therefore members of the 'underclass' will have severely limited access to all of them. This means they will be confined to their homes with little to break up the daily tedium except radio or television.

'Television is my only luxury. I couldn't do without it. It would be so boring.'
(An elderly woman living on a state pension and income support,
The Independent, 20 September 1989)

Poverty is much more than simply a lack of finance. It is a poverty of experiences also. Life in the 'underclass' will be dispiriting and depressing, and how many feel they will ever escape from such an existence?

Members of the 'underclass' are deprived of being able to take a full part in social, political and economic life. They are *marginalized*. As we have said earlier their marginalization is *fixed*. The majority of its members are *trapped*, and this condition is likely to last for the rest of their lives.

'The existence of an underclass casts doubt on the social contract itself. It means that citizenship has become an exclusive rather than an inclusive status. Some are full citizens, some are not . . . If some have no stake in the society, the society puts itself at risk. It becomes defensive and, in the end, closed. Extending full citizenship rights to all is therefore the main task of social policy.'
(Dahrendorf, R., *New Statesman*, 12 June 1987)

For the sake of the well-being of every member of our society, the existence of the 'underclass' – of a sector of the population cut off in many different ways from mainstream social life, should not be allowed to continue.

The future

'The rest of us continue on our spending spree while (just occasionally) Toxteth burns.'
(Saunders, P., *Social Theory and the Urban Question*, 2nd ed., 1986, p. 335)

There is much talk of the increased affluence of a large proportion of society 'trickling down' to those not so well off. It is true that many people, including members of the working class, have come to enjoy better living standards. However, by its very nature the 'underclass' is cut off from this 'trickling down' of financial prosperity. Unlikely to find paid employment and dependent upon state welfare benefits, members of the 'underclass' are trapped on a fixed income, the real value of which has declined, and may well decline further in the future.

It is a profound indictment of many of those in authority in our society today that the 'underclass' are coming to be seen more and more as a threat to social tranquillity. Rather than eradicate the social and economic conditions which has brought the 'underclass' into existence, they are merely viewed as a *control problem*, provoking the solution – we must 'toughen-up' on law and order. One further example of '*blaming the victim*'.

Class and the social carer

We have become accustomed to seeing advertisements for jobs in social care which state that the employer is an 'equal opportunities employer'. These adverts usually say that the employer will take on people regardless of their *gender* and *race*. Less often *disability* is mentioned, and still less frequently *sexual orientation*. *Social class* is never mentioned at all. Employers do not have equal opportunities policies which state that members of the 'working class' are welcome to apply, let alone members of the 'underclass'!

Why should this be? It is difficult to come up with a clear answer to this question. Social class does not appear to be treated with the same importance or urgency as the other factors we have mentioned. Perhaps a key to the answer is to be found in a general awkwardness or embarrassment in British society towards class. Although we know that our society is deeply divided along class lines, many people do not like to acknowledge this. They choose to ignore it, as if this will diminish its significance. Others might find the mere mention of class in a job advertisement actually offensive. Many people like to render class invisible, to push it into the background.

What should our reaction as social carers be to social class? First, we should acknowledge that our own social class position will frequently differ from that of our clients, no matter in what specific field we work. The quality of life we enjoy, our life-style and material well-being, will usually be more privileged than that of our clients. Many field social workers and probation officers will have completed a professional training course in higher education, they will, therefore, have benefited from a vocational education course at a higher level than the average person in our country.

Second, such privileged life experience may well have implications for how well we can have empathy for, and have knowledge and understanding of those who become our clients. The trapped position of a member of the 'underclass' will not usually accord with our own more flexible situation. We are not subject to the particular stress and depression that being in such a position can engender.

Third, an awareness and knowledge of social class is imperative if we are to be effective social carers. We must attempt to understand the client in her or his social class and cultural context. This will inform our practice and ensure that we do not fall into the trap of *blaming the victim(s)* of the social class system – the victim(s) of *structural inequality*. Thus our understanding, awareness and empathy will be enhanced.

In increasing our awareness of social class, we will be better placed to see *communalities* of experience between clients who share a common social class position. We can attempt to raise our clients' own awareness of this situation and thereby help them not to be defeatist or blame themselves overmuch for their own predicament where this is a direct cause of structural inequalities or other social factors beyond their control.

Sometimes this is summed up as a way of *empowering* the client – helping the client to take more initiative in regard to their situation and become more pro-active. This is of great importance if we believe that it is their very lack of power over their own lives and situations which is the main effect of our client's frequent marginalization. It is also important that this empowerment (dealt with more fully in the final chapter of this book) is real, and leads to definite, progressive change, rather than being merely fine-sounding rhetoric.

Turning from the individual social carer to the agencies for which they work, it would be encouraging to see social class, along with other factors such as gender and race, included in their equal opportunities policies and recruitment advertising. As we indicated earlier, the issue has been ignored or conveniently avoided. It is extremely important for a balanced social care work-force, that members of social classes lower in the scale are recruited, along with more people from minority groups in our society. A predominantly middle class social care work-force dealing with a largely deprived clientele, leads to an unhealthy situation which reflects the 'powerful-powerless' divide in our society. Social care should be in the forefront of moves to radically change this situation for the better.

Exercises

1. Using the three major class analyses discussed in this chapter, place yourself in what you consider to be your relevant social class position. Give the reasons for so placing yourself.

2. *Social mobility*   Go back three generations (to your great-grandparents) and place each adult from the different generations in what you believe to be their relevant social class positions. Again use all three analyses; Marx, the Registrar-General and Goldthorpe. Now trace the pattern of social mobility, whether upward, downward, or unchanged. Account for changes in this pattern.

3. Where in the social class structure would you place the following personnel in the caring services:

> Nursery Nurse/Nursery Officer
> Home help (home carer)
> Receptionist
> Fieldwork social worker

Ward sister
Officer-in-charge, residential home for children
Occupational therapist
Home help/care organiser
Education welfare officer
Senior social worker
Probation officer
Care assistant/officer, residential home for the elderly
Registered general nurse
Chief Probation Officer/Assistant Chief Probation
Officer

4. Read the following poem.

Another thing about the English middle classes
Is how they hate their children.
Those under fifty, and more still, those under forty
They instinctively hate their own children
Once they've got them.

At the same time, they take the greatest possible care of them
– Nurses, doctors, proper food, hygiene, schools, all that –
The greatest possible care –
And they hate them.

They seem to feel the children a ghastly limitation
– But for these children I should be free –
Free what for, nobody knows. But free!
– Awfully sorry, dear, but I can't come because of the children.

The children, of course, know that they are cared for
And disliked.
There is no means of really deceiving a child.

So they accept covered dislike as the normal feeling between people
And superficial attention and care and fulfilment of duty
As normal activity
They may even, one day, discover simple affection as a great discovery.
Middle-Class Children from *The Complete Poems of D.H. Lawrence* ©
1964, 1971 by Angelo Ravagli and C.M. Weekley, Executors of the
Estate of Frieda Lawrence Ravagli. Used by permission of Viking
Penguin, a division of Penguin Books USA Inc.

i) Is the poet's message based entirely on prejudice, or is there some truth contained in it?
ii) Is disadvantage experienced by people from *all* social classes? If so, what forms does it take?

5. *Media study*   Make a selection of national daily and Sunday newspapers, e.g. two tabloids and two more 'serious' papers. Read them carefully and try to ascertain which social class they might appeal to most. Give reasons for your judgements.

Questions for essays and discussion

1. How far is it true that the middle class undertake social work and the working class carry out social care?

2. Britain is becoming increasingly a classless society.
3. Regardless of income, wealth, home and share-ownership, social class is largely determined by a person's life-style.
4. Social class is a more important factor than a person's race or gender status.
5. Poverty is only one deprivation affecting members of Britain's 'underclass'. What other forms of deprivation do they suffer?
6. In order to be an effective social carer, should you be from the same social class background as your client(s)? Give reasons for your answer.

Further reading

Academic
Field, F., *Losing Out: The Emergence of Britain's Underclass*, Blackwell, 1989. An up-to-date account of the development of an 'underclass' in Britain, along with possible ways of eliminating it.
Goldthorpe, J., *Social Mobility and Class Structure in Modern Britain*, Clarendon Press, 1980. An academic account of a very large research project into the modern development of social class in Britain. Covers social mobility and the ways in which it has occurred.
Marshall, G., Newby, H., Rose, D., Vogler, C., *Social Class in Modern Britain*, Hutchinson, 1988. The Essex University Project which generally rejects the idea that social class is no longer significant in Britain.
Marx, K., Engels, F., *The Manifesto of the Communist Party*, Foreign Languages Press, 1975. Originally commissioned by the Communist League, an international workers organization, in 1847. A readable introduction to some of Marx's key concepts in his analysis of capitalist society.
Saunder, P., *Social Class and Stratification*, Routledge, 1990. An analysis of social class in modern Britain, unusually sympathetic to a variety of 'New Right' perspectives.
Townsend, P., Davidson, N., (eds.), *Inequalities in Health (The Black Report)*, plus Whitehead, M., *The Health Divide*, Penguin, 1988. Two major reports in one volume. Explores the connection between ill health, poverty and social deprivation.

Other literary sources
Bleasdale, A., *Boys From the Blackstuff*, Hutchinson, 1985.
Grossmith, G. and W., *The Diary of a Nobody*, Penguin, 1965.
Lawrence, D.H., *Lady Chatterley's Lover*, Penguin, 1990.
Orwell, G., *The Road to Wigan Pier*, Penguin, 1989.
Sillitoe, A., *Saturday Night and Sunday Morning*, Paladin, 1990.
Tressel, R., *The Ragged-Trousered Philanthropists*, Panther, 1965.

Films or plays
Gilbert, L., *Educating Rita*. UK, 1983.
Ivory, J., *A Room with a View*. UK, 1985.
Loach, K., *Kes*. UK, 1969.
Mowbray, M., *A Private Function*. UK, 1984.

3 Women, gender, inequality and sexism

The difference between women and men

At the beginning of a mixed student seminar discussion group the tutor posed the question, 'What is the difference between women and men?' For a long while there was silence among the 20 or so sociology degree students until one brave young woman eventually spoke up. 'Err . . . I know the difference but I can't quite put my finger on it!' The tension was broken and laughter ensued.

But what was it that this student was trying to articulate? And why did her colleagues have such difficulty answering such a seemingly straightforward question? The answer is of course that it was not an easy question. Defining the differences between women and men is not easy because of the confusion surrounding that which is 'natural' and that which is socially defined as being appropriate for females and males. In other words the difference between *sex* and *gender*.

The age old debate about how much human behaviour is derived from innate factors and how much is a result of social conditioning cannot be settled in these pages. Suffice to say that there are distinct biological differences between women and men and there are observable differences in the way they live their lives.

The biological differences are determined at conception. *Sex* is the word used for the classification of the species into either female or male; females alone can give birth and suckle children and males have a different hormonal and genital structure from females. *Gender* is the word used to describe social and personality differences between women and men; it refers to that which society defines as masculine and feminine.

Although it is normally assumed to be so, gender need not necessarily be related to sex. For example, in our society usually only women are seen wearing skirts; it is considered a 'feminine' mode of dress. Yet in other societies, Sri Lanka, for example, both men and women wear wrap-around sarongs in their everyday life; there is no notion of masculinity or femininity associated with this form of dress. However, the kilt is a symbol of masculinity when worn by men in Scotland or Ireland, because of its connotations with honour and bravery.

Unlike 'sex' which is a relatively stable characteristic, 'gender' is a more variable concept defined differently between societies and within the same society over time. For example, in some tribal societies it is deemed masculine to wear ornaments whilst the women are shaven headed and unadorned. In other societies women do all the agricultural and other heavy work and so these heavy duties are considered feminine tasks.

In modern industrial society it is claimed that the basic differences between women and men have been greatly exaggerated. It is argued that a woman's biological capacity to reproduce and provide nourishment for her offspring has restricted women's role generally to the care and socialization of children. As it is only women who can give birth and naturally feed children, the care and upbringing of young children has been defined as feminine.

Social roles are defined by society but, because they appear to stem from biological differences between women and men, they are also claimed to be 'natural' and therefore appropriate; consequently child birth and child care have been inexorably linked. The essential biological differences between women and men have tended to divide society unequally in terms of women and men's labour, power roles and expectations.

Gender role stereotyping

Consider the following variation on an old riddle. A father takes his son for a ride in the family car. Unfortunately the car becomes involved in a crash and the boy is injured. He is immediately taken to hospital whereupon he is rushed to the operating theatre. On looking down and seeing the boy's face the surgeon cries, 'Oh my goodness! My own son!' What relationship is the surgeon to the boy?

The solution will be quite straightforward for some of you, notwithstanding its context within this chapter. Others of you should be forgiven for not establishing immediately that the surgeon is in fact the boy's mother. Society's stereotyped image of a surgeon is not female (it is more likely to be a white, middle-aged male). This is not to say that women are incapable of performing the work of a surgeon; rather because the work is associated with high status, scientific precision, responsibility and the world outside the home, it is firmly entrenched within the male domain.

Various attributes are commonly associated with women and men; they are considered to be either *feminine* or *masculine*. Have a look at the following list of adjectives and see if you think they can be applied exclusively to women, exclusively to men or equally to either sex:

> Tender, artistic, sporty, sensitive, handsome, secretive, mean, vicious, pretty, emotional, submissive, strong, flirty, feminine, neurotic, creative, practical, dominant, ambitious, self-confident, home-orientated, masculine, entertaining, hilarious, tearful, sexy, flatterable, egotistical, nagging, caring, aggressive, warm, boastful, appearance-oriented, independent.

In fact all of the above qualities may be applied equally to either women or men although traditionally most are associated more firmly with one of the sexes. The crudest stereotype portrays men to be strong, aggressive, logical and confident, while women are portrayed as sensitive, caring and timid. These are harmful images of both women and men because they limit individual growth and development. Stereotypes restrict the fulfilment of our human potential. Unfortunately they are powerful images which often affect people from the moment they are born.

Gender processing

Gender processing begins from the moment of birth when baby girls are traditionally covered in pink blankets and boys in light blue ones. Initially the parents and immediate family are the child's primary socializing influence, but as the child grows and interacts with the wider social world other people, such as relatives, neighbours, nursery or other day care staff, siblings, peers and the media, contribute to the child's understanding of her or his social role. At every stage the child is subject to beliefs about how females and males ought to behave based on society's prejudicial notions of femininity and masculinity. Eventually by the time a child has reached the mid-teens she or he has a good idea of what is expected by society.

Studies have shown that babies are treated differently according to their sex: for example, it has been established that there is a tendency for mothers to breastfeed boys for longer periods than girls. Even this action, whether it is done unconsciously or not, tends to reflect an inclination to foster independence and responsibility in girls (later to be the principal care givers) whilst tolerating dependency in boys.

That children internalize society's expectations of them is apparent in subtle behavioural differences between girls and boys at a very young age. An observation of a nursery class of children getting ready to go into the playground, where it was raining, indicated differences displayed by girls and boys in carrying out the simple task of putting their coats on. Whilst the girls were generally seen to attempt to get their coats on, struggling with awkward buttons in the process, the boys more often than not sought assistance.

It is hardly surprising that boys act in this way. Consider, for example, the world through a young boy's eyes receiving a rather stereotyped traditional upbringing: he develops a primary dependency relationship with his mother who feeds and cares for him most of the day. He sees very little of his father who is out for much of the time. Even when his father is not at work he may still be unavailable, he may be absent, tired or 'recuperating' from his work outside the home. The child will be used to having his needs attended to largely by his mother. If the boy attends a nursery or playgroup setting he will observe that it is predominantly women who care for the children. When he ventures outside to the doctor, the shops or the hospital he will again see mainly women in the role of receptionists, servers and carers. His picture of men is likely to be very different because he sees them in the more 'interesting and exciting' social roles of builder, transport driver and policeman.

Susie Orbach (1978) in her book, *Fat Is a Feminist Issue*, claims that within the family girls are instilled with an inferior sense of self. She argues that mothers tend to hold back their daughters' desire to be autonomous and self-directed. Instead, from an early age a young girl is guided to put her energy into taking care of others. At the same time boys are taught to accept emotional support without learning how to give this kind of loving in return. She suggests further that in some cases this imbalance in a girl's upbringing may later manifest itself in the development of depression or, in extreme cases, one of the various eating disorders such as bulimia or anorexia nervosa. As women struggle with their need to be themselves against the pressure to create and maintain a body shape desired by the male dominated outside world, they are

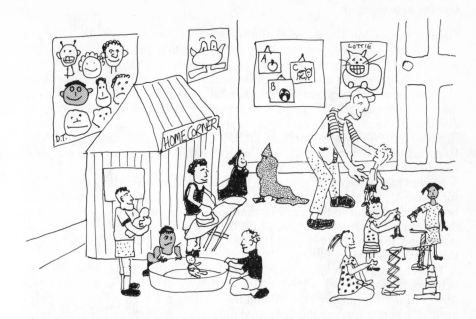

Staff gender and the activities children are permitted to take part in can serve to either reinforce or break down stereotypes.

particularly prone to such diseases. The consequences for boys, who Susie Orbach states do not learn to return the emotional support they are given, is that as men they are unable to give emotionally. This inability to relate on an emotional level inevitably becomes a major contributory factor to marital and partnership breakdown. According to NSPCC worker, John Roberts, 'social workers are often confronted with the inherent sadness men convey in not being able to reach out to other men (or women) with their own feelings and in not being able to share their insecurity and vulnerability' (*Community Care*, 25 August 1990, p. 22).

Women and depression

Many more women than men suffer depression and whereas single men are more prone to depression than married men, married women are more likely to become depressed than their single counterparts. One explanation for this is that the traditional housekeeping role is so poorly regarded by society that it represents an insufficient challenge to a woman's intellectual capacity. Consequently, those women confined to the home are more likely to break down than those who have paid jobs or are engaged in stimulating experiences.

Brown *et al.* (1975), in their classic study on women and depression carried out in Camberwell, highlighted the contribution to women's depression made by the absence of emotional support from their partner. They point out that many women fail to receive the closeness, mutual trust and opportunity for expression of feeling they need from a relationship. They identified four main contributory factors towards depression in women. These were the loss of mother in childhood, having three or more children under fourteen living at home, the absence of paid work and the lack of a close, confiding relationship. Apart from outside employment all these vulnerability factors are class related. For example, '43 per cent of working class women had three or more children living at home compared to middle class women; 9 per cent of working class women had experienced the loss of their own mother in childhood compared to 3 per cent of middle class women and only 37 per cent of younger working class women enjoyed a relationship of high intimacy compared to 75 per cent of middle class women.' They add that 'social structural factors are certainly at the root of some of the events that we call severe and that they partly explain their greater incidence amongst working class women' (p. 279).

Shere Hite confirms the frustration felt by women towards men regarding their unwillingness to share their feelings. In her study *Women and Love* (1988) she canvassed the opinion of 4500 women on their ideas about love and sex. She found 98 per cent of the women in her study 'wanted more verbal closeness with the men they loved; they wanted the men in their lives to talk more about their own personal thoughts, feelings and plans and to ask them about theirs'. For most women their best friends were women; this was the person with whom they chose to share their intimate secrets. Men too turned to women when they needed to be close to someone.

Men and socialization

There is much in the socialization of men that discourages them from express-ing their feelings. Pressure on them to always appear strong and in control in front of others means that they learn from an early age to hide their true feelings. 'Big boys don't cry', is a clear message throughout childhood which is reinforced in books and other forms of popular culture. The lyrics of the 1980s song *Boys Don't Cry* by The Cure is just one example. Another can be found in the earlier sentimental classic by Elvis Presley *Old Shep*. Tears finally come to a small boy, who is forced to shoot his dying dog, only after a great struggle.

Formaini (1990) discusses the narrow definition of masculinity to which society expects boys to conform. One of the 160 men on which her study was based explained what this definition of masculinity entailed. 'If I am a little boy, I have to cut off everything that means being a little girl. I don't cry anymore, I keep a stiff upper lip and I pretend to like games even if I am terrible at them and I am stoic and all that sort of stuff' (p.9).

Formaini comments 'Giving up feelings is a very heavy price to pay for one's masculinity. Without feelings, it is very difficult to make the kind of decisions that men need to make, whether the decision concerns personal relationships or something else' (p.11).

Signs of emotion and expressions of tenderness are often interpreted as weakness and are rarely admitted to by men to other men, except perhaps obliquely through jokes. Consequently, many men find themselves locked in an image conscious macho world built on bravado, banter and outward signs of success – a world in which they compete more easily than they relate.

The physical expression of feelings for most heterosexual men is restricted to acts of aggression or acts of horseplay, or it is ritualized in social situations, for example, at football and rugby matches. The typical male greeting involves the formal handshake or the slapping of palms; rarely do men freely wrap their arms around one another. In contrast women are more spontaneous; they touch each other more readily and kiss or hug one another when they meet. Gay men are generally more able than other men to express their emotions; they too touch and kiss more easily and have done much to break down the rigidity of the unfeeling male stereotype.

That so many men are unable either to own to or express their feelings and to communicate at a more intimate level, has detrimental consequences for their partners and for the children. By avoiding a deeper expression of what they feel, they also do themselves great harm by denying an essential aspect of their lives.

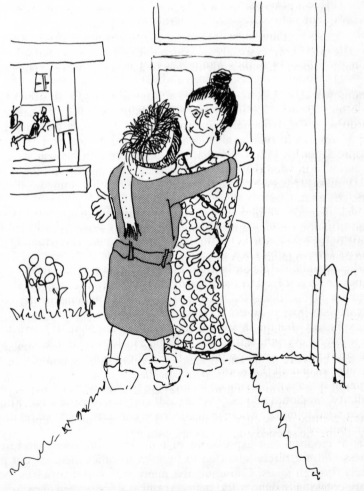

Women tend to be more spontaneous than men in the way they touch each other.

Education

Girls and boys can be seen to be treated differently within the education system in this country. Traditionally boys have been guided towards the science-based subjects whilst girls have been encouraged to study the arts and humanities. The potential academic ability of girls and boys is essentially the same, although minimal differences have been recorded at different ages. At the 16-year-old GCSE stage girls in fact achieve slightly higher results than boys. Yet at the A-level stage, two years later, they comprise only 47 per cent of entrants (Equal Opportunities Commission, 1989). This may be explained in some way by the fact that there is less emphasis on girls to achieve academically; their need for social credentials and future career prospects is not considered as vital as it is for boys. This is evident too in the allocation of YTS places. According to one study carried out by the Equal Opportunities Commission, girls were placed disproportionately on clerical, retailing and caring schemes whilst boys dominated the information technology schemes, in spite of the fact that the supervisor found girls to be more adept than boys (ibid.).

It is noticable that applicants for social care courses are almost exclusively female. The more general social care courses attract the interest of some young men, but once selected, male students may feel under pressure to complete the course.

A young working class man on a nursery nurse course was forced to leave after the second term. He had survived the banter from his friends and the awkwardness arising from belonging to a class of 24 female students. He was also coping financially on a small educational award. However, he succumbed to pressure from his father who had not been keen on his son starting the course and who insisted that he should start earning money and find a proper job. It is unlikely that such pressure would be placed on a young woman under the same circumstances.

The lack of male social care and nursery nurse students detracts from a balanced situation where young men and women can learn from each other. It also contributes eventually to the maintenance of the disproportionate representation of women in all fields of social care.

Over recent years, in response to the Sex Discrimination Act (1975), schools and colleges have developed policies in order to combat gender-based inequality. Educational materials have been scrutinized for their sexist content and where identified have been replaced by newly created non-stereotyped materials. Deliberate efforts have been made to break down the traditional gender association with subject areas; girls are being encouraged towards the sciences and boys are being encouraged to develop skills in domestic science, biology and office practice. Whilst these policies represent progress it must be remembered that sexism is so firmly entrenched in our society that significant change can only be gradual. Fig. 3.1 demonstrates that girls are still widely under represented in science subjects and boys are under represented in cookery, domestic science and child care subjects.

Sexism

'If sexism makes life difficult for successful and aspiring women, it makes the quality of life available to poor and powerless women almost intolerable.'
(Campling, J., *Learning the Hard Way*, 1986, p. **xi**.)

Sexism is firmly entrenched within our society ranging in degree from the overt to the subtle. A clear form of sexism would be where someone is denied admittance or membership to a club or premises on the grounds of her or his sex; for example, the current practice at Lords, the headquarters of the MCC and the English cricket establishment, to refuse admission to women members in the pavilion. More subtle instances of sexism will include the veiled put down which occurs in everyday conversation, when women are referred to as 'dear', 'love', or 'pet' by men with whom they might not even be familiar. (It should be noted that in some areas such words are used in a non-gender specific way in order to convey endearment.)

As well as being evident in ordinary interactions between individuals, sexism can be seen to be institutionalized in the practices and procedures of different organizations. Indeed there are many similarities between racism and sexism in this respect, but whilst racism is directed against a numerical minority in Britain, sexism is principally directed against women who currently make up 51 per cent of the population (OPCS, 1990).

The word sexism was coined by analogy to racism to denote discrimination based on gender. Originally sexism referred to prejudice exclusively against the female sex. It is now used in a broader sense to indicate the stereotyping of both females and males on the basis of their gender. Strictly speaking both sexes are affected by sexism, but it is women who suffer most. 'This is because sexism does not merely encourage an artificial segregation of the sexes: it perpetuates the notion of male superiority' (ILEA, 1985, p. 4). That is to say sexism is directed primarily against women because men hold power disproportionately within society.

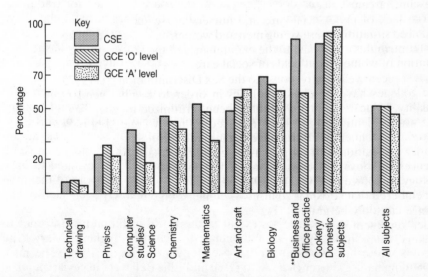

Fig. 3.1 Females as a percentage of entrants in selected subjects for CSE, GCE O' level and A' level summer examinations 1985. (Reproduced from *Women and Men in Britain: A Research Profile*, HMSO, 1988, p. 13.)

Patriarchy

We live in a patriarchal society: the word patriarch means male head of family or father, but when it is applied to society it is used to imply male domination. Men hold a disproportionate amount of power in society and so many of the rules, institutions and values of society support the notion of male superiority and reinforce the corresponding subjugation of women.

Consider the overwhelming presence of men in official positions of power in this country. They currently make up 94 per cent of the House of Commons and dominate almost as completely the House of Lords. They predominate in the higher echelons of the Civil Service, the armed forces, the police, the judiciary and the legal and financial institutions. Not only is this the position now but it has been established for as long as those organizations have existed. Men's power in the past helps them maintain notions of superiority today.

The Hansard Society Commission on 'Women at the Top' found that Britain lagged behind many European countries in the number of women holding senior positions in political, public, industrial and commercial life. It argued for example that only a handful of judges were women compared with more than a third in Holland and France (*Guardian*, 26 January 1990).

Academic institutions are male dominated. Much of what is studied relates to male activity. History has been written largely by men about men. The majority of ideas relate to the actions of men. The fact that most buildings were designed by able-bodied men accounts for the neglect of the principal needs of women and disabled people. Until the last few years no public buildings had specific accommodation for baby feeding and changing nappies, and this necessary provision is by no means widespread. Few buildings today have easy access for parents with prams or heavy shopping and many remain a barrier to disabled people. In the domestic sphere, the space allocated for traditional women's tasks such as cooking, washing and cleaning has been marginalized. Kitchens, bathrooms and washrooms, for example, often occupy a relatively small area compared to other rooms in the house. Only recently has it been generally acknowledged that these tasks are better performed within space and light.

What is valued as great art is almost exclusively male. Most women have either been denied the opportunity to fulfil their artistic creativity and so make a significant contribution to history; or when they have had the opportunity, their work has often been marginalized, trivialized or, in some cases, misappropriated. For example, the now acknowledged work of the seventeenth century artist Artemisia Gentileschi was appropriated and claimed to have been performed by men for a long time. Until recently the work of the artist Gwen John, which is now highly acclaimed, was completely overshadowed by that of her brother Augustus.

The same is true to a lesser extent in the world of literature. In order to compete intellectually in male-dominated Victorian England, Mary Ann Evans wrote her books under the pseudonym of George Eliot. The male sounding names Currer Bell, Acton Bell and Ellis Bell were necessary *nom de plumes* used by Charlotte, Anne and Emily Brontë in order to publish their poetry. Today women's impact in the world of literature is still restricted. Despite the work of the Women's Press and other publishing organizations, newspapers are still male dominated and tend to review books mainly by male authors. In late 1989 the *Guardian* produced a twelve page literary supplement under the heading 'Christmas Books'. Eighteen people had contributed to it and every one was a man. A similar feature was carried out by the *Observer* at the same time, in which just six out of twenty-four books reviewed were written by women. Not only were the majority of books reviewed male dominated, the actual reviewers themselves were almost exclusively male. This reflects what Nicci Gerard, deputy literary editor of the *Observer*, calls 'the influence of the metropolitan elite,' who run newspapers. She could not account for why the male editors continue to ignore women as authors. She said, 'I think mostly they don't know they are doing it, in the same way that men don't see that all the pictures in the art gallery are by men. But women notice' (*Cosmopolitan*, May 1990).

Women and the media

The media tends to reinforce the unequal position of women in society in two ways. It reflects existing inequalities, so that it depicts women predominantly in their caretaking role and renders them invisible in more socially powerful positions. It further distorts the view of women, since it is largely controlled by men and there is an over emphasis on what women look like. As Susie Orbach points out, 'the media present women either in a sexual context or within the family, reflecting a woman's two prescribed roles, first as a sex object and then as a mother' (1978, p. 61). Images of women are often stereotyped in a limiting way which does not reflect the true diversity of women's lives. Newspapers, cartoons, films and television often depict women as having negative characteristics, of having a narrow and specific range of interests and as being almost always white, heterosexual and able-bodied.

The media does not always aim to inform. Often it seeks to dramatize or to entertain in order to increase circulation or obtain more viewers or more listeners. In doing so it creates distorted images: its sensationalized emphasis on 'perverts' and 'sex maniacs' and 'monsters' helps perpetuate the myth about the limited range of men capable of being involved in child or partner abuse. The lack of black women's prominence in the media, except for their misrepresentation as victims or social misfits, contributes to their general invisibility within society. Furthermore the media's representation of 'idealized women' to which other women are expected to conform causes distress and offence to many women.

Over the past few years more women presenters have appeared on television, which reflects to a certain extent their improved access to positions within the media. However, it needs to be pointed out that womens' images are still a significant factor, and that they are up against the dual barriers of sexism and ageism. In a letter to the *Guardian*, a reader wrote, 'There is still too much of what Anna Ford called body facism, i.e. female presenters and reporters have to be attractive, have good if not perfect figures, be young, i.e. up to fortyish. Male presenters can be any age, figure or hair colour.' Another reader added, 'I want to see fat women reading the news and presenting documentaries . . . over half the women watching are size sixteen plus' (2 April 1990, p. 22).

Language and male domination

Language plays a major role in informing us of how society views women and men. There are many aspects of contemporary English language which reveal prejudicial attitudes; for example, the use of pronouns, word order and forms of address. Each helps to reinforce the dominant social values. Everyday language can be seen to support the status quo, i.e. the subjugation of women and the dominance of men.

One clear injustice with regard to language is the requirement for females to declare their marital status. Women are addressed as 'Miss' or 'Mrs' depending on whether or not they are married, but men, for whom Mr is the general courtesy title, need not reveal whether they are married. This situation has been mitigated to some extent in the past 20 years with the adoption of the non-specific female courtesy title Ms, although it is often wrongly used only to describe single women, thereby defeating the point of its intended usage. A further inequality is in evidence when, after marrying it is the woman who is conventionally expected to surrender her family name and adopt that of her husband.

Another example of the way in which contemporary English tends to demean the importance of women is in the continuous use of the pronoun 'he' in a general sense when 'she or he' would be the correct words to use. For example, one may read in a text book, 'When the child goes into care special attention is paid to *his* personal requirements in order that *he* is not too traumatized by the move away from home.' 'His or her' or 'he or she' could easily be substituted in the above sentence thereby rendering the true meaning and giving females and males equal footing. It is not only the apparent clumsiness of 'he or she' nor the grammatical incorrectness of 'they' when referring to the singular which encourages the use of this narrow form of expression; it is another instance of the general invisibility of women in society reflected in daily language usage.

The use of the word 'man' in the generic sense, to mean all human beings, is another example; words like mankind and manslaughter help to maintain the domination of men. The adopted relatively recent use of neutral words such as 'chair', 'ploughperson's lunch' and 'post person', however ridiculous they initially sound, represent a breakthrough and help promote social change. Generally words associated with men carry positive connotations, such as craftsmanship and sportsmanship. Fewer positive female-based words easily spring to mind, examples include 'sisterhood' and 'motherhood'. The fact that there are many more derogatory slang and swear words associated with females than with males is evidence of basic misogyny; and while there is a word for men who hate women there is no such equivalent word in the dictionary for women who hate men.

It is not only the meanings of words which betray male domination but the way people interact and the way in which language is used. Consider the following extract from the beginning of Peter Smith's book *Language, the Sexes and Society* (1985), which shows how in subtle ways use of language in everyday encounters serve to perpetuate male dominance.

Several years ago a well-known feminist author was interviewed on British television about her new book on language and the sexes, in which she argued forcefully that language is a man-made product, designed by and for the male half of the species to the neglect and exclusion of women. Her interviewers, besides the male programme host, were three male academics, two of them full professors of English. I had read her book myself, and was keenly interested in what she had to say as I was in the early stages of writing this book. I was to be surprised and disappointed, however, for the great majority of the words uttered in the 15 minute interview were spoken by men. In fact, although I did not take accurate measures, I estimated at the time that the author spoke for less than her democratic share of three minutes, much less than one might have expected under the circumstances. This did not seem to be due to the author's unwillingness or inability to contribute to the conversation – she had after all written the book. Moreover, I knew her to be a very intelligent and articulate person. I also noticed that she was interrupted in mid-sentence at least twice, although she was in her thirties and had completed a PhD, she was addressed by her first name by the host and other interviewers alike, and even at one point as "my dear", unlike the others, who were always addressed by their formal academic titles.

(Blackwells, 1985, p. 1)

Similarly school girls who had experienced an experimental two year single sex mathematics class were also able to remark about the way they were inhibited or put down in the classroom by boys. 'I think it is better with all girls – you are more confident – less frightened. If you get an answer wrong the boys laugh at you.' 'I prefer single-sex maths groups because when you get a question right all the girls say "that's good". In a mixed group the boys say "Oh! that's easy – anyone could have done that". (Cohen, 1988, p. 50)

The Women's Movement

The impact of the modern Women's Movement which flourished during the 1960s and 1970s was considerable, leading to a more widespread public acknowledgement of the position of women in society. The movement is often referred to as 'Second Wave' feminism, to distinguish it from the political struggle carried out by the suffragettes and suffragists during the end of the 19th century and early part of this century. Today, the Women's Movement, although still influential, is largely fragmented, embracing as it does a wide range of feminist opinion.

During the 1960s and 1970s, groups such as 'Women's Aid', 'Women Against Violence Against Women', and the women's peace groups were founded. Other action-based groups concerning issues such as abortion, education, trade unions and the media were formed and women campaigned both locally and nationally in order to heighten public awareness and to improve basic services. Political magazines established at this time, such as *Spare Rib* and *Feminist Review*, continue today to oppose male domination. As a result of the Womens' Movement, traditionally marginalized issues which had always been important in women's lives, such as child care, reproduction and work outside the home, were brought into the centre of political debate.

The Equal Pay Act 1970 was passed in order to establish equality between women and men and it became illegal to pay a woman less than a man for the same work. Despite the intention behind this legislation, women still receive generally lower incomes than men. In 1986 women's average gross hourly earnings were 74 per cent of that of men. If the effects of overtime are included, the average gross, weekly earnings was 61 per cent of men's. These figures relate partly to the fact that women are still predominantly employed in occupations which are less well paid.

The Sex Discrmination Act 1975 set up an independent statutory organization, The Equal Opportunities Commission (EOC), based in Manchester, and relating to England, Scotland and Wales (Northern Ireland has a separate commission). It's principle duties are:

1. To work towards the elimination of discrimination on grounds of sex in employment, education and consumer services and on grounds of marriage in employment.
2. To promote equality of opportunity between men and women generally.
3. To keep under review the working of this Act and the Equal Pay Act 1970 and when they are so required by the Secretary of State or otherwise think it necessary, draw up and submit to the Secretary of state proposals for amending them.

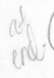

The impact of the Sex Discrimination Act can be seen in the declarations of equal opportunities statements and formal practices of many public organizations which are beginning to have an effect. However, it has to be said that the Women's Movement generally and the legislation which was passed during its most active stages has not yet resulted in profound social change.

Women and work

The principal reason women have for seeking paid work is the same as it is for men – that is, to earn money in order to provide for themselves and any family they may have. There are other non-financial benefits to be obtained from work outside the home and these vary from occupation to occupation. In the more skilled areas of work, these may include a sense of satisfaction, intellectual fulfilment, career progression or a chance to develop personal and social skills. Not all jobs are stimulating, in fact, the majority are mundane and repetitive, but employment outside the home at least offers women a source of independence, a chance to relate to other people, and to feel they are contributing to society. There have been several major studies on the debilitating effects of unemployment. The majority of these have focused on men. A study by Cochrane and Stopes-Roe (1981) showed that women in employment had fewer symptoms of depression than women not in paid work.

Many women and a small number of men choose not to work in order to remain at home so that they can look after their children. They find this work sufficiently stimulating and engaging. Other women may work outside the home part-time or on a job share basis, and spend only a part of their week exclusively looking after children. Not all women want to spend all their time looking after children and doing domestic duties. It can be an isolating and debilitating existence, particularly for single parents on low incomes. It has been established that many more women would work if there existed better provision of child-care services for the under-fives.

Women are now just over 43.4 per cent of the country's work-force and their proportion is growing. According to the Government's White Paper, *Employment for the Nineties* (1988), the number of women in the labour force will

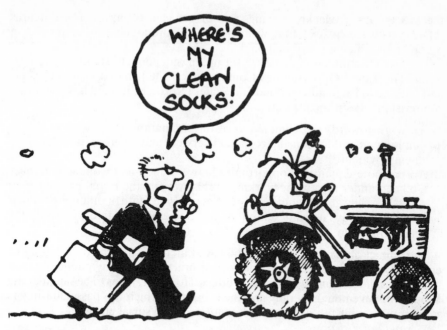

(Reproduced with permission from Spellbound Books, 23–25 Moss Street, Dublin 2).

increase. Two thirds of labour force growth between 1983 and 1987 was made up of married women and by 1995 the projected increase in size of the female labour force is some three-quarters of a million; over 80 per cent of the total.

Women have not always had such access to work outside the home. It took the First and Second World Wars to begin to break down the myth that only men could do certain types of work. The wars meant that everyone had to do her or his share regardless of gender. Vacancies created by the call of the armed forces meant that women were needed in a whole range of occupations including munitions, public transport and work on the land. By the end of the war the expectation was that women would give up their jobs and returned to their homes. Not all women did so but the prevailing social attitude and governmental policies were opposed to the majority of them remaining economically active. Today over 50 per cent of all married women are now engaged in work outside the home compared to 20 per cent in 1951 and 10 per cent in 1921 (Cohen, 1988).

Although women represent a large and increasing proportion of the work-force, working outside the home still involves discrimination against them. Women can be seen to be discriminated against in two ways: vertically and horizontally.

Vertical discrimination refers to discrimination within the same occupation. For example, within the teaching profession women can be seen to be dis-proportionately represented in the lower paid basic grade teaching posts and correspondingly under represented in positions of seniority, such as headships

Table 3.1   Age, gender and average salary of primary[a] schoolteachers and special schoolteachers in the UK, 1984–85[b].

	Age (Nos in 000s) Under 30	30–39	40–49	50–59	Over 60	Annual Salary
In primary schools						
Men	3	18	10	8	2	10 805
Women	24	49	50	35	2	9 337
In special schools						
Men	1	2	2	1	–	11 497
Women	2	4	4	5	–	9 939

a) Includes nursery schools and classes. b) *Education Statistics for the UK*, 1986 Edition, HMSO. *Note:* Annual average earnings, April 1985, non-manual workers:[2] Men £11 700, Women £6 958. Reproduced from Cohen (1988), *Caring for Children*, Commission of the European Communities.

and senior teaching posts. Table 3.1 shows the average salary of primary and special school teachers.

Horizontal discrimination refers to discrimination across all occupations and shows women to be over represented in certain lower status, largely service-related jobs, whilst they have a restricted access to other more prestigious or better paid occupations.

Women are concentrated in relatively few occupations. A substantial proportion of the female labour force is clustered in the clerical sector which employs nearly one-third of women and only 7 per cent of men. The other large concentrations of female workers are in the service sector groupings of catering, cleaning, hairdressing and other personal services. This sector employs a total of 23 per cent of women but only 4 per cent of men (Department of Health, 1990).

The main professional areas of employment for women are in the fields of health, welfare and education which employ 15 per cent of women and 5 per cent of men. In contrast, the range for men is more evenly spread, the two greatest concentrations being in managerial (13 per cent) and metal and electrical manufacture and repair (17 per cent). Over three times as many men as women are self-employed. Only 20 per cent of GPs and 13 per cent of hospital consultants are women, although this should change now that women form nearly a half of all medical students. In a city salary survey carried out in London in May 1990, it was shown that nearly four in every five of the most highly paid jobs in the city are held by men and very few women have jobs which command a salary above £20 000.

Inequalities in pay

Table 3.2 shows that despite the passing of the Equal Pay Act and the Sex Discrimination Act during the 1970s, the average gross hourly earnings for women continue to be significantly lower than those of men.

In 1986 women's full-time average gross hourly earnings were 74 per cent of men's, a difference of 26 per cent. Surprisingly the gap was slightly greater than 10 years earlier, having narrowed significantly from 1970 to 1977 but widened

Table 3.2 Average gross hourly earnings (pence per hour), excluding the effects of overtime, of full-time employees aged 18 and over, 1970–1986

	1970	1974	1975	1976	1977	1978	1979	1980	1981	1982	1983	1984	1985	1986
Men	67.4	104.8	136.3	162.9	177.4	200.3	226.9	280.7	322.5	354.8	387.6	417.3	445.3	481.8
Women	42.5	70.6	98.3	122.4	133.9	148.0	165.7	206.4	241.2	262.1	287.5	306.8	329.9	358.2
Differential	24.9	34.2	38.0	39.5	43.5	52.3	61.2	74.3	81.3	92.7	100.1	110.5	115.4	123.6
Women's earnings as % of men's	63.1	67.4	72.1	75.1	75.5	73.9	73.0	73.5	74.8	73.9	74.2	73.5	74.0	74.3

Source: *New Earnings Surveys 1970–1986.*

again in the late 1970s and the early 1980s. These figures do not give the complete picture of the inequality since they are gleaned from statistics of people in full-time work: a large proportion of women work part-time. For example, in relation to the hours of work of parents with children under the age of 10 years; 42 of women work part-time and only 6 per cent of men (*Social Trends*, 1987, **17**, HMSO).

Part-time work is by tradition poorly paid; 'In the UK 80 per cent of part-time workers earn less than the Council of Europe's decency threshold of 3.25 p per hour' (Cohen, 1988). Furthermore, part-time work often excludes benefits such as sick pay, annual leave and other arrangements customarily associated with full-time employment. A House of Lords Committee (1985) which examined the problems of part-time work commented:

> 'Part-time employees, while contributing significantly to the development of the economy and to the flexibility of the productive system, are, as a group, still behind their full-time colleagues in regard to wage rates, access to training and promotion and the provision of other benefits. This is both economically self-defeating and socially unacceptable, not least when it reinforces types of discrimination, such as that between male and female employees'.   (p. 72).

Women are forced into part-time work arrangements mainly because of their other responsibilities of caring for others and running a home. Figure 3.2 shows that the hours which women work are strongly influenced by the presence of dependent children. In 1985 over two-thirds of women with dependent children worked part-time.

Child care

Although there is a growing tendency for men to take more of a share in the care of children, the responsibility rests predominantly on the shoulders of women. It is still women who sacrifice career opportunities by withdrawing from the labour market for long periods to look after their children; it is women who reduce their paid working hours in order to be available for children outside school hours and it is women and not men who are most likely to take

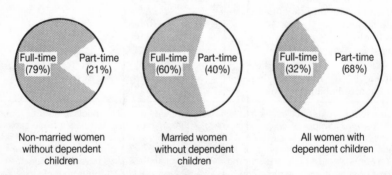

Non-married women without dependent children

Married women without dependent children

All women with dependent children

Fig. 3.2 Working women by family status and full or part-time employment in the UK, 1985. (Reproduced from *Key Facts Part III Employment*, HMSO, 1989, p. 41.)

time off work on the occasions when their children are sick and both mother and father are working.

It is largely owing to the lack of adequate child-care facilities that women are forced to sacrifice themselves in this way. With proper state-funded day-care facilities available, women would be freer to decide their own involvement in the labour market. At present the UK has less publicly funded child-care services than any other EEC country except Portugal. France has 95 per cent of children in publicly funded child care, Italy has 80 per cent, Germany 60 per cent and the Netherlands 50 per cent. Britain has 44 per cent which means the majority of parents in this country are forced to make their own child-care arrangements. Consequently, most families rely on relatives or neighbours to provide informal care for their children. Table 3.3 shows the child-care provision available in this country.

It can be seen that local education authority nursery classes or nursery schools and primary schools provide a high proportion of the places available for children under the age of five years. However, children need to be three years old before they can start. Further, the places are often part-time and unavailable during the school holidays. Nursery schools and classes are entirely paid for by the state and of course are normally very stimulating settings for young children. For this reason places are sought after by parents. However, since there is no statutory requirement for local authorities to provide education for children under five years, except where the child has a stated special need, vacancies depend on where the family lives and the political commitment of the local council.

Table 3.3 Non-parental child-care provision for under-fives in the UK, 1985

Type of provision	No. of[a] places	% of population aged 0–4 for whom this type of provision is available
LEA nursery class or school	338 541[a,b]	9.4
LEA primary school	295 202	8.2
LA day nursery	32 964	0.9
Registered childminder	144 908	4.0
Private and voluntary day nurseries	27 533[c]	0.8
Private schools	35 000[a]	1.0
Playschools	468 945	13.0
Nannies, au pairs, etc.	30 000[d]	0.8
Relatives	Not known[e]	–
Non-registered childminders	16 000[f]	0.7

a Figures for LEA nursery classes and schools, for private nursery schools and for LEA primary schools refer to number of *children attending*, rather than places, i.e. totals include substantial numbers of part-time pupils. b Predominantly 3- and 4-year-olds. c Includes some non-registered nurseries. d Derived from findings of 1980 Women and Employment Survey: 4 per cent of all working mothers and 6 per cent of mothers working full-time use this form of childcare for under-fives. e 47 per cent of all working mothers use this form of childcare for under-fives. f Recent research suggests that 20 per cent of childminders are not registered. Reproduced from Cohen (1988), *Caring for Children*, Commission of the European Communities.

Local authority day nurseries represent slightly less than 1 per cent of the total day-care provision and so is clearly unavailable to many families. Day nurseries have been forced to place priorities on their intake and allocate according to the child's social need: children at risk are given priority, and socially disadvantaged children are accommodated whenever it is possible. This practice has served to alter the function of day nurseries to some extent and also to create a stigma for women who take their children there.

Today there are fewer day nurseries than there were at the end of the Second World War, nearly 50 years ago. At the start of the war in 1939, there were only 14 day nurseries but as the war progressed there was a dramatic improvement in child-care facilities, particularly in the number of day nursery places. Within three years there were 1345 day nurseries offering 60 000 places to young children. Shortly after the end of the war in 1945, many of these newly created places were closed down as it was no longer deemed necessary to assist women to remain in work outside the home. Women had to wait until the 1960s when job opportunities became increasingly available again before there was an expansion of day-care provision, but the immediate post-war level of nursery places was never matched. Today there are roughly half as many public day nursery places available as there were in 1945. According to Tom White, National Children's Home Director of Social Work, 'Parents of Britain's 3.5 million under-fives are chasing less than 750 000 day-care places. Only 0.3 per cent of school children are being cared for in an after school scheme'.

In recent years there has been an increase in the number of work-place nurseries mainly in the public sector, in hospitals, town halls and colleges. These 'on-site' creches have obvious advantages to parents who work in the establishments, yet they are not numerically significant enough to provide many parents with alternative child care. In 1988 there were 100 work-place nurseries, 20 of which were provided by private companies. By 1990 there had been a great expansion within the private sphere as companies took the lead in attracting and keeping their female staff. In the budget of the same year, tax was finally lifted from work based nurseries so that it was no longer treated as a 'perk' for the company and employees could now obtain creche facilities at a reduced and more realistic cost. All other forms of day care involve parents in some expense and this in itself can be prohibitive; some mothers have to calculate whether it makes economic sense to take on a job because, in addition to having to consider the ordinary work-related expenses of travel, food and clothing, they need to calculate the cost of having their child or children looked after during the time they are at work.

Most working parents in the UK use child minders although not necessarily those registered and approved by the local authority. A recent report found that while 80 per cent of parents used child minders only 3 per cent believed it to be the best provision (Cohen, 1988). Play groups continue to be the main source of part-time day care. Au pairs and nannies offer support to children of high income families only. Owing to the expense involved in child care much of the existing provision discriminates against working class women and black women. In some areas these women have retaliated and have developed their own community nurseries or have pressurized councils into assisting them.

With proper day-care facilities many more women who wish to work would be able to do so. There would appear to be a clear correlation between participation of women in work outside the home and the availability of adequate child care provision. For example, in Denmark, where the level of public child care provision is high, 75 per cent of mothers with young children are employed, whereas in the UK which, as we have seen has a relatively low figure of child-care provision, the proportion is 28 per cent (*Hansard*, House of Lords, 21 June 1989, col. 263).

Women as informal carers

In addition to the fact that women are primarily responsible for the care of young children in our society, they are also the people most likely to be involved in caring for an elderly or otherwise dependent relative. In fact there are more women caring for dependent relatives than there are women looking after children under the age of 16 years. Hunter Davies, writing in *The Observer* on 13 November 1988, described his part in looking after his mother who was suffering from Alzheimer's disease. 'I admit I did little except pay the endless helpers and moan when they did not turn up, or cut corners when it was my turn. My sister and my wife carried and cared most. Women do. No that's not sexist. That's looking coldly around the planet.'

Caring for a dependent relative can be a full-time activity. Some may need attention 24 hours a day. Support services do exist and are provided by the local authority Social Services Departments but the availability of these highly demanded services vary from region to region. Limited financial assistance is also available through the Department of Social Security (DSS) in the form of attendance and mobility allowances. For many people however, this support is meagre in comparison to the personal sacrifices many carers have to make.

On a personal level, because of their commitment to the person being cared for, some carers may forego the opportunity of developing other loving relationships. It is common for a woman to devote a great many of her younger years tending to the needs of a dependent adult and, because of the demands involved, ultimately subjugate her own needs. Caring for others can be an isolating acitivity since it usually takes place within the relative's own home and physical caring tasks and the associated routines are often very time consuming. In addition a carer's need to be private may also be threatened:

'My husband has never been the same since he was in hospital with atrophy of the brain. He follows me everywhere all day, knocking on the bathroom door when I go to the toilet. There is no hiding place. I feel I am losing my mind. This happened only a year after my mother died aged 98 here at home, confined to bed for many years. I need to get a break, but so-called nursing homes here cost £200 per week at least, and I have no money. There is nowhere else for him to go, even for a few days . . .'

(*Guardian*, 10 December 1984, p. 10)

Whilst some carers undoubtedly derive satisfaction from the position they are in, a prolonged, isolating, caring relationship can psychologically undermine a women's confidence in other social situations because of her withdrawal from society in general. Various studies have highlighted the debilitating effect of unemployment including the psychological harm experienced by those who become isolated in their own home. These studies have almost exclusively focused on the plight of men who are out of work. Less attention has been paid to the many women who are similarly isolated from the mainstream of society.

It is a mistake to believe that all carers find themselves in the caring role as a result of their own choosing. They may volunteer to provide care but this is often done so as to avoid the unsatisfactory alternatives. Society quite firmly places the burden of care on women's shoulders. The principle is so deeply institutionalized that women may perform the task primarily because they need to avoid the guilt they would otherwise be made to feel.

Caring for relatives is not exclusively performed by women: men too are carers. Studies have shown that men are more likely to be involved when they are looking after wives who have become dependent. This arrangement does not normally require a dramatic shift in the living situation. In the case of parents being cared for by their children it is usually the daughter who responds to the demand for care. This situation is also true for the in-law relationship where a wife or partner is more likely to provide care for their father- or mother-in-law than any of her husband or partner's brothers. Furthermore, men are less likely to be involved in a caring relationship where the dependent person is suffering from any form of incontinence.

Women and violence

'Most women have painful emotional and/or physical experiences of coercion. It is merely one of the ways in which women's subordination is enforced, privately in the home, or publicly on the streets, in workplaces and in state departments.
Spare Rib, February, 1990

Within our society women constantly face the threat of or experience actual physical violence from men. This may range from verbal harassment to physical abuse, leading ultimately to rape or murder. It may take place in any setting, at work, in public spaces or more commonly, within the home. Much of it goes on undetected since, for a number of reasons, it does not get reported to the police. The precise extent of violence that women have to contend with is unknown; however, it is clear that many women can expect to be sexually or physically abused either as children or as adults in their lifetimes.

Sexual harassment is a common experience for women. The National Association of Local Government Officers (NALGO) has encouraged its members to seek advice from union officials if they experience what they consider to be harassment during their working hours. The Union's guidelines (1989) offer the following interpretation, 'it can be looks, gestures, touching, leering, obscene comments and suggestions. Flirtations, shouting as you walk by, teasing, chatting up, constant invitations, kissing you, sexual assault, rape, showing you or talking to you about pornography, 'phoning you at home and threats of bribery'. NALGO add, 'It can be done at home, in public, or in private'. Whatever form it takes, sexual harassment can make women feel offended, embarrassed, degraded or humiliated and in a work setting can deleteriously affect a woman's work and may actively damage her career or promotion prospects.

Outside of work women are exposed to physical and sexual abuse in everyday public settings, even within populated surroundings. In August 1989, Leah Geller wrote to the *Guardian* about how she had been sexually molested on a crowded tube train in London, telling how 'in appealing for support from fellow passengers – not a single pair of eyes would acknowledge the incident'. She described her assailant. 'He was about 6 foot 2, and was wearing an expensive, blue pin-striped suit. He was about 40, his dark hair greying. His face was distinct with sharp facial features'. She added, 'What I saw, or see in retrospect, was an image of arrogance and power' (2 August 1989).

Learning The Hard Way (Campling, 1989) contains the contributions of 57 mainly working class women and their struggle to survive and achieve in a male-dominated world. The following extract underlines the everyday nature of abuse to which women are subjected by men in public places:

> I was sitting in the pub with my women friends. Mistake number one. Never take up men's space – especially in large numbers (there were three of us). And never approach the pub on your own.
>
> At first the banter was innocuous and wildly original. 'Hello darlin'. What's a nice girl like you doing out on her own?' (Apparently my friends were invisible.) 'Let's have a bit of service here.' 'Isn't anyone going to serve the little lady?' (Is this the chivalry I've heard so much about?)
>
> 'Wot's the matter?' 'Lost your voice?' 'Thought you ladies didn't know how to keep your mouths shut' he laughs. 'Nice pair of knockers' another one joins in. 'Bet she could show us a thing or two.' A hand reaches for my breast, another clutches at my thigh.
>
> 'Fuck off you arseholes' I shout with some degree of terror and go back to my seat at the table. Jenny gets the drinks by going next door into the lounge and standing by an old man with a stick, who looks harmless enough. He beams on her breasts and allows his arm to brush against hers. Could be an accident. (Am I becoming paranoid?)
>
> Meanwhile back in the bar, Sir Lancelot (the 'chivalrous' one) and Neanderthal Eddie (his Oppo) amble over to our table. By this time we are the centre of attention with every male eye fixed on the fun.
>
> 'Wot's the problem girls? We're only trying to be friendly. Wot you talking about? Maybe we might have a few thoughts on the matter.'
>
> 'Look – why don't you just piss off' says Pam (who is braver than me) 'and leave us alone'.
>
> 'Leave you alone. I wouldn't touch you with a barge pole you ugly bitch.'

(Macmillan Publishers, p. 6)

According to the writers of the book, such instances are one of the consequences of the proliferation of the image portrayed in advertising, the media and in pornography: women are sex objects and they are permanently sexually available. So that men, 'however insignificant and undesirable', feel entitled to pass sexual comment and make judgements on women.

It is very difficult for women to go out unaccompanied to pubs or to the cinema or the theatre without attracting unwarranted attention or harrasment. Walking through the city centre or waiting to use public transport can be unsafe. Because of their fear of violence, many women remain at home, particularly after dark. As a consequence their social lives are curtailed, especially the lives of those women who do not have partners.

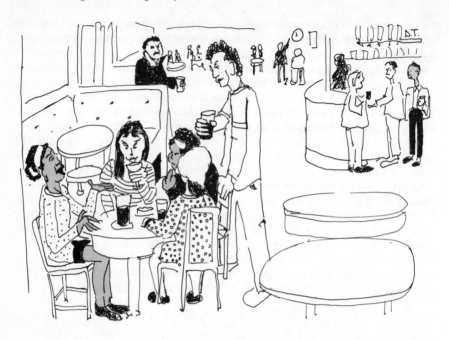

Men commonly feel entitled to invade women's public space.

In addition to the violence against women that takes place in public there is
the abuse of women which is carried out within the home. As already
mentioned, not all of this is reported, however, it is estimated that 30 per cent
of relationships involve some degree of physical violence. Furthermore, statistics show that one-half of women murdered in the UK are killed by men with
whom they have a current or former relationship (*Observer*, 28 May 1989,
p. 36). It is common for women who experience violence from their male
partners, initially at least, not to do anything about it; they neither report it to
the authorities nor attempt to leave their partners.

Women may not want to report abuse to the police or to the Social Services
because they are mistrustful of these organizations and fear the consequences
of reporting domestic violence for themselves or their children. Many are
concerned for their partner, whom they do not want to get 'into trouble', either
through fear of reprisal or for reasons of compassion. Some abused women still
love their violent partners and hope to enable them to change. Others are
emotionally dependent on their violent partner because they have become
systematically isolated and now regard their man as the only person in their
world. Another reason why women are loath to report incidents of partner
abuse to the police is that they feel that they will not be sympathetically treated.
The police have often been very reluctant to become involved in 'domestics', as
incidents of violence in the home are known, and women do not feel confident
of being helped. In a survey carried out by the Northern Ireland Women's Aid
Federation, 62 per cent of women interviewed were dissatisfied with the way
the police dealt with their cases and 95 per cent said that there are times when

they had needed police help but had not contacted the police. (ibid.) Widespread fear of the police makes black women particularly reticent to seek police help. In *The Hidden Struggle – Statutory and Voluntary Sector Responses to Violence Against Black Women in the Home* (1989), Amina Mama states that when domestic violence is directed towards black women the police often fail to act. However, it must be said that some police forces are beginning to take domestic violence more seriously and endeavouring to respond more appropriately to reports of its occurrence. In June 1987 the first domestic violence unit in Britain was started in Tottenham by two women police officers, Colette Paul and Annette O'Reilly, and this practice soon spread to other units within London.

Despite the danger to themselves, some women are reluctant to leave their violent partners. They may feel guilty and somehow responsible for what is happening to them. Other women will have strong religious or cultural reasons for not wanting to leave their partners; they may fear disapproval within their own communities, or may be morally opposed to breaking marriage vows. Whatever personal reason lies behind a woman's reluctance to leave a violent home, a major obstacle faced by most abused women is the absence of a realistic alternative. The houses of friends or relatives can only be a temporary solution. Women's refuges are grossly underfunded and numerically insuficient; referrals to London Women's Aid alone rose to 6341 in the year ending June 1988 – a 37 per cent increase. Moreover, there are only 300–400 bed spaces for women in refuges in London.Local authority temporary accommodation is also sparse and often substandard, particularly in major cities. The long wait faced by abused women for permanent council housing persuades many of them to return home though their lives may even be threatened. Of the 7217 calls to the London Regional Office of the Women's Aid Federation during the period of June 1988 to June 1989, 2324 were classed as requests for advice and 4893 were referrals for accommodation (Womens' Aid Federation, 1989). The problem of finding a new home is more difficult for black and Asian women who may face racism. Mama points out that it took between 18 months and three years for the black and Asian women in her London-based study to obtain permanent rehousing. She says that black women's access to public housing is severely circumscribed because many are ignorant of the provision available, some are unable to speak English properly and are put off by the bureaucratic process and the fact that structural racism mitigates against them. Lai Ha's plight illustrates this. She is 'a middle-aged Chinese woman who does not speak English, and lives like a slave in her abusive husband's house. She is his third wife and sees that the second wife is still homeless after a year and a half on a local authority waiting list' (Mama, 1989, p. 101).

Women and pornography

It is not possible to establish an absolute causal link between pornography and the incidence of male violence against women, although many people feel that a close correlation exists, and that violence does not occur in isolation from the rest of society. That 'hard porn' in particular leads automatically to violence and/or rape has never been scientifically proven and would be very difficult to establish conclusively. However, it is strongly felt that since pornography reduces women to sexual objects, it degrades and dehumanizes them and allows men to perceive them as being always sexually available. Against this it is argued that pornography acts as a release for men and dissipates potential aggression. Soft pornography certainly is viewed by many to be harmless. Mr Robert Adley MP said in a House of Commons debate, 'If a man gets hot and steamy, these pictures act as a release not a stimulation to rape' (*Observer*, 16 March 1986). Another MP, Mr Peter Temple argued, 'Everyone should be free to look at page three, we are not in the business of petty censorship. These pictures are amusing' (ibid). Both men were speaking in the debate following the first reading of Clare Short's Indecent Displays Bill 1986 which unsuccessfully sought to ban sexually provocative pictures of women.

Just as there is no overall agreement on the effect of pornography on its users and the rest of society, exactly what constitutes pornography is not universally agreed upon either.

The Campaign Against Pornography and Censorship (CAPC) defines pornography as, 'the graphic, sexually explicit subordination of women through pictures and words, that also includes one or more of the following: women portrayed as sexual objects, things or commodities, enjoying pain or humiliation or rape, being tied up, cut up, mutilated, bruised or physically hurt, in postures of sexual submission or servility or display, reduced to body parts, penetrated by objects or animals, or presented in scenarios of denegration, injury, torture, shown as inferior, bleeding, bruised or hurt in a context which is sexual' (*Guardian*, 15 February 1990). This rather comprehensive definition would include all representations of women ranging from 'hard porn' through to 'soft porn' including what have become known as 'page 3 pictures' of partially clad women which are to be found daily in certain tabloid newspapers.

Pornography needs to be distinguished from erotica, although for many people there will always be a thin dividing line between the two. *Erotica* has been defined by the CAPC as 'sexually explicit materials premised on equality'. For example, non-violent, non-degrading explicit sex scenes in films may be considered erotic rather than pornographic when they are the product of the relationship of the people involved. Although the attention of the camera, whether it zooms in, lingers or withdraws in order to allow the viewer to make the choice, can itself determine whether something is presented as pornographic or erotic. Erotica, whether it is depicted in books, pictures or films is generally considered to be healthy and/or stimulating since it is not based on a distortion. Pornography, as the CAPC point out, is less about sex and more about power. 'It reflects and reinforces inequality and injustice, manipulating sexist and racist stereotypes and perpetuating the power men have over women.'

The CAPC is concerned with challenging the acceptability of pornographic images. 'Images which silence women and children by denying them a personality, images which perpetuate the myth that "women are asking for it" when they are harassed, abused and raped; images which portray enjoyment of violence, images which are often an actual record of the rape of, or violence against women and children. Images which enable men to perceive women and young girls as sexually available.' These images are all around us. Hard pornography is readily available in local shops and soft pornography permeates the whole of the media and advertising industry to such an extent that the degradation and dehumanization of women is institutionalized. The images and representations reflect women's unequal status in society.

Pornography also exploits men because it peddles the idea that men can control and possess the women portrayed in the magazines and films. According to Ian Warwick of the Sheffield Men's Awareness Project, 'Brought up in a world where men are supposed to be strong and independent, sex brings fear of vulnerability. Pornography reasserts our security and identity. Perhaps this is why pornography more often leads to masturbation than to intercourse. While masturbating a man can control his own sexual pleasure, unaffected by the sexual desire of his partner.' A similar sentiment was expressed by Peter Baker in a letter to the *Guardian*, (8 May 1990), 'Teaching me that women were essentially objects for my own lustful purposes and that good sex was quick, impersonal and purely penetrative, pornography helped prevent me from easily forming permanent relationships with real women.' Ian Warwick adds, 'that within pornography, nowhere do men express tenderness, love and caring, nowhere do men experience closeness, warmth or the feeling of being loved'.

Women and social care

As we have already established it is women who undertake to perform the majority of paid care. Ninety per cent of nurses are women as are nearly all home helps and infant teachers. Within social work itself, most workers are female: 80 per cent of staff in elderly people's homes, 75 per cent of those who work in children's homes and the majority of field workers and medical social workers are women. However, senior and managerial roles are more commonly performed by men. So, whilst the grass-roots care is carried out mainly by women, policies and decision making is generally shaped by men.

One consequence of this is that social services policies are often based on society's dominant male values and operate against the interest of women. Women's propensity to act as carers has often been exploited by Social Services Departments (and Social Work Departments in Scotland) who have failed to support women in caring situations regarding their role as 'natural', whereas they have been more inclined to support a man in similar circumstances. Consider, too, the general inadequacy of the allowances normally paid to foster parents; the assumption being that fostering is no more than an extention of domestic labour. A foster mother's motivation would be considered suspect if she sought reward for her work over and above the cost of the child's upkeep. Lesbian mothers and black women have understandable reasons to fear intervention from white, male-dominated social work organizations.

The average woman now spends more years caring for a dependent relative than she does on the care of her children. The community care proposals for the 1990s and beyond have been based on the assumption that women will continue to perform their traditional roles. This is in part a reflection of the masculine ideology that distinguishes caring as being non-work and set apart from paid work outside the home.

Not only do women make up the majority of social carers, they constitute the bulk of social work clientele. The situation is almost completely reversed within the probation service which is largely staffed by men who work predominantly with male offenders. The probation service works mainly at the 'soft end' of the penal system and deals mainly with 'perpetrators' rather than 'victims' and therefore involves an element of social control.

The situation is different in Scotland where there is no probation service as such and the work is carried out by Social Work Departments. Consequently, more women than men are involved in work with offenders because there are more women social workers.

There are several reasons why women form the majority of social work clients, some of which have already been discussed. Owing to the responsibility society has bestowed on women – to be primarily concerned with the care and well-being of others, many women present themselves at Social Service Departments (and Social Work Departments in Scotland), because of, or on behalf of, other family members. They may seek help with their children, for a dependent relative or for the whole family. Women too, as we have seen, are more likely to experience mental illness in its various forms and to be victims of domestic violence and may need help because of this.

Women's lower earning potential or inability to obtain paid work, owing to domestic commitments, means that they are more likely to experience material deprivation and the effects of poverty. Consequently they may require social work support. Indeed, the fact that more women are on fixed incomes, either as pensioners, amongst whom women are the great majority, disabled people or because they are on income support, as single parents, or that they are on low incomes owing to the lowly regarded nature of the work they do, means that they are more likely to need support from welfare agencies.

Jalna Hanmer and Daphne Statham in their book, *Women and Social Work – Towards a Women-Centred Practice* (1988), suggest that social work directs itself towards recognizing the fact that it is essentially a female-dominated profession and that women, both as workers and clients, can draw strength from this. They feel that within social work it is important that more women reach positions of authority in order that they can have an influence on policy. Furthermore, they feel that policies could be made which emphasize the similarities women have with one another and that the division between worker and client should be minimized. Instead of being seen as 'elderly', 'disabled' or 'mentally ill', female clients would be seen as women first. Women clients would thus be empowered by the corresponding lack of stigma and by their closer association with their helper.

Conclusion

This chapter has focused on the unequal position of women in society. We have seen that women are undeniably structurally disadvantaged and that they have less access to privilege, power and life-chances than men. Whilst women's position within society has improved over the past 25 years or so, owing mainly to the increased awareness brought about by the resurrection of the feminist movement in the late 1960s, progress has only been gradual; women remain fundamentally oppressed. As carers it is important that we recognize this fact in order that we are better able to support our female clients and colleagues.

We have examined the socialization process and highlighted the instances and effects of sexism at both the individual and institutional level. We have seen that much of the contribution women make to society goes unrewarded (it is undervalued and is often taken for granted) and that further, this negative attitude towards women is deeply engrained within our culture. However, in more recent years there has developed a more respectful representation of women, as well as a greater acknowledgement of the contribution they make to society and the difficulties our society creates for them. In an interview with Murray Davies in the *Daily Mirror* (29 March 1990), Glenda Jackson talked about why she was giving up her acting career in order to become a Labour candidate in the next election. She had recently been selected to represent the Hampstead and Highgate constituency. In answer to the question, 'Why choose an actress?' she answered, 'I'll tell you why. Because to be an actress, I have first to be a woman. I have been a daughter, sister, mother, wife, a shopper, a cleaner, a gardener, a home economics expert, a driver, a dress-maker, a cook, a nanny and a professional career woman. It would be very difficult to find a man who had done all that.'

The growth of feminine scholarship, the research and publicity carried out by such organizations as the Equal Opportunities Commission and the National Council for One Parent Families, and the positive attempts made by some voluntary and statutory social care agencies to integrate women more centrally into their organizations has contributed to women being more visible and more valued.

Exercises

1. *Who are the 'dinner ladies?'*
Observe the differences in gender roles in your place of work or college. Make a list of all the occupational positions within your establishment, either full or part-time, and divide those done by females and those performed by males. Consider the status related to all the posts. Include administrative, domestic, kitchen and caretaking staff and all social care/teaching and management staff. What conclusions do you draw? (You could extend this study from your own place of work to include the whole agency).

2. *Community resources*
Investigate within your own community the number and range of community resources and provisions available exclusively for women (or ethnic minority women). Comment on your findings and suggest why it is important that women should have separate provision from men. Consider other areas where community provision could be made more available to women.

3. *Pornography versus erotica*
Each member of the group should select a few items from the media (pictures, 'news' stories, cartoons, video extracts) or from literature (stories or poems) or from art (paintings, drawings or postcards). With the help of some of the information in this chapter, try to categorize these items along a continuum between acceptable and unacceptable images – either as 'pornography' or 'erotica'. Discuss your reasons with other members of the group.

4. *Team meetings*

One problem in team meetings is that some people, often men, tend to dominate discussions, either by constantly interrupting their (female) colleagues or by talking over them. Plan how you would raise this as an agenda issue for your next meeting and try to produce constructive suggestions on how the team members can create an environment where everyone can be heard and will feel safe to express themselves in their own style.

5. *Who does what at home?*

The 1980s reputedly saw the emergence of the 'new man' – a partner willing to do an equal share of domestic and childcare tasks. How true do you think this is of most families? Who normally does the work in your home? Is it still structured along sexist lines? Make a table of the various domestic duties and estimate the time spent by males or females on those jobs within your household over a short period.

Questions for essay or discussion

1. What can be done in order to attract more men into social care/nursing? Why do you think it is important that more men become involved in this field either as paid workers or volunteers? What possible long term consequences would there be should more men become involved in social care?
2. What can be done in order to enable women to feel safe outside the home on their own after dark?
3. Men are 'sexist' by their very nature and it is impossible for them to change?
4. The feminist movement in Britain has not fully represented and reflected the history and interests of black women in this country.
5. Social care and social work students on work placements and student nurses should be able to ensure that they are supervised by someone of the gender of their own choosing.
6. How far does a lack of confidence and poor self-image contribute to the absence of women from the more senior managerial positions within social care or social work?

Further reading

Academic sources

Cohen, B., *Caring for Children – Services and Polices for Child Care and Equal Opportunities in the UK*, Commission of the European Communities, 1988. A comprehensive and detailed study on child care, equal opportunities and the position of women in society.

Hanmer, J., Statham, D., *Women and Social Work – Towards a Women-Centred Practice*, BASW Macmillan, 1988. A book which clearly outlines the relevance of gender to social care, emphasizing what women social carers have in common with women clients, as well as what divides them.

Hite, S., *The Hite Report – Women and Love*, Penguin, 1987. A comprehensive survey about what women want from close relationships, what they expect from their partner, what actually happens in their lives, and how they feel about love.

Mama, A., *The Hidden Struggle – Statutory and Voluntary Sector Responses to Violence Against Women in the Home*, London Race and Housing Research, 1989. A London-based detailed account of black womens' experience of violence, homelessness and the response of the voluntary and statutory 'caring services'.

Oakley, A., *Sex, Gender and Society*, Gower/Maurice Temple Smith, 1972. A classic study attempting to establish the 'real differences between men and women' and whether they are culturally or biologically determined.

Ungerson, C., *Policy is Personal – Sex, Gender and Informal Care*, Tavistock Publications, 1987. A study of informal carers, looking at the reasons why women, in particular, care with reference to a small number of case studies.

Other literary sources
Collins, M., *Anger*, Womens Press, 1987.
Emecheta, B., *Second Class Citizen*, Fontana, 1987.
French, M., *The Womens' Room*, Abacus/Sphere Books, 1978.
Hall, R., *The Well of Loneliness*, Virago, 1982.
Plath, S., *The Bell Jar*, Faber and Faber, 1990.

Films and plays
Campion, J., *An Angel at my Table*, 1990.
Friel, B., *Dancing at Lughansa*, Faber, 1990.
Greenwald, R., *The Burning Bed*, US, 1984.
Scorsese, M., *Alice Doesn't Live Here Anymore*, 1974.

4 Racism, black people and discrimination

Introduction

Racism is an immensely complex subject and one which perhaps, more than any other, is likely to evoke strong feelings whenever it is raised. People may feel strongly because they have experienced and continue to experience the effects of racism in their everyday lives, or they may feel angry simply because of the social injustice of racism. Some individuals may feel threatened and act defensively whenever the matter is mentioned for fear of their own actions being criticized or condemned. Yet others will remain confused and uncertain about an issue which they feel to be inflated in importance since it has barely touched their lives.

Before we go on to look at racism and the various definitions associated with it, we need to acknowledge as a starting point that Britain is a racist society and has been so for centuries, and that racism is evident at both the individual level and in society as a whole.

This chapter aims to examine the complex issue of racism in as simple a way as possible in order that we can try to understand the phenomenon and consider its influence within society today. We can also try to understand our own position as individuals and see how racism affects us and those for whom we care.

Discussion of some of the terms used

Throughout history attempts have been made to classify human beings into groups; as certain racial types distinguishable by their physical characteristics, cultural patterns and modes of behaviour. It would seem that the aim of such classification was to demonstrate that one *race* or group of people was in someway superior to others and to justify or facilitate the creation of a structural hierarchy.

Superficial differences do exist between people but these are nothing more than indicators of how the human race has adapted to the various climatic surroundings during the evolutionary process: for example, dark pigmentation offers the skin more protection against the sun and is consequently a characteristic of those people whose ancestors lived in hot countries. Observable physical characteristics have no other significance and there is no evidence that one race of people is in any way superior to another.

The very concept of 'race' is in fact imprecise as there can hardly be such a thing as a pure race given the increased mobility of people throughout history. For a pure race of people to exist today it needs to have led a very insular and self-contained existence; in a vacuum, isolated from an ever expanding and increasingly interdependent world. All 'races', therefore, are made up of a mixture of different people and the notion of a pure race is not valid. However the term 'race' remains a powerful social concept which is widely understood and used.

Racialism and racism

Generally these two words are considered to be interchangeable and in everyday usage convey broadly the same meaning. However one of the key organizations that represents the interests of ethnic minority people in Britain, the Institute for Race Relations, distinguishes between them. *Racialism* refers to individual prejudiced beliefs and behaviour. Any individual who pre-judges another person on the grounds of her or his skin colour or cultural differences and acts accordingly is considered to be a *racialist*. *Racism* refers to the situation where racialist views are interwoven into the structure of society so that society's major social, economic and political institutions systematically perpetuate the philosophy of racial superiority. *Racialism* then refers to individuals and *racism* refers to the way in which society is structured and operates. Despite this distinction, however, the words racialist and racist are commonly used interchangeably to describe individuals in everyday speech.

Not everyone's definition of racism will accord with that of the Institute for Race Relations. In fact there is a wide diversity of interpretation. A common and strongly held view is that *racism equals prejudice plus power*. In other words racism is a combination of individual racial prejudice and society's support. In Britain today the political, legal and economic institutions are staffed in the main by white men and some white women, so that social policies reflect the ideas of the white majority and the 'black perspective' is largely absent. The practices and procedures of so many of our organizations are consciously or unconsciously racist in that they operate unfavourably towards and therefore discriminate against people from ethnic minorities. As we shall see this accusation applies to all the caring services, as well as to business and industrial institutions. At the same time it needs to be pointed out that genuine attempts are now being made to counteract racism within these various organizations.

According to the above definition it would be impossible for a black person to be racist in a white dominated society. Correspondingly, a white person could not be racist in a black dominated society. This is because the structure and institutions of a society reflect the dominant ideology of the majority people. However, the problem with the definition 'racism equals prejudice plus power' is that it implies that *all* white people in a white dominated society are automatically racist despite any attempts they make towards combating their own racism. It is true to say that all white people who are brought up in Britain, are almost bound to be racist to a certain extent because of their conditioning. They have been subjected to a socialization process which values white skin colour more highly than black. This is not to say that white people have chosen to be racist; rather the process is much more subtle and occurs subconsciously during their formative years and is reinforced throughout their lives. In order to combat this process white people need to make a conscious effort to eradicate racism within themselves and to oppose it within society. Daphne Statham, Director of the National Institute for Social Work, represents a stance commonly held amongst white people. 'My position is,' she said, 'that however liberal I like to see myself, having been brought up white and benefiting from that status, I must be racist. It is my response to try to overcome it in my job and in my relationships with other people. I make mistakes and I have to learn from them' (*Social Work Today*, 9 November 1987).

Further, as an ideology racism has been used in many different societies to support the oppression of various minorities at different stages throughout history. At its most extreme the practice of discrimination and persecution has led to genocide; a clear example in recent history being the wholesale murder of millions of Jews, gypsies and other minorities by the Nazi regime during the Second World War.

In today's world, racism is most starkly apparent in the apartheid structure in South Africa, where black people are denied many basic human rights and are forced to live in restricted townships and suffer extremes of deprivation while the minority white people have almost exclusive access to privilege and power. In Britain, racism is clearly not so extreme nor always so blatant, yet it is still prevalent.

Blackness and whiteness

The words black and white are not really accurate when they are used literally to describe skin colour, for few people could properly be described as either black or white given the extensive gradations of skin colour. Most people fall somewhere inbetween. However, for the purpose of classification *black* normally refers to those people whose family origin is African or West Indian (Afro-Caribbean) and *white* refers to people of European (or North American) descent; *Asian* includes the people who originate from the sub-continent of India. Within Britain, apart from the Chinese and Irish, minorities are not generally regarded as being sufficiently numerous to be categorized by themselves, and so for convenience they are included in one of the above categories.

This form of classification is obviously very crude and unsatisfactory, not least because it obscures the enormous cultural diversity between people of the same country, let alone those between people of different countries. The term 'Asian' for example can be seen to be a blanket term, which broadly covers identifiable groups of people but includes a range of countries such as Bangladesh, Hong Kong and Sri Lanka; a range of religions such as Sikhism, Buddism, Christianity and Islam; a range of languages such as Urdu, Gujarati and Sinhalese, and an infinite variety of other customs and styles. Similarly, as Dudley Rhodes, a Barbadian, was quoted as saying, 'There are a number of black people here who come from a variety of islands, and to lump us together as one group who have got the same causes and the same difficulties is insulting, is denying my culture, is denying my heritage' (*Social Work Today*, 9 November 1987).

To some extent the term *ethnic minority* was introduced in recognition of the great variety of different cultures. Ethnic minorities are thus all those groups of people whose land of origin is not the host country. It must be remembered that 'minority' is only a relative concept: a Pakistani becomes a member of a minority only when she or he settles outside of Pakistan, and that globally speaking white people are in fact a minority.

In Britain, when we talk of racism we are almost exclusively speaking about discrimination based on skin colour, since this is the most visible difference between people. This is not to say that racism is not directed at other minority groups, including e.g. Irish, Jewish, Polish and Greek people and others. However, it is agreed that their experience of racism, though similar, is less severe than that of black people because of their closer physical similarity to white people. Their language and cultural differences are not immediately apparent from external observation. For example, a white Irish person with a regional accent may not face discrimination until after she or he has spoken.

Since the 1960s the word black has been used to convey a more positive identity of people of Afro-Caribbean origin. 'Black Consciousness' and 'Black is Beautiful' are two examples of positive statements of blackness made during this period. Similarly, the word 'Asian' now serves to distinguish further between black people and provides a more distinct identity for people from the Indian sub-continent.

As well as the examples listed above, there is yet another use of the term 'black'. It is used in a wider political sense as an umbrella term to describe all those whose life chances are reduced in an equivalent way to those who are non-white. In this way white-skinned Irish or Polish people, for example, could be considered 'black' on the occasions when they are discriminated against in the job market or a housing situation. In this generic sense black is synonymous with the term ethnic minority.

According to Banda Ahmad, Director of the Race Equality Unit – Personal Social Service, at NISW: 'For those who define themselves as black:

- It is a declaration of struggle for equality and justice.
- It is an acknowledgement of similar experience of racism and racial discrimination in Britain.
- It is a challenge to white perceptions of blackness being inferior and getting rid of negative connotations.
- It is redefining white definition of black, which has historical links with slavery and colonialization.
- Above all, it is a positive statement.'

(*Social Work Today*, 11 May 1989)

Tokenism

Organizations may be accused of being tokenistic when they appoint a member of a panel or employ a worker who is black merely in order to give the impression of balance, where the change is superficial and does not represent full implementation of equal opportunities policy.

Origins of racism

The roots of racism are to be found in the past. Furthermore, clear influences in the development of racism can be traced in the English language itself, as well as the justification of supporting the practice of the African slave trade and the policy of imperialism.

The English language

Throughout English literature and within the English language there has been a long held association between the word 'black' and something which is intrinsically bad: the devil, black magic, blackmail and black-ball. This is illustrated in the following anecdote in which a black military bandsman was strolling down the Strand during the seventeenth century when he was accosted with the question: 'Well, blackie, what news the devil?' He knocked the questioner down, remarking: 'He send you that – how you like it?' (quoted in Fryer, 1984, p. 88).

Whiteness on the other hand, has stood for 'goodness', 'virtue' and 'cleanliness'. Clear examples of the association of 'white' with 'purity' are to be found throughout literature. Take for example, Shakespeare's use of such associations in Othello. The Duke summarizes the character of the dark skinned noble Othello thus:

> . . . 'far more fair than black'

and again, later in the play, Othello agonizes over Desdemona's supposed unfaithfulness:

> 'I'll have some proof. Her name, that was as fresh
> As Dian's visage, is now begrimed and black
> As mine own face.'

In his emphasis of the beauty of Desdemona he says:

> 'It is the cause. Yet I'll not shed her blood,
> Nor scar that whiter skin of hers than snow,
> And smooth as monumental alabaster.'

Images associating the colour black, darkness and the night, the devil and evil abound throughout Shakespeare and other works, both before and after. They have their origins in early medieval beliefs and the symbolic use of darkness and light in the Bible.

Given this link with medieval superstition, it became possible to ascribe these negative connotations to dark-skinned people when they were first encountered in large numbers. Similarly the idealized, flattering associations with whiteness could just as easily be internalized by white people and so contributed to the feelings of superiority necessary for racism to take root and flourish. Racism thus found its earliest expression in our existing language. It was to deepen with society's involvement in a lucrative slave trade and subsequent colonialization.

Slavery

The system of slavery met the needs of an expanding British economy for a period of 150 years, spanning the seventeenth to the nineteenth centuries. The buying and selling of black women and men was a profitable business; it formed part of a sophisticated triangular trade arrangement between Britain, Africa and the Americas (Fig. 4.1).

On the first leg of the journey Britain shipped manufactured materials such

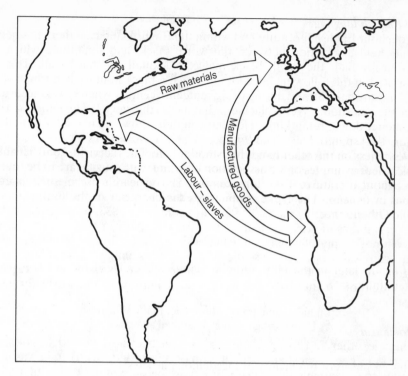

Fig. 4.1 The slave triangle.

as tools and textiles to Africa. These goods were sold in exchange for young Africans who were then transported to the West Indies and the Americas in order to work on the new sugar and cotton plantations. The traders only took the healthiest of the African people, the youngest and strongest, in the interest of maximum profits. The harrowing, overcrowded conditions which the slaves had to endure were so severe that many failed even to complete the journey. Those who did survive were sold to plantation owners and forced to work long hours and undertake arduous tasks. Devoid of their basic human rights, the slaves were kept in chains and subjected to the whims of their masters.

The product of their labour, mainly sugar and cotton, was then shipped back to Britain to meet a growing demand. Some slaves were bought back to Britain and sold into servitude to wealthy families, where owning a black slave denoted elevated social status.

The whole system, based on the treatment of human beings as commodities, as things to be bought and sold, generated huge profits for all those concerned in the trading. These profits made a considerable contribution to the later industrial development in Britain, particularly in the expansion of the ports of Bristol, Liverpool and London. Any guilt stemming from those who acknowledged or were involved in this inhumane and degrading practice was off-set by the material gains it produced.

> I own I am shocked at the purchase of slaves,
> And fear those who buy and sell them are knaves;
> What I hear of their hardships, their tortures, and groans
> Is almost enough to drive pity from stones.
> I pity them greatly, but I must be numb,
> For how could we do without sugar and rum.
>
> (Cowper, W., *Pity for Poor Africans*, 1788, cited in Fryer, P.,
> *Staying Power – The History of Black People*, Pluto Press, p. 39)

For the system to have been tolerated and to have lasted so long, it needed some form of moral justification; this was supplied by racism – the belief that Africans were inferior to white people. They were regarded as barbaric, even sub-human, capable of only dull, menial work and needing to be enslaved and manacled because they could not be trusted with their own freedom.

Slavery was officially made illegal in this country in 1833, by which time the lives of millions of Africans had been destroyed. African slavery came to an end but not simply as a result of righteous indignation; by this time there had been many slave insurrections, the system was becoming less profitable and there were easier gains to be had elsewhere. The owners of capital turned their attention to the exploitation of other countries in the world through colonialism.

Colonialism

Alongside other European countries, Britain became involved in colonial expansion: the conquest and exploitation of other countries. Britain was in a position to expand and develop a vast empire because of her powerful armed forces: military superiority implied cultural superiority and Britain was able to repress cultures far older than her own. Colonial expansion took place in three main ways.

In the first, the British invaded, settled and imposed their authority on the host country pushing aside the native people. One consequence of this action apparent today is the disaffection felt by the Maoris in New Zealand or the Aborigines in Australia, who are now minorities in their own countries and whose cultural heritage, ancestory and relationship to the land has been all but lost in the wake of the establishment of a white, European-based culture. Theories of white superiority justified wholesale slaughter of many indigenous peoples.

In other instances, in countries like South Africa and Zimbabwe (formerly Rhodesia), the original inhabitants remained the numerical majority, but the British and other Europeans settled, having eventually defeated the native peoples and taken their land. The indigenous people were then used as cheap labour and the ruling whites used force to maintain their position of privilege.

The third and most common form of colonialization occured in countries like India and the West Indies, where the British did not settle in large numbers but instead ruled the countries from afar. Britain became known as the mother country and at the height of the Empire ruled over one quarter of the world. It was so vast that it was claimed that the sun never set on the British Empire.

Colonized countries were rich in raw materials and cheap labour which was exploited by Britain. Opponents of colonization point to the economic dependence with which many former colonies are left; their economies having changed

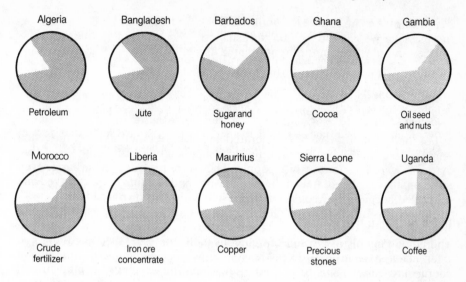

Fig. 4.2 Dependency of developing countries. Proportion of income derived from one product (dark shading). (Adapted from *Patterns of Racism*, Institute of Race Relations, 1982, p. 40). Developed countries such as the USA, USSR, UK and South Africa etc. derive their export income from a wide range of products. Less than half of the export income of these developed countries comes from 15 products.

from self-sufficient agricultural communities to economies dependent on the international fluctuations of their main cash crop (Fig. 4.2). Supporters of the process of colonialization point to the great benefits bestowed on the developing countries; road and rail networks, the establishment of legal and political institutions and commercial systems. If benefits did accrue, they did so not as a result of altruism; they were incidental, a consequence stemming from activities generated by the pursuit of profit.

The legitimization or moral backing for colonization was initially supplied by the church. Black and Irish people were considered 'heathens' and 'savages' in need of enlightment and civilization. Later came the scientific or pseudo-scientific explanations aimed at justifying white supremacy; some scientists measured skulls in order to try to demonstrate differences in the brain capacity of black and white people. Others focused on the proportions and shape of the skull and the nose in order to establish intellectual superiority between 'races'. They were not successful. A more recent study carried out by psychologist, Arthur Jensen, tried to prove that white people had higher IQs than black people. His results were discredited because amongst other things they took no account of environmental factors.

It may seem a little surprising in a discussion on racism to have devoted so much time to issues of the past. The significance of this lies in the effect that past attitudes with their roots in centuries of slavery and colonization have on our present lives. The racism of the past permeates our culture today. It is in everything we come across; the books we read, the lessons we receive at school, the message we get through the newspapers, magazines, TV, films and the policies and practices of different organizations.

> "If you want to understand British racism – and without understanding it no change is possible – it is impossible even to begin to grasp the nature of the beast unless you accept its historical roots. Unless you see that 400 years of conquest and looting, centuries of being told that you are superior to the 'fuzzy-wuzzies' and the 'wogs', all leave their stain on you all: that such a stain seeps into every part of your culture, your language and your daily life: and nothing has been done to wash it out."
>
> (Salman Rushdie, The New Empire Within Britain,
> *New Society* 9 December 1982)

Black people in Britain

There is a long history of black people living in Britain. Early records make reference to black soldiers in the Roman army of occupation. However black people have always been a minority in this country and still are today.

Post-war settlers

It was not until comparatively recent times that black people have been coming to this country in any large numbers. The arrival of the 'Empire Windrush' on 22 June 1948 brought 492 Jamaicans, described in one newspaper as 'five hundred pairs of willing hands'. This marked the beginning of a period of increased black immigration to this country, made possible for several reasons including the passing of the 1948 Nationality Act which granted British citizenship to all members of the existing and former British colonies. Some say the Act was introduced in gratitude to the colonies who had helped during the Second World War. Others argue that black people were invited primarily to meet the needs of a growing economy. After the devastation of war, the economy picked up through the 1940s and continued to grow throughout the 1950s.

In response to the need to find workers, particularly for the essential services, the Conservative Government of the time decided to recruit from abroad. The recently established National Health Service and London Transport, for example, canvassed directly in Jamaica and other Caribbean islands. The advertisements themselves eulogized the nature of the work and the prospect of life in Britain. It was hardly surprising then that many West Indian people took up the challenge and welcomed the opportunity of full-time work and the chance to escape the poverty and high unemployment in their own countries. Over the years people from other countries, particularly the Indian sub-continent and East Africa, also came to Britain to seek work and to flee the poverty or political uncertainty of their own lands. All immigrants at this time, as Commonwealth citizens and British passport holders, were entitled to come to Britain to live and work. Furthermore, they were encouraged to do so by the government.

In the minds of many of the immigrants, the trip to Britain was a short-term venture to enable them to save money and support their families back home and so improve their basic standard of living. Whatever had attracted them to

Britain and whatever they had been led to believe, it is doubtful they expected to encounter racism on the scale that met them.

> I love me mudder and me mudder love me
> We come so far from over de sea,
> We heard dat de streets were paved with gold
> Sometime it hot and sometime it cold.
>
> (Zepheniah, B., *I Love Me Mudder*, in *The Dread Affair-Collected Poems*, Arena, 1985, p. 36.)

Early difficulties

Immigrant black people faced a number of difficulties when they came to this country. Housing was expensive and rented accommodation was often denied to them on the basis of their skin colour. Notices saying 'No blacks' or 'No Irish' were commonplace. After all, only a few years earlier, in 1943, the Captain of the West Indies cricket team, Sir Learie Constantine, had been refused accommodation at the Imperial Hotel in London on the grounds that his colour may offend the other guests. In successfully suing the hotel, he did however set a precedent and made some inroads into the operation of the 'colour bar' which had been a major issue for some time. The 'colour bar' is a term referring to the prejudicial exclusion of entry to various private facilities on the basis of colour. It was used by the owners and proprietors of hotels, golf clubs, night clubs and guest houses.

Black people were similarly openly discriminated against in the job market despite the fact that many were skilled workers. They found work mainly in the more menial and lower paid occupations. As a consequence of these factors there was a strong tendency for black people to settle in the poorer industrial towns and inner city areas. In a sense they continued to remain cheap 'immigrant' labour.

Once established in these deprived and physically decaying areas, the new immigrants were then associated with these surroundings and blamed for the squalor that was truly society's neglect. This association fuelled the racist argument that black people created the decay and decline of certain districts. Furthermore, a worsening of the economic conditions, a rise in unemployment, and an unresolved and deepening housing crisis exacerbated relations between black and white people.

Black people were obvious and visible targets for the anxiety felt by white people about job and housing shortages and an easy and convenient scapegoat for the social dissatisfaction of the times. This insecurity was fanned by politicians and the press. Most famous was the 'rivers of blood' speech made in 1968 by the former Conservative MP Enoch Powell. In his speech he alluded to impending racial violence and the 'swamping' of British culture by 'foreigners'. This theme has periodically been restated, notably by Margaret Thatcher, who referred to 'swamping' in 1979 and more recently by Norman Tebbit MP, who in 1990 questioned the loyalty of black British people with the infamous cricket test speech. He argued that people of Caribbean, West Indian, Indian, Pakistani and Sri Lankan origin would rather support the cricket teams of these countries than England and thereby insinuated a lack of 'Britishness'.

The government responded to the difficulties faced by black people in

Britain by attempting to give them some form of protection through the passing of race relations legislation. At the same time government intervention caused hardship to the black community through a series of immigration laws which restricted the entry of black people into Britain in a way which could hardly have been envisaged in 1948, and thereby reinforced the idea that black people were a problem.

Race relations

The rights of all minorities were formally recognized by the passing of the Race Relations Acts of 1965 and 1968; these were later replaced by the 1976 Act. This legislation sought to make all forms of racial discrimination illegal. The 1976 Act distinguished between 'direct' and 'indirect' discrimination.

Direct discrimination consists of treating a person, on racial grounds, less favourably than others who are or would be in the same circumstances. For example, in November 1982 a young man of Granadian origin with a medical disability was refused a flat he had been invited to view by the Ealing Housing Department on the grounds that 'you blacks play loud music' (Commission for Racial Equality – CRE, 1983, p. 46).

Indirect discrimination 'consists of applying a requirement or condition which, although applied equally to persons of all racial groups, is such that a considerably smaller proportion of a particular racial group can comply and it cannot be shown to be justifiable on other than racial grounds'. For example, in July 1978, the headmaster of Grove Park School, Birmingham, refused to relax the school's uniform rules to allow a 13 year-old Sikh boy entering the school to wear a turban. The boy was therefore unable to enrol (ibid., p. 45).

It was one thing to outlaw overt racist practice, it was another thing to eliminate it completely. Some people felt that the Race Relations Acts increased racial tension rather than decreased it because somehow black people were seen by some whites as being favoured. Another criticism was that the Acts dealt only with overt racism and had no power over the more subtle forms.

Immigration laws

The Government itself has been charged with racism over its immigration policies. A series of Acts passed in 1962, 1967 and 1971, culminating in the 1981 Nationality Act, have redefined the status of the former British Commonwealth Citizens and systematically restricted the rights of black people to enter Britain.

According to the Joint Council for the Welfare of Immigrants (JCWI), 'In 1987, a Canadian national had a 1:4,876 chance of being refused entry at the UK port. For an Australian, the figure was 1:2,361. The New Zealander faced odds of 1:1,640. However, a Caribbean national had a 1:193 chance of refusal' (JCWI, 1990, p. 11). The JCWI also state that 'refusals of Caribbean nationals have reached epidemic proportions. By 1985, one in every 40 Jamaicans seeking entry to the UK was refused: in other words, each aeroplane arriving at a UK airport from Kingston or Montego Bay was likely on average to contain three or four Jamaican citizen passengers who would be denied entry to the UK and face summary return' (ibid. p. 4).

The immigration laws have created undue hardship for many black families as members have been subject to excessive delays whilst their applications to come to Britain are processed. In extreme cases, some Asian women suffered the indignity of having to undergo vaginal examinations in order to establish the validity of their claims to enter Britain – a practice stopped in 1979.

At a press conference following the report of the Joint Council for the Welfare of Immigrants, Jeremy Corbyn, Labour MP for Islington North said, 'It's disgusting the way non-white arrivals to the UK are treated. These people are put through long delays and a series of long interviews, often after coming on long flights' (*Guardian*, 18 July 1990). The 1981 Nationality Act dispensed with a 900 year right of *ius soli* (the right of soil) the automatic right of a child born on British ground to be a British citizen.

It can be seen from Table 4.1 that in most years since the early 1970s, there has been a net loss of population in Britain. In other words, during this time more people have left this country than have entered it. The years 1985 and 1986 are the exception to this but the net gain of residents to the United Kingdom can be explained by an increase in migration from the European Community and 'other foreign' areas (*Social Trends* classification). Primary immigration from the Caribbean ceased as long ago as the 1960s. Today most black immigration is of a secondary nature; that is immediate relatives joining a family who have already settled in this country.

Racism and inequality today

It is possible to confirm that we live in a racist society simply by looking around us. That is not to say that we will witness clear instances of racial abuse; rather we need only consider the lack of prominence of black people in society. In other words racism is characterized by the absence of black people in positions of power and authority in our society. In some ways this reflects their general social class position as well. It is well known that working class people are not in positions of power and authority.

It can be seen in Tables 4.2 and 4.3 that black people number nearly two and a half million and represent 4.3 per cent of the total population. By the laws of average you would expect this percentage to be reflected in all occupations. This is not the case.

At the general election in 1987 a record number of four black MP's were returned to the House of Commons out of a total of 654. The only previous election of a black MP, Shapurji Saklatrala, was over sixty years ago. At local government level the situation is similar with very few black councillors. Top civil servants, bank managers, bishops and managing directors are almost exclusively white and male. Within the caring profession there is an under representation both in teaching and in social work, most noticeably at management level: less than 2 per cent of probation officers, 1 per cent of police officers and 1 per cent of prison officers are black. In November 1989 there were only 426 black police officers in the Metropolitan Police force. It was estimated that 'London needs ten times as many officers from the ethnic minorities to reach the proportion of black people in the capital. About 90 per cent of black officers

Table 4.1 Migrant flows[1]: by age and citizenship (UK)

Thousands

	British	Old Common-wealth	New Commonwealth and Pakistan (NCWP)		European Com-munity[3]	Other foreign	All countries
			Indian sub-continent[2]	Other			
Into the United Kingdom							
1971	92	17	19	17	13	41	200
1976	87	16	23	19	12	34	191
1981	60	11	22	14	10	36	153
1985	110	19	17	18	20	48	232
1986	120	16	18	16	35	46	250
Of which aged:							
Under 16	26	1	7	2	1	11	48
16–24	27	9	4	6	18	11	76
25–44	50	4	5	6	14	21	101
45 or over	18	1	2	1	2	3	25

Out of the United Kingdom

1971	171	13	6	11	14	26	240
1976	137	15	4	10	15	29	210
1981	164	13	3	13	13	26	233
1985	108	12	4	12	10	28	174
1986	132	19	3	10	10	40	213
Of which aged:							
Under 16	22	2	–	1	4	9	38
16–24	28	2	1	3	3	9	45
25–44	57	12	1	5	3	18	98
45 or over	24	2	1	–	1	4	32

Balance (net movements)

1986	– 12	– 3	+ 15	+ 6	+ 25	+ 5	+ 37
Of which aged:							
Under 16	+ 4	– 1	+ 7	+ 2	– 3	+ 2	+ 10
16–24	– 1	+ 7	+ 3	+ 3	+ 16	+ 2	+ 31
25–44	– 8	– 8	+ 4	+ 1	+ 11	+ 3	+ 3
45 or over	– 7	–	+ 1	– 2	– 7	+ 3	

1 Excludes movements between United Kingdom and Irish Republic.

2 India, Bangladesh, Pakistan and Sri Lanka.

3 Excludes Denmark and Irish Republic in 1971, Greece in 1971 and 1976 and Spain and Portugal in all years except 1986.

(Reproduced from *Social Trends*, 1988, with permission of the Controller of HMSO.)

Table 4.2 Population: by ethnic group and age 1984–86

Percentages and thousands

Ethnic group	Percentage in each age group					Total¹ all ages (= 100%) (thousands)	Percentage UK-born	Percentage resident in English metropolitan areas
	0–15	16–29	30–44	45–59	60 or over			
Ethnic group								
White	20	22	20	17	21	51 107	96	31
All ethnic minorities	34	28	20	13	4	2 432	43	69
of which								
West Indian or								
Guyanese	26	33	16	19	6	534	53	81
Indian	32	27	23	13	5	760	36	66
Pakistani	44	24	17	12	2	397	42	66
Bangladeshi	50	20	14	15	1	103	31	79
Chinese	28	28	28	11	5	115	24	52
African	26	31	27	12	4	103	35	75
Arab	17	40	28	10	5	66	11	62
Mixed	53	27	11	7	3	235	74	58
Other	28	25	30	12	4	119	28	63
Not stated	29	24	18	13	17	691	68	37
All ethnic groups	21	22	20	17	20	54 230	93	33

1 Population in private households.
Source: Labour Force Survey, combined data for 1984 to 1986 inclusive, Office of Population Censuses and Surveys
(Reproduced from Central Statistical Office, Social Trends, 1988, p. 26, with permission of the Controller of HMSO.)

Table 4.3 Estimated size of populations of minorities in the UK, 1951–1985

	1951	1961	1971	1981	Average 1983–5
Number (1000s)	200	500	1200	2100	2350
Percentage of population	0.4	1.0	2.3	3.9	4.3

(Reproduced from OPCS, 1986.)

are at the lowest rank of constable' (*Guardian*, 20 November 1989). Nationally the situation is no better. 'These are only 3 black women police officers with a rank higher than PC in the whole of England and Wales. All of them are sergeants . . . there are just two black superintendents, one chief inspector, and twelve inspectors' (*Today*, 13 October 1990, p. 5).

At the other end of the occupational scale unskilled jobs are disproportionately undertaken by black people. Visitors to London need only travel on public transport, visit the museums and art galleries and shop in the supermarkets and fast-food centres to have this confirmed. When it comes to unemployment, studies have shown that black people are roughly twice as likely to be unemployed than their white contemporaries (Fitzgerald, 1989). In 1985, unemployment for white people was 10 per cent; for ethnic minorities as a whole it was 20 per cent (West Indians 21 per cent; Indians 17 per cent; Pakistanis and Bangladeshis 31 per cent).

With regard to the younger age group, reports have shown that black people are disproportionately represented on Youth Training Schemes, although they are less likely than white youths to be on the more prestigeous employer-led schemes – those with the greater employment potential (ibid.).

In October 1990, a Government sponsored report carried out by researchers at the University of Sheffield claims that 'many more young Asians complete education and training courses after 16 than young whites, but they have only half as much chance of getting a job as white students with equivalent qualifications'. The report suggests that racism and stereotyping dominate employer's recruitment policies. 'Black and Asian job applicants spend longer periods unemployed and are less likely to secure the best jobs' (*Independent on Sunday*, 28 October 1990).

> Inglan is a bitch
> dere's no escapin' it
> Inglan is a bitch
> y'u haffi know how fi suvvive in it
>
> well me dhu day wok an' mi dhu nite wok
> mi dhu clean wok an' mi dhu dutty wok
> dem seh dat black man is very lazy
> but if y'u si how mi wok y'u woulda sey mi crazy
> (Lynton Kwesi Johnson, *Inglan is a bitch*.
> Reproduced with permission from Race Today
> Publications.)

These disturbing figures are evidence of what is termed *institutional racism* i.e., the employment organizations responsible for recruitment (the political parties, legal organizations, the caring services and the voluntary agencies) are discriminating against and failing to meet the needs of black people in our society because of their practices and procedures. Institutional racism is sometimes referred to *camouflaged racism*, meaning that it is not open and visible but concealed in practices and procedures.

The education system provides further evidence of institutional racism. Studies have indicated the tendency for Afro-Caribbean children, in particular, to under achieve in school. Several reasons have been put forward for this; the main reason is believed to be the low expectations from teachers. White teachers have in some cases stereotyped black children as having potential for sports but not academic subjects. For example, Anat Arkin, writing in a newspaper, cited the case of Dionne Ferdinand, a graduate of Leeds University.

'At school Dionne was encouraged to take CSE's rather than O'levels and to concentrate on sport. When she told her careers officer of her ambition to become a barrister, she was advised to think about working in a factory instead.'
(*Guardian*, 30 January 1990)

Some children of West Indian descent have been further handicapped by the linguistic difficulty of having to acquaint themselves with standard English whilst using a form of Patois in their own familiar surroundings. Another distancing element is the fact that most teachers are middle class and black children are over represented in the working class.

The Swann Report (1985) found that there was a clear relationship between the achievements of minority groups and their social and economic conditions. Asian children were shown to perform better than West Indian children in British schools and this was explained in part by the fact that they were not quite as socially and economically deprived as West Indian children. Furthermore, Asians (except for Bangladeshis) performed as well as whites who were less disadvantaged. This was attributable to the supportive family structure.

The content of the school curriculum is itself often racist, with history, for example, being taught from a Eurocentric viewpoint; glorifying white British individuals and successful global conquests. Everybody who has passed through an English school has heard and learned to admire the great dedication of Florence Nightingale, but how many have heard of Mary Seacole, a black nurse who received the Crimean medal for her outstanding services to nursing on the battle fields only to die in obscurity? Similarly, how many have heard of the social and political contribution of the Chartist, William Cuffay, Shapurji Saklatrala, a Communist MP or Claudia Jones, the political rights campaigner?

Not only is the contribution made by black people in the past ignored or played down, but black people are conspicuously absent from text books in all subjects: Anglo-saxon names are mainly used and white people feature in the illustrations. Consequently, black children have a dearth of positive *role models*, that is, people whom they can look up to and identify with.

Another areas of social disadvantage includes housing; black people are

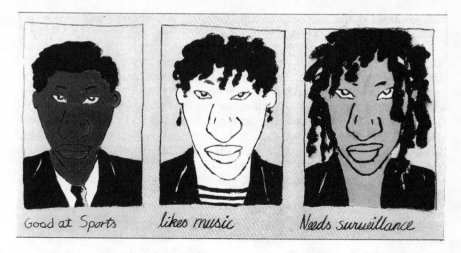

Good at Sports   likes music   Needs surveillance

UK School Report by Tam Joseph. (Published by Leeds Postcards.) The faces are painted red, white and blue from left to right.

known disproportionately to experience conditions of poor housing. (Bad housing conditions often correlate to other areas of disadvantage and low educational achievement.) With regard to various health studies, it has been shown that black people are more likely to be prescribed tranquillizers than white people and are more likely to be 'sectioned' under the Mental Health Act. Other studies show that black people are more likely to go to court on arrest than whites and more likely to receive a custodial sentence. They are also more likely to be held in custody and to be refused bail.

The effects of racism

'I say I'm a black person who lives in Britain. Although I hold a British passport I still don't say I'm a British citizen. I will only say that when I believe I'm treated justly and get fair treatment from this society.'
(John Fernandez, college lecturer and a Goan who has lived in Britain for over 20 years, *Asian Times*, 3 March 1989)

The influence of racism is felt at a very early age. Young children are aware of the differences in colour between themselves and other children and soon recognize which colour is more highly valued by society. There have been examples of young black children scrubbing themselves 'in order to become white'. This point was made by the CRE who state in *From Cradle to School* (1989), 'We know from research evidence that by the time they enter primary school, white children may well be on the road to believing they are superior to black people. Black children may believe that society is not going to show them the same respect and esteem that white people receive.' The CRE add: 'such attitudes are not innate, but learned. What is learned before the age of five in race relations is therefore of critical importance to the stability of the next generation and to society as a whole.'

For this reason it is vital that playgroups, nurseries, childminders and schools oppose the dominant culture and message of society and provide young children with surroundings which instil equal tolerance and respect for all cultures. There are many ethnic minority children in various childcare settings who do not see themselves or their culture reflected in their surroundings. All children need positive cultural images and role models and to have their history acknowledged and identity respected. Particular requirements concerning dietary needs, skin and hair care, religious and other cultural needs have to be met, and all festivals have to be acknowledged and celebrated. Much of this is already firmly integrated into the day to day structure of nursery and school provision.

In some cases, where all the staff and children are white, objections have been raised to the development of anti-racist practises on the grounds of it being inappropriate. Such objections miss the point of anti-racism. Children are growing up in an increasingly diverse, multi-cultural society. As individuals all children need to cherish and respect their own cultural heritage and be open to embrace the rich diversity of other cultures devoid of any artificial notion of inferiority or superiority. As the CRE point out, 'it is important to acknowledge that racism damages all concerned; black children may internalize racist messages while white children too are limited by a narrow, ethnocentric environment which denies them the opportunity to develop positive attitudes towards other people and ways of life. Being proud of one's culture is not the same as believing it to be superior.'

The task facing those working with the under-fives is to recognize and eliminate discrimination and to maximize each child's motivation, 'by encouraging her or his sense of being included, personally, racially and culturally in all aspects of the learning experience'. This is important in order to avoid 'another generation of white children developing a belief that they are superior or somehow more British than their black peers because of a very narrow, old fashioned notion of what being black means'.

Individual racism takes many forms, ranging from looks, verbal abuse, assault and in some cases even murder. Racism is an ongoing threat to all ethnic minority members in Britain and occurs in everyday situations. According to Brian Jacobs, 'For minority groups racism is something which is part of everyday life and it is they, therefore, who are best placed to understand the full implications and effects of it.' Some black social care students from Kilburn College discussed its routine occurrence. Samantha spoke of how a white female shop assistant, whose hand she had inadvertently touched whilst paying for her purchase, unselfconsciously withdrew her hand and wiped it against her overall. Eloise cited a similar example of being rudely forced away after offering assistance to an elderly white woman who had stumbled. Another student, Ramone, feels angry when each time she goes into a department store or large shop and she is immediately singled out and asked 'Can we help you madam?' while other shoppers are free to browse and shop at their own pace. This was a common occurrence for many black women in the group. So too, was the experience of being the subject of a lengthy security check, even for cheques made out for very small amounts. They also talked of instances where white women were seen to clutch their handbags closely to themselves in the presence of a black person. Hannah, who came to Britain in 1956, felt that racial prejudice had diminished. She remembers the signs 'No Blacks, No Irish' and the difficulties she had in obtaining basic living accommodation when she first came to this country. She talked, too, of her initial puzzlement at the behaviour of young white boys who would approach her and ask her the time. When she looked at her watch and told them they would go away disappointed. She later discovered that young English boys expected her 'as a black woman' to look at the sun in order to find out the time.

For other black people racism still has an everyday reality. It means being at a job interview and knowing you will not be chosen, or having a vacant seat next to you on a crowded train. For one young man, Andrew, 'it is something I can feel the moment I enter a room'. The effects of everyday racism can be debilitating, as Jocelyn Mignott says:

'I get tired of people calling me coloured because they feel it sounds better than black. I get tired of being the only nice black person people have ever met. I get tired of being mistaken for someone else. Take a good look at black people – we don't all look the same. I get tired when relatives of my residents look through me and search for a white officer. I get tired of people who think that to be white is "normal". I get tired of people who pay lip service to the abhorrence of racism yet fail to confront it in their every day lives.'

(*Social Work Today*, 28 March 1988, p. 28)

Racial violence

According to the Home Affairs Committee in its *Report on Racial Attacks and Harassment* (1986), 'The most shameful and dispiriting aspect of race relations in Britain is the incidence of racial attacks and harrassments'. Sir Peter Newsman, in his preface to the CRE report, *Living in Terror* (1987) adds that 'racial attacks on members of ethnic minorities are increasing, not only in areas where they are well represented, but also in areas where their numbers are low'.

Racial attacks are not a new phenomenon: rather their scale and number is. Some attacks occurred during the early part of this century in the dock areas of some of Britain's major cities. Violence between white people and black people flared up again in the inner city areas in the late 1940s. In the 1950s there were clashes between white and black youths, some of which were so serious (including the ones at Nottingham and Notting Hill in London) that they were referred to as race riots. The 1960s and 1970s saw the 'Paki bashing' phenomenon led by gangs of white skinheads. The 1980s saw a number of horrific racially based acts of violence against black families. In 1986, an Asian boy was stabbed to death by a white boy at a school in south Manchester because he was of Pakistani origin. At the inquiry into racism and racial violence in Manchester schools, a senior teacher told the panel in evidence that he saw 'nothing wrong with the word "Paki"', because it was simply an abbreviation of Pakistani'. This is a clear example of institutional racism within a school.

A study carried out in Newham in 1986 found that one in four of Newham's black residents had been the victim of some form of racial attack during the previous 12 months (London Borough of Newham, 1987). Of the 1550 incidents of racial harassment there were 774 cases of insulting behaviour; 188 cases of attempted damage to property; 175 cases of attempted theft; 174 cases of threats of damage or violence; 153 cases of physical assault and 40 cases of damage to property.

This situation is not isolated. 'Few areas in Britain can now be regarded as completely safe for black residents . . . racial attacks have taken place in areas such as middle-class Hendon and in Shrewsbury in rural Shropshire' (Gordon, 1986). Evidence is also cited from Glasgow where more than half of the 50 people interviewed said they had suffered racist graffiti on their homes and almost half said they had been racially abused (Scottish Ethnic Minorities Research Unit, cited by CRE, 1987).

These figures could well be an underestimate, given the possibility that many incidents have gone unreported through fear of reprisal or lack of faith in the agencies which are meant to support the victims.

Two short histories reported to the Commission for Racial Equality are described below.

Case 1 – South London Local Authority

Mrs A was an Asian single parent with four children, aged 11 months (twins), five years and eight years. She lived with her uncle in a two storey council flat which she had moved into in 1983.

Mrs A and her family began to experience extreme racial harassment three months after moving into the flat. She had no friends or relatives in the borough and hers was the only black family in the block. The neighbours were openly hostile to her, slamming doors in her face, for example, and when the children went out to play they were verbally abused and physically assaulted. Sometimes they were tied to railings and left there. They even had their hands tied behind their backs and were put in the large communal dustbins and left, their clothes having been removed first. The whole family were continually abused and chased on their way to shopping, etc. The children sometimes had their heads banged against walls by 10- to 14-year-old white youths. Mrs A and her twin babies were spat on when she asked them to stop.

During 1985 the harassment became very frequent. Mrs A's milk bottles were smashed and pushed through her letter box almost daily, her door was urinated on regularly, lighted material was put through the letter box on five occasions and eggs were frequently broken through the letter box. All the tyres of her car were slashed on one occasion and her windscreen wipers were broken. Eggs were also frequently broken over the car.

A group of white adult men, after drinking in a nearby pub, would abuse the family verbally and throw stones, bottles etc. at Mrs A's bedroom windows, sometimes until 1 am. They would also bang on her front door at these times and shout racist abuse.

Eventually, Mrs A's family were moved in February 1986, and experienced racial harassment in their new flat. Mrs A's condition deteriorated and she then applied for a mutual exchange and moved to another London borough.

Case 2 – North Western Local Authority

A family with two children moved into their house and within a few weeks the incidents began. The mother and children were verbally abused, stones were thrown and there were obscene and abusive 'phone calls. These forms of harassment continued for some months.

The perpetrators then started on the family pets; the children found their cat dead and skinned on the doorstep; a second cat had its tail broken; and a third had its face smashed in with a hammer. In addition, the family's car, parked outside their house, was repeatedly vandalized. A local community organization working in the area has taken up the case with the police and the local authority.

Changing relationships between black and white people

During the 1960s there was an expectation that black immigrants would *assimilate* themselves into the established British way of life in the way immigrants to Britain had done throughout history, i.e., black people were expected to fit into the existing social structures.

By the 1970s, this emphasis on assimilation was recognized as a denial of the value of the contribution black people made to society. Within educational settings particularly, the importance of people's cultural backgrounds was being recognized and incorporated under the umbrella of multi-cultural education. Children learned to appreciate differences in food, dress, music, customs and religious festivals. The effect of multi-cultural education generally increased the awareness of people about the rich cultural diversity of modern Britain. However, it did not appear to lead towards a decrease in racism. Put simply, informing people about 'saris, samosas and steel bands' was not confronting the institutional racism of society.

The 1980s saw a change of emphasis and the development of anti-racism as an approach aimed at addressing the institutions and organizations within society which by their very practices and procedures deliberately or unwittingly perpetuate racism. Many organizations have now made anti-racist statements. In addition to making any racist act a punishable offence, by examining such issues as staff recruitment and selection and scrutinizing working procedures, organizations are able to rid themselves of those practices which hitherto worked towards excluding black people. Colleges with an anti-racist policy will, for example, monitor the ethnic origin of students and compare these with the population of the catchment area, consider the ethnic background of the staff at all levels within the hierarchy and see how this reflects the local population. Educational materials are examined for their possible racist influence and with the purpose of ensuring that there are positive black images which black students can relate to. Anti-racism is after all about social justice. It seeks to eradicate institutional barriers to equality of opportunity to all British citizens whatever their skin colour.

Equal opportunities

Owing to the under representation of black people in local authority and voluntary services, many public bodies have sought to redress this balance by implementing equal opportunities policies. Such policies recognize that be-

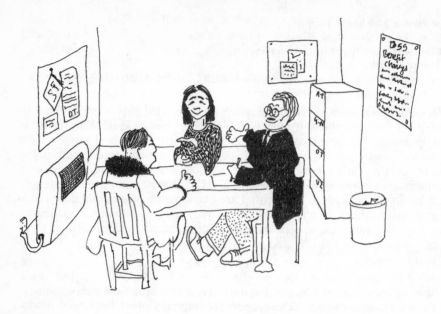

Having knowledge of another language and of another culture is a positive attribute to any social work organization.

longing to an ethnic minority is in itself a positive attribute particularly when the nature of the work concerns working with ethnic minority communities. Membership, knowledge and understanding of another culture, as well as proficiency in one of Britain's several living languages other than English, is of great value to any organization wanting to work closely within the community. With regard to staff recruitment, less emphasis may be placed purely on academic qualifications and relevant life experience is sought after and acknowledged. Professional standards remain the same but in a situation where, for example, four candidates for a job were equally qualified academically and only one was a member of an ethnic minority, that person would be offered the post in recognition of her or his additional value to the organization. *Positive discrimination* can be considered as a development of equal opportunities which concentrates on equality of outcome. The principle allows an organization to discriminate in favour of a recognized disadvantaged group. For example because of the disproportionate under representation of professionally qualified black social workers, a college may set out to recruit a certain percentage of its CQSW/Dip SW students from ethnic minority groups. This means that a black person and a white person could be equally suitable for a place on the course but the offer would be made to the black candidate in accordance with the general policy.

The media and black people

'When you are lying drunk at an airport, you're Irish. When you win an Oscar, you're British.'

(Brenda Fricker, Actress, *Observer*, 5 May 1990.)

The media, in particular television, plays an important part in portraying that which our society values. It reflects as well as creates images. With regard to ethnic minority people many of these images have been, and remain, very negative. Some impressions of black people are grossly stereotyped in cartoons, or they are portrayed as subjects of 'jokes', or they are disproportionately associated with 'trouble'. This type of presentation is not balanced with positive associations and neither are black people commonly depicted in responsible authoritative roles. There are very few programmes provided for minority communities, except during off peak hours, and even then these programmes are often directed at an English speaking audience. Twitchin (1988) points out:

'We live in a multilingual society. But this fact could not be derived from watching TV or listening to the radio. There are over 12 languages, other than English, that are spoken in England by a very large number of people. These languages are Chinese, Arabic, Punjabi, Urdu, Bengali, Gujerati, Hindi, Polish, Italian, Turkish, Greek and Spanish.'   (p. 45)

However, the situation is slowly improving as television companies become more aware of their responsibilities towards all groups in society. But until they operate true equal opportunity policies they will continue to marginalize black people to a nation which watches an average of 27 hours television per week.

Black people and social care

It is now widely recognized that both Social Services and National Health Service provision have in general failed to meet the needs of the black community. In 1978, the report of a joint working party made up of the Association of Directors of Social Services (ADSS) and the CRE stated that the response by Social Services Departments (SSD) to ethnic minority communities was 'patchy, piecemeal and lacking in strategy'. More recently in 1989, studies carried out by the CRE, based mainly on areas of high ethnic minority population, showed that not all local authorities had fully committed themselves to equal opportunities in service provision; policy implementation was still in its early years. In other words there had been little advance in the eleven years between the two reports.

That services have not effectively reached black people is evidence of institutional racism. By and large the policy of SSDs and the NHS has been shaped by white, middle class males who comprise the majority of senior and higher management positions. Within Social Services ethnic minority people are grossly under represented at the decision making level. In 1990 there were

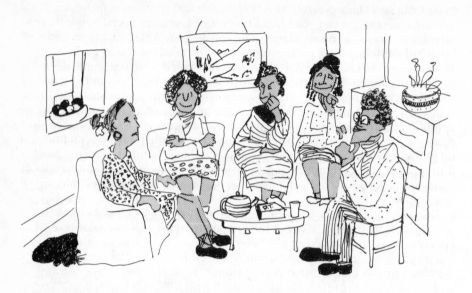

Black people have sought support amongst members of their own community as a
positive response to the lack of adequate social provision.

only two black male directors of social services and no black women directors.
Black people are under represented throughout the fieldwork sector and at the
managerial level within residential and day care work. Members of ethnic
minorities, particularly women, are more commonly employed in the more
basic social care roles of care assistant/officer, home carer and home help. This
situation is paralleled within the Health Service, where much of the basic care
and domestic work is carried out by black women and once again black people
are less directly involved in decision making.

Institutional racism within the NHS is evident in the way that black people
are treated the same way as white people: because of this there is very little
knowledge about diseases specific to black people and a reluctance to
encourage research in this field. This is most clearly illustrated in the case of
genetically transmitted diseases such as sickle cell disease, which until recently
has always been regarded as a rare tropical disease of little significance in
Britain. There are in fact many sufferers of this disease amongst people in
Britain: an estimated one in 200 people of West Indian or African origin (Sickle
Cell Society, 1987).

Many black carers are themselves subject to individual racism in the form of
racial abuse which is sometimes directed against them by patients or clients.
Sometimes this coincides with society's racism if the management of an
establishment have failed to acknowledge the existence of racism and therefore failed to developed strategies for its elimination. In such circumstances a
black worker may be tempted to ignore abuse rather than voice her or his
objections and risk being labelled a trouble maker. When an establishment
implicitly condones racial abuse, an employee with the reputation of a trouble

maker can find this adversely affects their job and promotion prospects.

Josie Durrant, former Assistant Director of Lambeth Social Services, now director of Focus, a social care training consultancy, refers to the 'decades of failure of the social work profession to meet the needs of black people' (*Social Work Today*, 17 October 1989). She adds that much serious damage has been done to black families, particularly Afro-Caribbean families, 'in the name of social work intervention'. The disproportionately high numbers of black children received into care and the large number of black youths sent to detention centres are evidence of the hard consequences which social control agency policies have had on black families. These policies have been founded on prejudicial assumptions about the ability of black families to cope. Cultural differences have often not been acknowledged or explored and differences in childcare practices have been stigmatized as being automatically inferior or inadequate.

Similarly, many black people have been mistakenly labelled mentally ill by white psychiatrists who have not fully understood the cultural context of their clients behaviour. This point has been well made by Roland Littlewood and Maurice Lipsedge (1982) whose study on ethnic minorities and psychiatry stemmed from a concern that people from, "Eastern Europe, the Caribbean and South Asia were often admitted to the hospital by their family doctors or by the police under a 'section' of the Mental Health Act – that is as involuntary patients. On arriving in hospital they frequently received the diagnosis of schizophrenia and were seldom offered psychotherapy, usually being treated with pharmaceutical drugs" (p. 45). The authors go on to say ". . . we then looked at how the schizophrenia diagnosis was being made and realized that it often conveyed a doctor's lack of understanding rather than the presence of 'key symptoms' by which this reaction is conventionally recognized by British psychiatrists. Patients appears to be unintelligible because of their cultural background" (p. 46).

More recently Alison Whyte (1989) has reiterated the point. She asks 'How can a white, middle class, male psychiatrist know how a young Afro-Caribbean man expresses grief or how an Asian woman deals with depression?' But she goes on to state that the answer is not simply one of educating psychiatrists about culture. The problem lies within the racism which permeates our society and what Errol Francis, Director of the Afro-Caribbean Mental Health Association calls 'the long route to the hospital'. 'The point at which a person is diagnosed,' he says, 'is the last port of call on this route.' If a person is socially disadvantaged and emotionally upset, then every contact with the police, the housing department, the DSS, social services and other agencies can compound their distress and eventually lead to mental illness (Alison Whyte, *Community Care* 20 September 1989).

Residential social services provision has also been seen to have ignored the particular needs of black people, although there are signs that this is being seriously addressed by the more enlightened authorities. As recently as 1988, The Wagner Report commented, 'we have, however, formed the strong impression that ethnic minority communities are almost without exception particularly ill served by the residential sector and that special provision for them in all its forms is in everyway inadequate and in many places virtually non-existent' (p. 11).

Some ethnic minority communities have learned to expect little support from welfare agencies owing to past negative experiences. Indeed, amongst some communities there is a deep-seated mistrust. There is also widespread ignorance of the range and type of services available. Language is sometimes a barrier to some people and they are not always reached by the information and publicity which is directed essentially at the white, English-speaking public. Amongst some cultures there is a great reluctance to ask for help even if the services available are known. This reticence may stem from pride, fear of losing self respect, or suspicion of white dominated organizations or a combination of these and other reasons. However, according to Jocelyn Mignott, officer in charge of a local authority old people's home, the biggest barrier to services reaching all those in need is the assumption held by the caring organizations:

> 'There is a racist orientated myth that should be written on the tombstone of every black, elderly person who dies, cold, alone and poor, unaware of the services which could have advanced their later years – they look after their own.'
>
> (*Social Work Today*, 24 March 1988.)

The assumption that ethnic minority communities are made up entirely of caring, close knit, extended families which do not need or require support, has meant that many SSDs have failed to make ethnically sensitive provision for the communities they serve. For example, despite the growing proportion of black elders in this country very few attend local authority day centres or

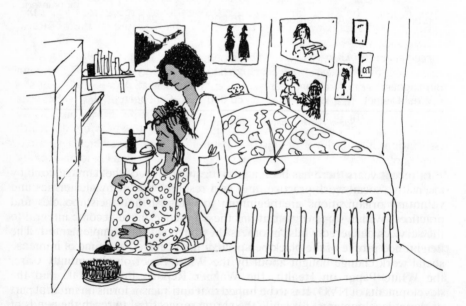

Black children in residential care must have their personal care needs met and their cultural identity reaffirmed.

elderly person's homes. They are often put off, partly by the absence of other black service users and partly by the predominance of traditional British activities and fare. Instead, many black elders have turned to the voluntary organizations, the church or local community groups in order to meet their specific needs.

The failure of many SSDs to recruit adequate numbers of foster carers representative of the community they serve has meant that many black and ethnic minority children have remained in residential care longer than necessary. Within institutional settings the needs of black children have often been neglected; for example, the need to receive proper attention regarding hair and skin care, to meet a dietary and cultural requirement and, above all, the need to have their ethnic identity affirmed and respected. Similarly, within foster placements many black children have suffered the disorientation of being brought up by white carers who, however loving, have not been sympathetic to their cultural needs (see Table 4.4).

Table 4.4 Resources for providing same race placements

Authority	Ethnic community	Size	Number of black/Asian fosterers	Size of family recruitment team
Tower Hamlets	Bangladeshi	55 000	1	5 posts approved but not yet appointed
Lambeth	Afro-Carribean	75 000	210	25
Waltham Forest, South District	Indian and Pakistani	6 000	12	5.5
Rochdale	Asian	20 000	3	3
Birmingham West District	Afro-Caribbean/ Asian	60 000	3 Asian 15 Afro-Caribbean	12

(Reproduced from *Social Work Today*, 22 February 1990, p. 8.)

In recent years there has been a growing awareness of the damage done by insensitive social work practice, and as a result of this many authorities and voluntary organizations are beginning to establish anti-racist policies and practices. Within some organizations these practices have become integral to the services delivered whilst in others they have yet to be implemented. The heightened profile of the black perspective has occurred at a time of immense social work change bought about by the White Paper on Community Care, the White Paper on Health, the Wagner Report, Project 2000 and the developments of NVQ. It is to be hoped that anti-racism forms an integral part of these developments, for while the caring services fail to reach the needs of all those people who make up society, they continue to discriminate against them.

Conclusion

We have seen that racism exists throughout society and it adversely affects the lives of black people daily in many varied ways. At its most extreme it takes the form of physical violence; at other levels it can just be 'felt' by the victims, in the manner in which they are treated and in the way they are looked at or addressed in everyday situations.

It is reasonable to conclude that everybody is to some extent racist given the influence of being brought up and conditioned by society. It is further suggested that in Britain white racism is the problem. However, it is too simple to suggest that racism is therefore solely a white person's problem. Dialogue between black and white people needs to continue and to be encouraged in order to allow change to occur. As carers, whatever our skin colour, we need to examine our own feelings and attitudes and consider what part we play in the maintenance of racism.

Exercises

1. Get into small groups of about four or five and discuss the similarities of your broad life experiences; the schools you have attended, the neighbourhood you grew up in and the friends you had, etc. Consider what you have in common. In particular, consider the first time you came across somebody of a different colour from yourself. How did you feel? Were you conscious of the difference in skin colour? Share these observations of the early events in your life with others.

2. Does your employer have an equal opportunities policy? If so find out where the policy is located and with regard to race:
- familiarize yourself with its contents
- consider its relevance to your organization
- find out how it is implemented and monitored.
Share your understanding of the policy and its implications with your colleagues.

3.
> 'Hospitals are frightening and confusing places for old people from any background; much more so if the staff cannot understand what you are saying and cannot make themselves understood; if you can't eat the food and your body is exposed and handled in a way in which you find shaming and distressing.'
> (Norman, A., *Triple Jeopardy: Growing Old in a Second Homeland*, 1985.)

Consider the sentiments expressed in the above statement and apply them to your own work setting. In your care team consider practical ways in which your establishment (or placement) can avoid inflicting such humiliation and distress.

4. Study your own organization. Find out the ethnic makeup of the community in which it is situated. Compare this with the proportion of ethnic minority people employed by your organization or college and the 'racial' mix of the service users or students. Note the level of employment with regard to status and responsibility.

5. With regard to any ethnic group, find out all you can about the following:
- Dietary needs and preferences

- Special hygiene habits
- Religious practices and festivals
- Practised social activities
- Range of lifestyles
- Traditional family structure
- Gender ascribed roles etc.

Questions for essay or discussion

1. African slavery and British colonialism are irrelevant to an understanding of racism in Britain today.
2. In Britain only white people can be racist, black people can only be racialist.
3. How can the caring services more effectively meet the needs of ethnic minority groups?
4. What can individuals regardless of their own skin colour do about combating racism?
5. Jokes about minorities are inevitable and harmless. They serve to lighten any potential discord between cultures.
6. Just as it is impossible for men to completely rid themselves of sexism so it is impossible for white people to eradicate their own racism.

Further reading

Academic sources

Ahmed, S., Cheetham, J., Small, J., *Social Work With Black Children And Their Families*, Batsford Ltd, 1986. A detailed examination of the experience of black families with regard to how they have been dealt with by the social services, with suggestions for future improvements.

Dominelli, L., *Anti-Racist Social Work*, Macmillan, 1988. A clear account of the value and need for anti-racist social work.

Fryer, P., *Black People In Britain*, Pluto Press, 1984. A comprehensive account of the long history of black people living in Britain, the difficulties they have had to overcome and the significant contribution they have made to society.

Institute of Race Relations, *Roots of Racism*, Volume 1 and 2, Institute of Race Relations, 1982. Easy to read and detailed examination of racism throughout the ages looking at slavery and colonization.

Institute of Race Relations, *How Racism Came to Britain*, Institute of Race Relations, 1982. A cartoon-style book giving a pictorial account of Britain's colonial past, and present day policies.

Jacobs, B.D., *Racism in Britain*. Christopher Helm, 1988. An up-to-date look at racism today and how minority groups have organized to defend their interests in a society that is so often hostile towards the notion of equality of opportunity.

Other literary sources

Angelou, M., *I Know Why The Caged Bird Sings*, Virago, 1986.
Lee, H., *To Kill a Mockingbird*, Pan Books, 1974.
Miller, A., *Focus*, Penguin, 1989.

Morrison, T., *Beloved*, Picador, 1989.
Ngcobo, L., *Let It Be Told – Black Women Writers in Britain*, Virago, 1988.
Walker, A., *The Colour Purple*, The Women's Press, 1990.

Films or plays
Clavell, J., *To Sir With Love*, UK, 1967.
Jewison, N., *Heat of the Night*, US, 1967.
Schmultz, O., *Mapantzala*, South Africa, 1988.
Van Peebles, M., *Watermelon Man*, US, 1970.

5 Other marginalized groups

5.1 Introduction

Society is divided along a number of other lines in addition to the three major ways already dealt with in detail. It is possible to be a member of a minority on grounds of age, health, disability, life-style or sexual orientation, as well as in other ways, while also being disadvantaged by social class, gender and race. Thus people may experience *multiple marginalization* because they are disadvantaged by being a member of more than one minority. For example a black, working class boy experiences discrimination in what is known as 'double jeopardy': first, from his colour and second, from his class position. Similarly the term 'triple jeopardy' can be used to describe the marginalized position of black elderly women, who are thereby discriminated against on the three grounds of race, age and gender. The term 'triple jeopardy' was coined by Alison Norman (1985) to describe the situation of black elders in Britain today. She says 'they are not merely in double jeopardy by reason of age and discrimination, as has often been stated, but in *triple* jeopardy, at risk because they are old, because of the physical condition and hostility under which they have to live, *and* because services are not accessible to them' (p. 1). To extend the point further, a gay, elderly, working class, disabled, black woman would experience discrimination on six counts. The opposite is also true of course – a heterosexual, young, middle class, able-bodied, white man has the most to gain from society.

In order to look more closely at some of the other ways in which society is divided, we have selected eight minority groups. The selection was not an easy task because there are so many marginalized groups. Only lack of space has prevented us from including sections on homeless people, unemployed people and 'informal' carers. It is known that over 300,000 people in England and Wales are registered as homeless with local authorities. This figure does not include the majority of single homeless people, many of whom sleep 'rough' in our towns and cities. The homeless represents a sizeable minority, but although it is not dealt with separately, the issue of homelessness is discussed in sections of this chapter as well as elsewhere in the book.

We recognize that unemployed people represent a sizeable group which in recent years has become almost an institution, so much so that it is taken for granted that unemployed people should exist in such large numbers. Although they are not dealt with specifically as a section in this chapter, they have been referred to throughout the book.

In the case of 'informal' carers there is a clear case for them to be considered as a separate marginalized, albeit varied, minority. As already mentioned, it has been estimated that there are over six million people looking after dependent relatives. However, because carers are central to the book, they are not dealt with here as a separate minority group; instead, they are integrated throughout the whole book.

All the groups discussed in this chapter are marginalized. We acknowledge that some may have chosen their life-style and may also have been aware that a partially 'marginal' existence might be the result of this decision – the obvious example is that of travellers. The majority, however, are victims of political, economic and social processes which result in their being treated as 'outsiders' by our society. Although free choice is a factor, once travellers have chosen their life-style the same excluding processes operate.

Such processes are prejudice, discrimination and stigma directed at the groups discussed by members of the wider society and by its institutions (including the Health Service, Education Service, Social Services Department, and Housing Department). A common consequence of these processes is that once society has *victimized* (or marginalized) the members of these groups, it then often goes on to *blame* them for their victimized or marginalized position. Consider the following examples.

First, unemployment has increased since the 1970's, partly as a result of the decline in large manufacturing industry. Many women and men who were nearing retirement age found it impossible to find alternative employment. Similarly traditional job opportunities were no longer available to school leavers. However, both young and old have been stigmatized and have frequently had to bear negative labels through no fault of their own.

Second, elderly people are also blamed for being victims of the ageing process. Because they are no longer economically active they are undervalued. Their past contribution to society is forgotten and their current contribution ignored. The fact that they require services is often resented by others and elders themselves can internalize society's image of them as 'burdens'.

Third, many people who experience mental illness do so as a result of the stress they experience in their personal lives. However, mental illness is often regarded as a sign of weakness or social failure and people who experience it are blamed because they do not appear to cope as well as others.

As mentioned earlier, marginalized groups fundamentally lack power. We have seen, for example, how stigma can only be attached to the less powerful by the more powerful. William Ryan (1976) has said 'The primary cause of social problems is powerlessness. The cure for powerlessness is power' (p. 250).

Power relationships fluctuate according to changes in the relationship between particular groups of people and the wider society. Today there is evidence of more public understanding and empathy towards minority groups. Furthermore, all of the groups we have selected have sought more power for themselves and adopted a more assertive profile. This has manifested itself in a number of forms: many self-help groups have been formed to promote their own particular interests; a great deal of publicity and informative material has been produced and there has been an increase in the use of the media; action has been taken to push for policy and practice changes, in order to influence the personal social services and other welfare agencies. Examples of such changes can be seen in the application of concepts of 'normalization' for those with learning difficulties; taking services to the homes of elderly people, instead of providing them mainly in residential settings; and an emphasis on greater user involvement and choice for all client groups. These progressive policy and practice developments have been officially endorsed by the Griffiths Report (1988), the Wagner Report (1988) and subsequent legislation involving 'Community Care'.

It is not the intention of this chapter to provide a detailed causation of the various disabilities experienced by some of the groups discussed. Neither does it attempt to discuss in any depth the ageing process or provide a detailed history of travellers throughout the world. Such material can be found elsewhere, and there are some indications in the 'Further reading' section at the close of the chapter. Instead, we have concentrated on the social effects of marginalization on those particular groups we have selected.

5.2 People with learning difficulties (mental handicap)

People with learning difficulties are marginalized in our society primarily because of their inability to learn as quickly and as comprehensively as others. This negatively affects how they perform everyday living tasks and correspondingly increases their dependence on other people. Their full social integration is hampered further by the predominance of myths and demeaning public stereotypes concerning people with learning difficulties.

The streotypes place undue emphasis on the less attractive aspects of behaviour displayed by some people with learning difficulties. This may include unusual mannerisms and inappropriate behaviour, such as dribbling, spitting or shouting, or standing too close or touching too familiarly. More extreme behaviour can include sudden and violent gestures and action. Stereotypes are reinforced and perpetuated because most members of the public do not have close contact with people with learning difficulties. They may only have seen people with learning difficulties *en masse*, either being transported by Social Services, or at day centres or in hospital wards, when their collective presence may serve to emphasize any strangeness.

With the exception of those individuals who have had a mentally handicapped person in their own family, most people in our society have had little contact with people with learning difficulties. As children they rarely shared classrooms, Sunday school lessons or parks and playgrounds with them and few now share their homes, work or social life with mentally handicapped adults. Little wonder that there is so much widespread ignorance about the needs of people with learning difficulties and so much embarrassment and apprehension amongst ordinary members of the public. Furthermore, the perceived social abnormality of mental handicap is reinforced by the media, which rarely focuses on people with learning difficulties except in controversial circumstances. They are not featured in ordinary everyday settings.

The description 'learning difficulties' or 'special needs' embraces a wide range of people from those whose disability is mild and barely discernable through to those whose condition is severe and with whom communication is often extremely restricted. It should be remembered that people with learning difficulties are as unique as ordinary people. Stereotypes only obscure this individuality. While society fails to recognize fully their needs as individuals, it also fails to acknowledge their capacity to enrich the lives of all of us.

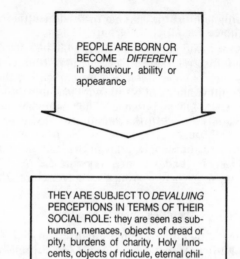

Fig. 5.1   How an initial handicap is made worse by the devaluing perceptions of others. (Reproduced from Brandon, D., Ridley, J., *Beginning to Listen: A Study of the Views of Residents Living in a Hostel for Mentally Handicapped People*, Campaign for People with Mental Handicap, 1985, p. 5.)

Much of today's misinformation and negativity towards people with learning difficulties has its roots in the past. Until the middle of this century, social provision was directed by the principle of 'out of sight, out of mind'. People with varying degrees of mental handicap were incarcerated in specially built, self-contained hospitals often situated in remote settings away from built up areas. Many spent the remainder of their lives in an institutional world, separate and well apart from the rest of society. Moreover, many mentally handicapped people were certified and admitted alongside the mentally ill, thus 'reinforcing prevailing stereotypes about the uniform character of madness' (p. 12, Wagner Report, 1988a). Fig. 5.1 outlines the process by which a person born with learning difficulties has her or his difficulties compounded by negative social attitudes.

Over the past 20 years, and particularly during the last decade, services for people with learning difficulties have undergone important changes. With the advent of principles such as *integration* and *normalization* the emphasis has been to recognize the individuality of people with learning difficulties and their right to live as normal a life as possible. The move has been away from institutional care towards care in the community. However, it is said that

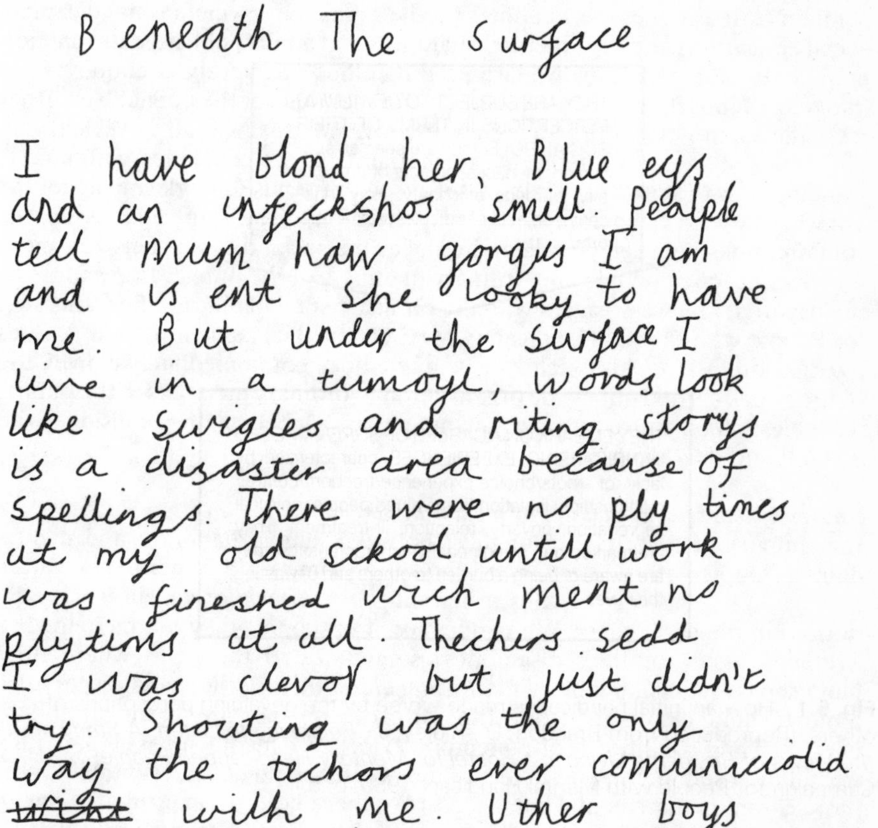

Beneath The Surface

I have blond her, Blue eys and an infeckshos smill. People tell mum haw gorgus I am and is ent she looky to have me. But under the surface I live in a tumoyl, words look like swigles and riting storys is a disaster area because of spellings. There were no ply times at my old sckool untill work was fireshed wich ment no plytims at all. Thechers sedd I was clevor but just didn't try. Shouting was the only way the techors ever comuniciolid ~~witht~~ with me. Uther boys made fun of me and so I beckame lonly and mishroboll. it was like being on a decert island lost and alone. Life was life and sckooll was sckool.

Fig. 5.2 Dyslexia is one kind of learning handicap. This piece, by Alexander Parsonage, was entered in the Dyslexia Institute's 'As I See It' Competition, 1989.

society disables people with learning difficulties more severely than their mental limitations do, and that what is required in order to make policy changes more effective is an accompanying growth in public tolerance and respect towards people with a mental handicap.

What are 'learning difficulties'?

The use of the term 'learning difficulties' has arisen as a more dignified, less stigmatizing alternative to the term 'mental handicap'. However, 'learning difficulties' is too vague a term to always convey its intended meaning; sometimes it needs to be qualified by the former title, mental handicap. A social education centre for mentally handicapped adults publicised its function as a centre for people with learning difficulties and received enquiries for 'language support' and 'maths lessons' from members of the public! Nevertheless, the use of the term forces us to recognize that we all have learning difficulties of some sort in our lives, whether they are concerned with understanding how to start a car, being assertive with friends or work colleagues, or knowing how to behave in new social situations. The term focuses on the common links between people and reduces the social distance between mentally handicapped people and ordinary members of the public. In response to the negativity now associated with the phrase mental handicap, the Campaign for People with Mental Handicap (CMH) changed its name in 1989 to Values into Action (VIA). Although its new name does not immediately convey the type of work carried out by the organization to ordinary members of the public, it enables VIA to move forward unhampered by a label that they consider to be 'hurtful and degrading'.

Causes of learning difficulties or mental handicap

It is important to briefly distinguish between mental handicap and mental illness. People with a *mental handicap* suffer some form of permanent brain damage. They have difficulties in learning, the effects of which are usually noticed in the early years. With education and support they can be helped to overcome some of their disabilities, sometimes to the point where their handicap is minimal. People with a *mental illness* on the other hand, experience a mental state emanating from stress or problems they are no longer able to control. Their condition is often temporary because mental illness is generally treatable or self limiting, although relapses can and do occur. Mental illness is more common than mental handicap: it is experienced by an estimated one in nine of the population at some stage in their lives. Some people have a predisposition to mental illness. People with learning difficulties may experience mental illness in addition to their mental handicap, but they are no more prone to it than ordinary people.

Mental handicap may be caused by a number of factors although the exact cause is often not known. Most people are born with their disability e.g. Down's syndrome but some acquire the condition during their lifetime, or following a viral infection, or by sustaining brain damage through injury. There is estimated to be between one and one and a half million people with a mental handicap in this country. Of these, the great majority have moderate learning difficulties only, and how far they go towards reaching their full potential will depend on the amount of love, stimulation and support they receive. All people with learning difficulties will be dependent upon others for assistance and support in varying degrees throughout their lives, as to a certain extent we all are.

Special difficulties for parents of children with learning difficulties

Some families are not able to cope with the unexpected extra demands and strain created by the arrival of a child with learning difficulties. Marriages may break down, possibly resulting in either the child being received into care, or one of the parents, usually the mother, being left with sole responsibility for the child's upbringing. Most parents, however, react positively to their situation and strive to provide their child with all the love and attention she or he needs. In reality they have little choice. Although their task is not entirely devoid of many of the essential joys of childrearing, it is often an isolating and debilitating struggle. Society's reluctance to share the responsibility means that the parents face a life long battle without respite.

'Don't tell me that it is always difficult being a parent – will *you* still be paying for babysitters when your children are 20, 30, 40 . . ?'
(Millerman, A., *Guardian*, 22 September 1989)

Those who become parents of children with learning difficulties need to make huge emotional adjustments as they endeavour to come to terms with the feelings brought about by a sense of overwhelming disappointment and loss. They may be counselled against having further children in case they produce another child with special needs. They may worry too about the social and emotional stresses that having a child with learning difficulties might have on any existing children. Parents may also experience guilt or shame at having produced a child with special needs because it is not seen as perfect by the rest of society. The situation is more difficult for families within some communities where having a handicapped child is seen to represent a divine punishment. The family will have to carry that added stigma.

Having a child with learning difficulties may mean that the family will be practically excluded from engaging in many of their hitherto cherished activities. The following extract is from an account of how an ordinary day to day event served to bring home to a mother the limitations of her handicapped twin daughters and the implications for the family's future. The children were approaching their first birthday; three months earlier they had been diagnosed as being severely brain damaged.

'Christmas shopping had to be done. Some niceties must always be observed. I braced myself and embarked on a trip to Habitat. A harmless enough venue I thought. What confronted me there was the moment that stands out more than any other moment in the last 13 years.

There, amid the glasses and the kitchenware, furniture and fancy goods, stood stark realization. Stretching high towards the ceiling was a large display of skipping ropes. Hundreds and hundreds of them. The perfect present for a little girl. I have never known a little girl who hasn't skipped at some time in her life. It's a simple activity totally devoid of class, status, age, wealth, culture, race or religion. As I looked at them they began to represent the entire life that we would have to say goodbye to: the fell walking that we had always loved, that would now only be possible with supreme physical effort and the help of others; the family outings that we'd dreamed of during pregnancy – trips to funfairs, zoos and the countryside, which would all now take on the proportions of a major expedition. Even nipping out to the shops was going to be a thing of the past. How could one person ever go anywhere again, on impulse, with two wheelchairs to push?

The total enormity of the situation hit me in the stomach like a bag of wet cement. I sucked in my cheeks, turned around and walked out as fast as I could. I didn't cry until I reached the car.'

(A. Millerman, unpublished)

Parents of children with learning difficulties will need support from friends and relatives more than most families, yet they are more likely to be isolated in this respect. For various reasons, including their own embarrassment, awkwardness and ignorance, friends and neighbours may be reluctant to visit or help out in a situation with which they are not familiar and where they do not always feel at ease.

Social provision, ranging from financial benefits, home conversion grants, special school arrangements and respite care facilities are available, to a varying degree, to families with children with learning difficulties. However such provision is often inadequate: it varies form region to region and is not always available from birth, and strict eligibility criteria excludes some families. The situation is obviously exacerbated when local authorities and voluntary organizations are forced to cut back on expenditure.

As children grow older the difficulties for the parents increase; the children become heavier and physically more difficult to manage, and they need extra support in coping with the changes brought about by puberty and adolescence. Whilst they are at school they are cared for. When they get beyond school age however, the responsibility for full time care goes back to the parents. In some cases residential care is necessary but for many families this is not appropriate. The Wagner Report (1988b) *Residential Care – A Positive Choice* recommends that: 'Education and training for people with mental handicap should aim at enabling them to live with minimum support in ordinary housing' (p. 7). Until appropriate provision is made available for all people with learning difficulties parents will continue to be plagued by their major concern – 'Who is going to look after them when I'm gone?'

Social provision for people with learning difficulties

Children

Children with special needs have a statutory right to education from the age of two until they are 19 years of age. Since the 1981 Education Act, every child who is considered to have special needs, including those with learning difficulties, has a right to be made the subject of professional assessment and have a statement drawn up outlining her or his needs. Furthermore, in order to encourage integration, children with learning difficulties should have their education provided, where possible, within mainstream education. The principle of integration has its detractors who feel that children with learning difficulties may miss the specialized support found only in special schools, and may experience a sense of failure in the larger mainsteam schools. However, it is argued that children with learning difficulties will benefit from experiencing ordinary schooling, albeit with special support, and an opportunity to grow up and make friends with ordinary children. Children without special needs will also benefit from exposure to people with learning difficulties from an early age.

Adults

As already mentioned, once people with learning difficulties leave school their parents face their most difficult times. Education is statutory but once it is over people with learning difficulties are entitled to nothing. The Disabled Persons Act 1986 recommends, but does not insist, that local authorities should define need and provide for it. Without a continuity of support the chances are that the progress and developments made in childhood may be wasted as people with learning difficulties deteriorate or lose their confidence. Very few are able to find work directly; an increasing number may be able to obtain a place on a Further Education course, although these are not always available; some will remain at home; others will seek places at social services day centres, again only where places are available.

The needs of people with learning difficulties have never been a great priority within the Social Service Departments and Social Work Departments in Scotland. Social services have tended to concentrate on their statutory work concerning children, their families and 'sectioning' the mentally ill. Services to people with learning difficulties and their families have been poor and the implication that people with disabilities are somehow less important prevails within the caring services just as it does within society as a whole.

The original aim of *Adult Training Centres* (ATCs) was to provide basic employment training skills and enable people with learning difficulties to eventually find work. Indeed, they grew out of occupation centres which were started following the First World War by voluntary organizations and some local authorities. Until quite recently they remained unstimulating places, their central activity being some form of dull, repetitive contract work such as packing, for which the trainees (as the service users were known) were paid very little. In recent years the move has been away from work 'training' towards 'social education'. *Social Education Centres* have been established, some of which have replaced ATCs, to enable people with learning difficulties to develop skills that will enable them to cope better with the requirements of everyday life. At the SECs, students with a wide range of learning difficulties may learn to prepare meals, do their own washing, receive a continued general education, practice arts and crafts, experience supervised shopping trips and undertake work experience placements. The centres work towards *self-advocacy* encouraging clients to make decisions and determine their own life-styles. Many of the students are able to achieve greater independence through being able to manage money and use transport and other community resources, and eventually they are able to live more independently in a sheltered flat or group home. Of course some people's learning difficulties are so severe that they will never reach such independence, but all targets they reach will enrich their lives and make caring for them easier.

It is argued that services for people with learning difficulties are too 'building-based' and that segregated provision reinforces too many misperceptions. For example, some people feel that day centres, which remain the mainstay of community provision, should be completely abolished. It is felt that more effort should be made to enable people with learning difficulties to become more integrated into the community in order to widen their basic choices. It is argued that colleges of Further Education are the right place for adults with learning difficulties to receive education and skills training in common with others in the population. In this way day centres are seen to operate against the spirit of normalization owing to their segregated form of provision.

Normalization

Although normalization is a seemingly straightforward concept it raises complex issues. Most importantly it begs the question – what is normal? This is, of course, relative and could be defined differently according to time, place and culture. There are also divergent individual interpretations of the word and therefore there is no overall agreement on precisely what is meant by 'normal'.

The concept of 'normalization' was developed in Scandinavia during the 1960s. It was originated by Bengt Nirje (1976) who defined it as 'making available to all mentally retarded people patterns of life and conditions of everyday living which are as close as possible to the regular circumstances and ways of life of society'.

This somewhat academic definition primarily refers to the treatment of people with learning difficulties in our society, although it has wider applications to a whole range of other groups including elders and people who are mentally ill. Essentially normalization improves the lives of people with learning difficulties and combats their devalued status by ensuring an existence as close to normal as possible.

The following figure shows how a vicious circle can operate to the detriment of people with learning difficulties. For example a person labelled 'mentally handicapped' and who has major learning and communication problems, nevertheless presents a very positive image if she/he is fashionably dressed, lives in a flat with a room-mate and has a paid carer and is productively

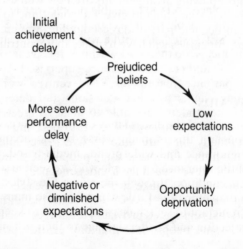

employed at a standard wage. The same person will be seen much less positively if she or he lives in a locked ward, is drably dressed, looks dirty and unkempt and spends each day idle except for 30 minutes of 'recreational therapy'. All of these characteristics – appearance, activity, living place and occupation, we can do something about. The principle of normalization urges provision which will increase the positive aspects of peoples' lives.

Normalization does not claim that people with learning difficulties are normal, or that they are not negatively valued by the rest of society. Some people, particularly parents of those with learning difficulties, are suspicious of the concept. They feel that its pure application can obscure their children's specific needs. Objections have been raised at the way some social workers have single mindedly pursued their ideals of normalization (client choice and participation in decision making), regardless of the person's stage of development. In an article published in *Community Care*, parents asked, 'Why can't social workers accept that our children are *not* normal?' Particular examples quoted were:

'Mary must be allowed to take responsibility for her money, even if it means she spends it all on bars of chocolate instead of replenishing an empty larder.'
'Philip must be allowed to go to the pub with his mates, even though he is liable to drink too much and become violent or have a fit.'

(Community Care, 8 May 1986)

Normalization does not seek to deny a person's stage of development, rather it purports that the style of service provision and the experience enjoyed by the recipients should be as close as possible to that of the mainstream community. According to Julian Hillman, writing in *Social Work Today* (13 April 1989), normalization requires that 'every one be entitled, as their potential allows, to be taught the skills and allowed the life style that our society values.'

There are many examples of good practice which have been inspired by the principle of normalization. These include various work schemes such as café and grocery delivery services which are exclusively run by people with learning difficulties. They have also formed their own theatre company. Finally many different forms of group living arrangements are now well established, recognizing that everyone has something to give and something to gain. The more such experiences can become part of day to day life, the greater the chance people with learning difficulties will have to make their contribution to the rest of society.

5.3 People with HIV/AIDS

The nature or progression of the disease may eventually necessitate some form of physical isolation and this is made worse by the accompanying social isolation. Fed by ignorance and widespread, media-based scaremongering, society has shown little tolerance for people who are seen in some way to have contributed to their condition through their own life-styles. Blame is more easily apportioned than empathy. Little wonder that so many people with the HIV infection are reluctant to seek help, and attempt to keep their condition secret for fear of rejection and further damage to their self-image.

'My parents did not know I was ill . . . I walked into their kitchen and told them . . . A couple of days later at dinner I was given a glass of sherry that had a piece of cotton round the stem . . . The plate was marked underneath with a cross.'

(Community Care, 8 June 1989, p. 18)

'. . . I repeated the facts of my friend's illness and could hear Dad trying to take it all in. Then, about an hour later, my father rang in a distraught voice, "Listen you shouldn't have that person staying in the house with you. I've been talking to your mother and we are both very frightened."'

(ibid, p. 16)

AIDS/HIV has only relatively recently become a major public issue. Very little is known about the precise origin of the disease, why it has spread so rapidly or why some people are more susceptible than others. Unfortunately one thing is certain, and that is that there is, to date, no cure. By September 1990 there were 14 723 reported cases of people living with HIV in the UK (Center for Disease Statistics, 1990). The actual prevalence is likely to be much higher; estimates range from 20 000 to 50 000. Because of the long incubation period of the virus, estimated to be as many as 10 years, many more people will become ill over the next few years.

What is AIDS/HIV?

Acquired: Something you have picked up not inherited.*
Immune Deficiency: Your body can not defend itself against illness.
Syndrome: The set of illnesses you get as a result.

*This is no longer true: pregnant women can pass the infection on to their newborn babies.

AIDS is caused by the human immunodeficiency virus or HIV. This virus attacks the white blood cells which help defend the body against disease. People with AIDS do not die from AIDS itself. They die from some other infection or disease their bodies cannot fight.

Antibodies are produced by the body in response to HIV. However, these antibodies do not seem to affect the virus. The antibodies can be detected in blood tests and if they are found they will indicate that the person has been infected. The presence of antibodies does not automatically mean that person will develop AIDS. Some stay well. Others will move through the infection and *eventually* die of AIDS.

AIDS includes a whole range of illnesses for which there is no medical cure. People with HIV may experience loss of vision (sometimes very rapidly), physical wasting and severe weight loss, constant fevers, persistent diarrhoea, heavy night sweats and other major physical changes. All these symptoms advance rapidly within a short space of time. Skin cancers and cerebral atrophy also occur.

How is the disease transmitted?

HIV, the virus that causes AIDS, only survives in human body fluids such as blood, sperm fluid (semen), vaginal fluid and breastmilk. (The virus has also been found in saliva and tears but in exceptionally small amounts and no-one is known to have caught HIV from saliva or tears.)

HIV can be spread in three ways, as outlined in CCETSW training guidelines:

By sexual contact with an infected person by unprotected, penetrative sexual intercourse (either vaginal or anal) which involves the exchange of semen and vaginal secretions. In this way men can infect men, men can infect women and women can infect men.

By exposure to blood or blood products. UK donated blood is now screened for HIV antibodies reducing the risk of transmission by blood transfusion to about 1:1 million. In the past people have been infected by blood transfusions. People who share needles, equipment or 'works' when injecting drugs are therefore vulnerable. Transmission by 'blood to blood' contact, through cuts, abrasions or skin lesions is extremely rare, with only a few instances world wide.

By mother to child. Infection can occur during pregnancy from an infected mother to her child and later, via breastmilk.

The majority of people who have contracted the virus in the UK have been gay men and bisexual men, injecting drug users, recipients of infected blood products, such as people with haemophilia, and babies born to HIV-infected women. In Scotland, 52 per cent of those who are HIV infected are categorized as injecting drug users. In the rest of the UK it is 8 per cent (*Scottish Drugs Forum*, 1990).

How is HIV not transmitted?

HIV cannot be transmitted by ordinary social contact; by touching, hugging, social kissing, sharing utensils or toilet seats. It is not passed on by animals or insects.

The Centers for Disease Control in the US has studied the families of those people infected with HIV. These families shared facilities such as toilets, baths, beds, crockery and cutlery. The studies found that apart from the sexual partners and children born to infected women . . . no-one in the families of more than 12 000 people with AIDS is known to have developed the disease (Connor, S., Kingman, S., 1982, p. 138).

Much of the publicity surrounding HIV has been damaging and has contributed to the stress already being experienced by those infected. It has also added to the wide spread confusion felt by the rest of the population. Harmful myths about how the disease is spread, and misleading stereotypes about people with the infection, have deepened the severe stigma felt by those with HIV.

The initial government advertising campaign carried out in the late 1980s, with its doom laden images of coffins and icebergs, did little to properly educate the public about the facts relating to HIV. A later campaign, which started in February 1990, was more effective and informative. Misinformation, however, has been rife. For example in November 1989, Lord Kilbracken announced that only one person in Britain had contracted AIDS through heterosexual sex. Tabloid newspapers followed this with headlines claiming 'normal' people did not get AIDS. In fact, according to the Health Education Authority in December 1990, 'In the UK over 600 HIV carriers had become infected through heterosexual sex' (*Observer*, 11 February 1990). Nevertheless much media intensity has been focused on gay people who have been blamed for the disease. This blame has facilitated the venting of other, more entrenched, prejudices against gay people and reinforced the marginalized position they have in society. Similarly the reputation of black people has suffered at the newspapers' claim that AIDS 'came from Africa' although Johnathan Mann, former director of the World Health Organization, maintains that 'on the basis of available information we believe that HIV is an old if not ancient virus of unknown geographical origin' (Global Programme on AIDS – The Global Impact of AIDS, WHO Summit 1988, Barbican, London).

In addition to coping with the physical symptoms of the infection, people with HIV need to combat social discrimination. There are recorded instances of people with HIV having their homes fire-bombed. They have lost jobs, friends and social privileges, and they are discriminated against financially by insurance companies and mortgage companies. Some MPs have called for a reversal of the community care programme suggesting that some former long stay psychiatric hospitals, currently being closed down, should remain open in order to cater for people with HIV. This was precisely the philosophy which led to the siting of the original mental hospitals in isolated geographical locations when they were built in the nineteenth century.

People with HIV do not normally need to be in hospital for long; they can live their lives in the community with varying degrees of medical support. When they are admitted into hospital they may be admitted into a side ward. According to Mike McCarthy this 'has a two fold effect; for some it may be seen as a punishment, for others it can be seen as helpful and a protection from outsiders' (*Social Work Today*, 5 May 1986, p. 19).

The effects of HIV on social care/social work
HIV creates a whole series of implications for social care/social work. It highlights issues, including those not normally openly discussed in our society, such as sex and sexuality, death, racism, lifestyles and disease, disfigurement and disability. All this within a climate of uncertainty save the knowledge that there is no cure at present.

Henry Davidson, a social worker with the Royal Victoria Group of Hospitals in Northern Ireland, describes his earliest experience of working with an HIV patient:

'The first person with AIDS in Northern Ireland died in this hospital in 1985. I worked closely and intently with him and his family for over a year. Together we weathered diagnosis, disclosure of sexuality, stigma, guilt, fear of disclosure, fear of infection and progression, through to repeated and unpredictable acute episodes of illness, with limited possibilities for treatment. This was further compounded by body change, physical disfigurement, rapid and severe mental impairment and the accompanying management problems that this imposed; isolation in the extreme and death.' He adds, 'The unrelenting traumatic effects did not cease with the death of the person. They continued for the family when making plans for the disposal of the body, registration of the death, leakage of information to the press, and fears for the family as a result of exposure to employers, friends and school. The stigma and trauma live on. With death, under other circumstances, pain becomes somehow more bearable. As the patient's mother put it, "Instead of getting better with time it only gets worse".'
(*Social Work Today*, 29 September 1988, pp. 11–13)

The way in which social work services respond to the development of HIV will have particular relevance to people with HIV living in Scotland. Whereas they form 10 per cent of the UK population, they include 15 per cent of those who are known to be HIV infected in the UK (*Scottish Drugs Forum*, 1990, p. 7). This over representation is due mainly to the fact that Edinburgh has the highest number of known HIV cases in proportion to its population. The continued practice of drug taking in certain areas of the city has undoubtedly contributed to the high numbers of HIV infected people. 'Edinburgh, the capital of Scotland, is in the unenviable position of having the highest proportion of intravenous drug abusers who are known to be HIV seropositive in any British city' (Morgan Thomas, 1990, p. 88).

As well as presenting a fresh challenge to social care/social work, HIV serves to highlight the importance of core social work principles; the need to 'respect' and to 'value', to maintain the client's dignity and be 'non-judgemental' is underlined by the nature of the disease. Furthermore, because of the many fundamental matters concerning the human condition raised by HIV, carers are being forced to examine their own attitudes with regard to death, sexuality, culture, lifestyle and other issues. This is necessary otherwise how can they be of assistance to those living with HIV?

5.4 Elders

> When I am an old woman I shall wear purple
> With a red hat which doesn't go, and doesn't suit me.
> And I shall spend my pension on brandy and summer gloves
> And satin sandals, and say we've no money for butter.
> I shall sit down on the pavement when I'm tired
> And gobble up samples in shops and press alarm bells
> And run my stick along the public railings
> And make up for the sobriety of my youth.
> I shall go out in my slippers in the rain
> And pick the flowers in other people's gardens
> And learn to spit.
>
> (Jenny Joseph, *Warning*, in *Rose in the Afternoon*,
> J.M. Dent and Sons Ltd., 1974, with permission)

The elderly members within our society form an increasing proportion of the population, yet they remain largely on the periphery, unable in many cases to enjoy the benefits of a developed society to which they have all made a contribution. There are, of course, many examples of elderly people living full and active lives well into their eighties and even nineties, but for those suffering ill health and/or financial hardship, old age is a struggle often spent in isolation.

In other societies, notably in the East in countries such as India and China and even many European countries, elders have a more important functional role, particularly within the family but also within wider society in general. They are respected for their age and are afforded responsibility and recognition, whereas in Britain, old age is seen primarily as a problem. Of course, there are certain difficulties associated with old age, including the likelihood of physical impairment and the possibility of mental deterioration, but these health issues are very much compounded by society's attitude towards its elders.

The ageing process starts at birth and slowly begins to accelerate when we are in our late twenties, when the first physical signs such as greying hair or facial lines begin to show, and early aches and pains begin to establish themselves. Most of us, however, become accustomed to having to live with a gradual diminishing physical capacity and by the time we reach old age we are psychologically adjusted to cope.

With regard to the mental state of elderly people, it is estimated that about 20 per cent of people over the age of 75 suffer from some form of senility: a disease involving degeneration of the brain cells often manifesting as confused behaviour. Correspondingly, this means that around 80 per cent of the elderly population are as alert as ever. Despite this fact elders are still generally stereotyped as confused geriatrics.

The mass media bear some responsibility for generating and maintaining society's attitudes to the elderly. On television and radio, in newspapers and magazines, elders are often portrayed as figures of fun; as harmless, confused, powerless human beings who are usually irascible, awkward and set in their ways. Rarely are they associated with serious issues unless they happen to be celebrities, or asked to perform important roles in dramas or to feature centrally in other settings. The world of advertising is obsessed with images centred around youth, good looks and conspicuous 'success'; elderly people are almost entirely absent save when they are needed to endorse pension schemes or insurance packages. News stories about older people tend to focus on them as victims, highlighting the occasions when they are robbed or attacked in their own homes. This in itself helps to convey an unnecessary feeling of insecurity to elders who are, in fact, statistically the least likely age group to be mugged or robbed.

A recent experiment carried out in New York over a three year period underlines now elders within society are not so much handicapped by their physical disabilities as by the attitudes and psychological barriers set up by other people. Pat Moore, a social scientist and researcher in her thirties, disguised herself as an elderly woman and roamed the streets of New York. She experienced being 'a young mind in an old shell' and became 'so intimidated by the attitudes of others [she] started to move aside to let people pass and began to say [to herself] "After all, old ladies have plenty of time don't they?"' During the experiment she would, as her normal self, go into the same social situations she had been in as 'old Pat', only to find she was treated more courteously and on a more equal footing by the same people who had abused and patronized her earlier (*Guardian*, 1 August 1989).

In Britain colloquial terms like 'old dear', 'old codger' and even 'pensioner' convey images of passivity and frailty. Within the health service elders are commonly mislabelled as geriatric even when the illnesses they happen to be suffering from may affect anybody and have nothing specifically to do with old age! The terms and words we commonly use in association with elders help perpetuate the stereotyped image of their dependency and perceived uselessness, and so deny their human validity.

Population

According to official figures, on 1987 there were 8.8 million people over the age of 65 in Britain representing nearly 20 per cent of the population as a whole (Age Concern, 1990). Those over 75 years numbered 3.5 million and those over the age of 85 numbered nearly three quarters of a million. This latter and potentially more vulnerable age group is increasing and is likely to reach 1 million by the year 2000.

Since few people of pensionable age are economically active, the majority are dependent on their fixed incomes for survival. These fixed incomes reflect a person's class position and life-long social status, consequently more women, retired manual workers and people from ethnic minorities experience old age in or on the margins of poverty. For those people who retire following many years of high earnings with related benefits such as membership of occupational pension schemes, job security, incremental pay rises, opportunities to save and property ownership, the risk of state dependency is minimal. For those who have worked in low paid occupations, experienced periods of unemployment and have been unable to save, retirement is a time of economic hardship and some experience inequalities in living standards more starkly than at any time in their lives. Britain's pensioners survive on the lowest pensions in Europe and for those without any additional financial resources everyday life remains a struggle. It has been calculated that, on average, 'Pensioners are dependent on social security benefits for 48 per cent of their household income on average (the remainder coming from savings, occupational pensions and small earnings), in contrast to 13 per cent for the average household in 1986' (Child Poverty Action Group – CPAG, 1988).

It is clear that our society values those people who are still working, because they contribute to the wealth of the nation more than those who do not, even if they have done so in the past. In this way elders share a common status with others who are unemployed. In retirement, people lack the legitimacy and purpose attributed to those who work. Low incomes are seen as one of the several inevitable consequences of old age to which elders are expected to adjust. It is recognized that older people are likely to suffer from hyperthermia and social isolation but these sufferings are attributed to their age and not to the fact that they may have insufficient incomes to heat or light their homes properly, or pay for telephone calls or travel.

Women make up nearly two thirds of the elderly population and are more likely than men to be poor pensioners; there were three times as many women as men who were entirely dependent on the state pension (old supplementary pension) in 1987. This can be seen to be a consequence of womens' average lower earnings throughout their lives, their interrupted work patterns and their longer life span.

The Social Security Act of 1986 both weakened the state earnings related pension and increased incentives to take out private pensions. The effect of this Act is likely to cause an increase in old age poverty in the future. Private pensions reflect inequalities in the labour market, and leaves those who have worked in low paid jobs or those who have worked intermittently to a bleak future of even greater poverty in their old age. Those who have had well paid secure jobs of course will have continued financial security after their retirement.

Lack of money is a major problem faced by many elders and in some cases the effects of this are worsened by the living conditions many of them have to endure. According to Age Concern, in 1986 people over 60 occupied 61.9 per cent of properties lacking basic amenities; 39.9 per cent of unfit properties and 35.3 per cent of properties in poor repair. This situation exacerbates still further the trials of those older people who live in isolation and suffer from loneliness. Again this is primarily a female issue as 80 per cent of those over the age of 65 who live alone are women. Over one third of elders live with spouse only, and a total of two thirds have as their principle helper someone who is over the age of 50. Many elders have no regular visitors at all except service and delivery people. Less than half have access to a telephone and the great majority live in households without a car.

Social provision

Support services exist for elderly people and are provided in the main by the Social Services Departments (Social Work Departments in Scotland) and the National Health Service. Services too are provided by the many voluntary organizations who specialize in working with older people, such as Age Concern, Pensioners' Link and Help the Aged, who, alongside other non statutory organizations, are responsible for much of the innovatory and developmental work being done to help elders. Despite the many instances of good practice in various social care settings within both the voluntary and the state run sector, the needs of the elderly population are not being met. Indeed the general disregard for older people by the public sector amounts to *institutional ageism*: where older people are denied the services that are provided as a right for younger members of society. It is expected that old people will be ill and suffer social deprivation.

Within the local authority Social Services Departments (and Social Work Departments in Scotland), attention and resources have focused by and large on other client groups, notably families with young children and cases of serious mental illness, where the departments have a pronounced statutory responsibility. Legislation concerning elders has either not been implemented or has been ignored because it is too costly to deliver. Generally work with elders has been viewed negatively by social workers who see older people in a stereotyped fashion as being without the potential for change. Social workers have ignored the great age differences of people over 65 and the tremendous variety of needs which exist even between relatively young elderly people and those who are very old. Instead there has been a tendency to see elders as an homogenous group for whom creative enabling intervention is not really possible. This attitude is reflected in those Social Service Departments where work with older people is undertaken mainly by unqualified staff or social work assistants and whose homes and day centres lack stimulation and imagination.

The low priority given by Social Service Departments towards elders has had an adverse effect on those who care for their relatives who have had to continue without support. The growing number of black elders have also suffered from inadequate services which have lacked sensitivity and appropriateness. As-sumptions about ethnic groups, such as the Chinese and Asians, not needing help because of support from their extended families have proved unfounded. Linguistic and cultural differences have meant that the up-take of services for many ethnic minorities has been poor. Black elders have tended to look to the voluntary agencies or self-help for social provision.

A similar situation exists within the National Health Service where less prestige is associated with working with elders; their routine requirements therefore are given a low priority. For example, long waiting lists are common for operations such as hip replacements, despite the enhanced quality of life this normally totally successful operation brings. Furthermore, older people are not seen as a priority for other general services such as counselling or occupational therapy, and as a consequence illness, depression and confusion often go untreated because they are considered normal and therefore expected in old age.

Older people who are disproportionately dependent on the health service do not have their needs met, and face inherent, ageist attitudes in both hospital and community settings. Working with elders is unpopular and largely considered to be unrewarding. Correspondingly investment and research into geriatric medicine is less likely to be funded than proposals from more prestigious health disciplines.

The fact that the health services in general are not geared to meet the needs of elderly people has been commented on by Alison Norman (1985).

'Individual practitioners from the various professions are often excellent, but overall the tendency is to grudge the time, trouble and resources needed to give elderly people genuinely equal treatment. Many GPs take little interest in their elderly patients and may indeed take them off their list if they need too much help. The acute wards of hospitals are often not geared to maintain elderly patients' physical and mental functioning at optimum level, so that the trauma of admission for treatment or an operation can be compounded by unnecessary confusion, incontinence and immobilization. Geriatric and long stay wards are usually in the oldest sections of the hospital building and are often relegated to another site away from the facilities and consultant supervision. The prestige of working with the elderly is low and it is one indication of racism in the National Health Service that – from consultants to nursing auxiliaries – an unusually large proportion of this workforce is of Afro-Caribbean and Asian origin. For elderly people living in the inner cities, the position is even worse. As the Black Report has shown, health services of all kinds are inadequate and overstressed, and here again, if a choice has to be made in the allocation of resources, the elderly will lose out.'

(CPA, p. 3)

The way elders are treated by the caring services underlines their marginalized position within society. If investment in our older people is viewed as short term and regarded as being less important, and resentment is felt over the need to use scarce resources on people who have already 'had their lives', society continues to deny enormous human potential by focusing on a chronological milestone.

5.5 Single parent families

Single parent families are not a social problem. However, they are often regarded as such by policy makers and the general public alike. The negative image of lone parent families stems in part from the long associated stigma of

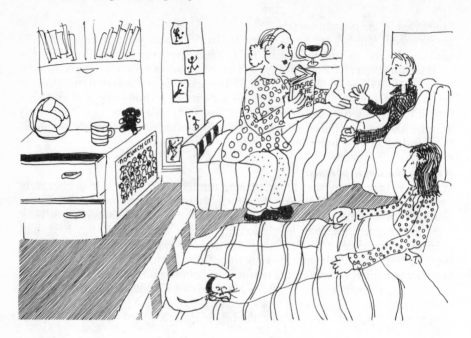

Single parents are often able to spend more time with their children than their counterparts in two parent families.

immorality that has been attached to unmarried mothers and their children. Earlier this century women who became pregnant outside of marriage were often classified as 'moral defectives' and admitted to mental hospitals. Since then other myths and prejudices have evolved concerning one parent families including young women deliberately becoming pregnant in order to obtain council housing, idle mothers living off maintenance and fatherless teenagers turning to drugs. Single mothers are often assumed to be permissive, therefore, it is thought, they are unable to discipline their children properly; lone fathers are thought not to be able to react emotionally towards their children.

Sue Slipman, Director of The National Council For One Parent Families, (NCFOPF – formerly The National Council for The Unmarried Mother and Her Child), writing in the National Council's Annual Report (1988) stated, 'The spectre of immorality, so potentially alive at our foundation (in 1918) still haunts the official and popular imagination, reaffirming the myth of one parent family life. There can be few areas of public policy making so dominated by prejudice and ignorance and so little informed by fact' (p. 5). The idea that lone parent families are a problem-ridden alternative to the 'normal' two parent family is harmful and creates difficulties for those who are members of lone parent families. It is more accurate to view single parents and their children as belonging to one of several existing and legitimate family forms, and one which, following the increase in numbers over the past twenty years, is here to stay.

Proportion of the population
Single parent families are on the increase. In 1971 there were just over 500,000 families headed by a lone parent; today there are over one million. Figures produced in 1986 (NCFOPF) showed that one parent families represented 16 per cent of all those households with dependent children and that one child in seven is in a family unit headed by a lone parent. Ninety per cent of these families are headed by women. Very few Asian families (less than 5 per cent) were headed by lone parents but the family form was common among people of West Indian or Guyanese origin (around 42 per cent).

Who are the single parents?
While it is true to say that an increasing number of women are deliberately choosing to bring up children on their own, their number remains small. Some women choose to have children and bring them up by themselves because they want to be independent of a relationship with a man. Often they have had negative experiences of men. Other women who want to be mothers may be part of a lesbian relationship; they are therefore able to form a different type of two parent family. However, the majority of people who become single parents do not attain their status by choice; it tends to be thrust upon them by a traumatic event, such as, death, divorce or separation. Approximately 80 per cent of single parents were married at one stage (NCFOPF, 1990).

Prejudice
Myths, negative media reports and other prejudices concerning single parents are common and do little to create understanding of the difficulties many of them face. Dr Rhodes Boyson MP aroused no sympathy for lone parents when, in 1987, he published his pamphlet entitled *The Defence of the Family*. He alleges that, 'Football hooliganism, riotings and muggings in the middle of cities are a product, in a large case, of the one parent family, where the father is not present and there's no pattern for boys of what controlled good manners is all about' (p. 2). His views were supported by one member of the public who wrote in a letter to the *Daily Express*, 'The complete two parent family with built in self discipline is the norm and always will be. Circumstances will always produce exceptions to the rule and these must have an equal place in society, but they must never be accepted as "normal".' (25 April 1987).

These rather extreme views of one parent families are based on a number of misconceptions. First, that all single parents are female, whereas there are over 100,000 lone fathers. Second, that children of lone parents get into trouble more frequently than children of two parent families *because* they are members of one parent families. There is no research that supports this view. In fact according to Penny Letts (NCFOPF), 'In over 60 years of working first with unmarried mothers, and then, since 1973, with single parents of any marital status, we have found that, "There is no evidence at all to show that a child being brought up by a lone parent is less able to grow up into a whole person than one from a two person home" (1983, p. 7).

It is tempting to feel that children from one parent families miss out by the absence of one parent and therefore lack an appropriate role model. However, it is argued that depending on a child's surroundings, good role models may be provided by other people in the family network such as grandparents, friends or others close to the family. Love, consistency and security are what children need and this *can* be provided by one person. Indeed, it is clear that many two parent families fail to provide children with the love and care they need. Some people feel that there are positive benefits for children of lone parents. A single parent writing in *Bringing Up Children On Your Own* (McNeil-Taylor, 1985), claims a distinct advantage to single parenthood: 'When you're on your own with your kids, something happens to you – you can give yourself entirely to them. If there are two adults in a family it is split down the middle with the adults in one camp and the kids in the other, but when you are a single parent you and your kids are all part of the one unit' (p. 141). Another parent stated in a letter to the *Guardian* on 31 January 1990 'Single parents live for their children. In a lot of ways they get more attention than children from two parent families.' The writer further added, 'I think there is less chance of them becoming juvenile delinquents.'

Lone parents differ in every case, just as all individuals differ. What they have in common is the sole responsibility for their children and a strong likelihood that they will experience social deprivation and live on or around the margins of our society. Poverty is experienced by the majority of one parent families.

Financial hardship

Most single parents of small children are not free to work, either full or part-time. In order to do so they would have to earn substantial amounts of money to cover the cost of child care, meet the extra costs of going to work and make up for the loss of any state benefit. Some parents are able to work part-time but a characteristic of part-time work is that it is low paid and rarely offers the benefits of full-time employment such as maternity leave, pension schemes and annual holidays. Part-time employees are also more vulnerable to redundancy. Single parents of older children are more able to find work but employment is again likely to be part-time. Lone parents often suffer discrimination in the job market where some employers are reluctant to employ parents with sole child care responsibilities. Consequently single parents are often forced to take jobs below their qualification or skill level. In 1986 18 per cent of single mothers worked full-time and 24 per cent worked part-time (NCFOPF, 1990). The majority of one parent families rely exclusively on state benefits and so experience a feeling of fixed dependency. In 1990 a total of 750 000 lone parent families were dependent on Income Support (*Community Care*, 25 January 1990). Of these only 1:5 were in receipt of maintenance from their former partners. Where this was received, it was automatically deducted from the single persons' benefit.

The absence of adequate state child care provision, the difficulties lone parents have in obtaining well paid work and the enforced reliance of so many on state benefit, means that the majority of single parents and their families face permanent financial hardship. In 1987 the average total weekly income for one parent families was calculated to be 36.7 per cent of that of two parent families. (After National Insurance and Income Tax were deducted, the amount one parent families had to spend was 41.6 per cent of that spent by two parent families.)

Table 5.1 provides a crude indicator of the material standard of living

Table 5.1 Percentage of households with certain durable goods (1987)

	All households	Man, woman, 2 children	One parent family
Car	63.4	83.1	25.2
Central heating	74.4	84.7	67.0
Washing machine	84.6	98.6	90.1
Fridge	97.6	99.6	97.3
Television	97.9	99.4	98.2
Telephone	82.5	86.8	58.4

(Reproduced from NCFOPF, *Key Facts. Family Expenditure Survey*, 1987, p. 5 with permission.)

experienced by the average single parent family as compared to their two parent counterpart.

The financial hardships experienced by so many lone parents results in their being less able to take part in life enhancing activities. They are less able to afford to be involved in leisure pursuits, to enjoy public entertainment or to go on holidays; such activities tend to be taken for granted by the rest of society.

Housing and living standards
Housing is another area where single parents and their families often experience difficulties and hardship. Approximately 6 out of 10 single mothers are in local authority housing (NCFOPF, 1990). Since the 1980 Housing Act, the availability of public housing has been reduced; much of the better housing has been bought by tenants exercising their right to buy. This has left only the more dilapidated and less desirable properties that councils have been unable to restore due to a lack of financial resources. Because of their desperate plight some lone parents are forced to accept accommodation in 'hard to let' properties or they are put up temporarily in hotels or hostels while they await more permanent accommodation. Lone mothers are particularly vulnerable to homelessness; some may be turned out of their home and some may find it necessary to seek refuge from male violence.

Stigma
Apart from experiencing material disadvantages, single parents and their children suffer the stigma of being seen as an incomplete family and therefore inadequate. Single fathers may not be considered to be capable parents. 'People are always telling me what is best for my son, especially the Headmistress. They think I haven't got a clue' (Single father quoted in *Double Trouble*, NCFOPF, 1983). Single mothers may be branded as failures because they have been unable to keep their man – the assumed goal for all women! – and doubt may be cast upon their ability to properly guide and discipline children on their own, 'The Headmaster told me that my daughter might not have the right kind of family background or kind of support to be able to cope in his school' (Single mother quoted in *Double Trouble*).

Martin Hughes who featured in a television programme called *Someone Like Me* (BBC, 18 March 1990), talked about his family experience since the death of his wife three years previously. He and his children struggled to survive, first on his redundancy and then on state benefit. He was unable to get a job as well paid as the one he had voluntarily given up to care for his sick wife. He felt society had treated him like '. . . the dregs of the tea-pot'.

Lesbian single parents arouse twice the disapproval both on account of their single status and their sexual identity. Often they are reluctant to seek help from the authorities because of the disapproval and hostility they fear they may be subjected to.

Over half of the children in care are from one parent families, but many single parents are suspicious of the formal caring agencies and may be loathe to admit they have difficulties coping with their children.

Isolation

Single parents are more likely than parents with partners to experience loneliness and isolation. Since the great majority of single parents do not work outside the home, they not only miss out financially, they also go without the social and psychological rewards a job could bring, such as regular contact with adults, a feeling of belonging and being needed, independence, stimulation and achievement of career goals. As previously stated general poverty prevents lone parents from playing a full role within society. Practical difficulties such as finding and paying for a baby sitter may prove prohibitive. Single mothers are more likely to be isolated than lone fathers because it is more difficult for them to go out unaccompanied. The streets are often dangerous after dark and in many social settings a single woman would feel conspicuously uncomfortable on her own. 'Like every other single parent there are a lot of negatives in my life. I get lonely, I get depressed, I feel sad when I see couples and feel superfluous at social gatherings.' Many parents lose confidence as a result of their isolation. Self-help groups, such as Gingerbread, have done much to highlight the position of one parent families and provide a focus for support and a chance to share their readily identifiable problems.

Children

As stated previously, there is no evidence that children of lone parents suffer emotionally or psychologically because they are brought up by one parent. One parent is fully capable of providing the love and security children need. Indeed a one parent family where there is concern for each member is infinitely more preferable to a two parent household characterized by discord and violence. However, many children from one parent families do suffer from the consequences of fixed poverty. Being part of a family with a low income precludes single parent children from enjoying school related activities. They are not able to afford school trips abroad, necessary sports equipment, music lessons, or have their own computer at home. Their education and life chances are correspondingly adversely affected.

Further, it must be remembered that 80 per cent of one parent families are formed as a result of marital breakdown caused by death, divorce or separation, and any one of these events is likely to have a traumatic effect on a child or children of the marriage. Despite the immediate relief children may feel following the break-up of parents who do not love one another, they are often left with confused feelings and divided loyalties. Children require time to adjust appropriately to the loss or absence of a parent.

Poverty is the main problem faced by single parents and their families. The great majority of lone parents are women and often a huge drop in the family's standard of living is experienced when it is the father who leaves a family. Some families start out headed by lone parents. What ever their origin it is true to say that the discrimination that lone parents experience and the regard in which they are held is closely related to the unequal position of women generally in our society.

5.6 Gypsies and travellers

'We do not want to be regarded as curios from some forgotten era; rather we want to be seen as ordinary people and to be treated as such.'
(National Gypsy Council in *Community Care*, 29 September 1988, p. 26)

About 1000 years ago the ancestors of the Romany-speaking peoples left India and travelled along trade routes used at different times by many other migratory nations. Historical documents show that some 200 to 300 years later they arrived in eastern Europe. By the end of the fifteenth century, they had been recorded as living in the British Isles.

The Romany language has an Indian base, but words were borrowed from every country through which they travelled. The fragmented language now has hundreds of dialects. Today Romany-speaking people live throughout the world. Many have intermarried with other peoples and enjoy a large number of diverse cultures. Only a minority of Romany-speaking communities in the world remain nomadic.

Thomas Acton (1974) has made academic studies of the Romany-speaking peoples and states that 'no definition of the term "gypsy" could even begin to command universal acceptance' and he speaks of the 'illusory image of the "true" gypsy' (p. 2). As far as he is concerned 'racial purity' is as much a myth among gypsies as among any people of the world. It is thought that the word 'gypsy' may be a corruption of the word 'egyptian'.

There are other groups of nomadic people in our society who do not call themselves gypsies. Some have been around for hundreds of years, but others, such as the 'teepee' people and the 'hippy' or 'peace convoy' have their origins in the 'youth movements' of the 1960s. The term which finds general acceptance amongst all such groups (including gypsies) is 'travellers' or 'travelling people'.

Language
Specific groupings of people are often associated with a native, 'secret' language which is private to a particular group. Those who prefer to be called 'English travellers' use what they call an 'Anglo-Romany' language. Irish travellers use the 'shelta' or 'gammon' language. The Anglo-Romany word for a non-traveller is a 'gaujo'. The language of travellers has a strong verbal rather than written tradition.

Life-style

'The gypsies are still on the road, and it is not assimilation that they are looking for. Society must not make this unreasonable demand of them.'
(Smith, M., *Gypsies: Where Now?*, Young Fabian Pamphlet no. 42, 1975, p. 19)

Clearly there is a great deal of variety of life-styles among travellers. Each travelling group's life-style will depend on a number of factors, which include historical and cultural traditions as well as economic status. Some travellers may be settled, either temporarily or permanently, on sites or even in ordinary housing. There is little if any truth in the image of a carefree 'life on the highways' with a pony grazing outside the caravan. Most travellers have to work extremely hard to make a living.

The majority of travellers are self-employed and are commonly involved in scrap dealing, road and path surfacing and general dealing, often in household goods such as furniture. Some travellers trade in horses but as work horses are not utilized today they often represent a side-line or a form of capital investment. Others are involved in 'casual' agricultural work.

The development of motorized transport has changed the pace of the traditional nomadic life-style of many travellers. Very few now have a traditional horse drawn wagon. Indeed, many are no longer nomadic in the strict sense. The majority live in comfortable, modern caravans with conventional facilities such as radio and television. Their leisure activities and forms of entertainment are not so very different from that of ordinary house dwellers.

Population

It is extremely difficult to say with any accuracy how many travellers there are in the UK. Numbers change all the time owing to a variety of factors. A nationwide census in 1965 produced a figure of 15 000 individual people, but it was suggested that this figure was a serious underestimate (HMSO, 1967). A government estimate two years later stated that there were 25 000 travellers. Present day estimates, believed to be more reliable, would put the number at around 60 000. There are approximately 11 000 caravans on sites in addition to an unknown number 'on the road'.

Marginalization – public reaction to travellers

Many of us will have seen signs displayed in the windows of some public houses which read 'No travellers'. This is a common example of the rejection of travellers by 'conventional' society. Following a court ruling in 1988 (Commission for Racial Equality v. Dutton) travellers are now protected from overt discrimination of this kind by the Race Relations Act (1976). The Commission for Racial Equality regards travellers as an ethnic minority group which must be protected against discrimination. It has taken up several cases of alleged discrimination.

Myths and legends, often of an unhelpful nature, are still perpetuated in our society, sometimes by travellers themselves but mostly by the antagonistic sentiments voiced by non-travellers. Such sentiments are usually based on fear and suspicion and stem from ignorance of travellers; they perpetuate prejudice and mythical stereotypes.

As recently as 1967, an official government report entitled 'Gypsies and other Travellers' quoted a rhyme which it stated 'children still repeat':

'My mother said I never should
Play with the gypsies in the wood.'

Although it decried the thought behind the rhyme, the report stated 'a popular legend still exists that gypsies actually steal children'. Legends and rhymes have traditionally been passed down orally throughout the centuries, but what is surprising is that some are still believed today.

The general perception of travellers by the public is poor. One of the chief culprits in maintaining this erroneous perception is the mass media. Virtually all of the stories carried in the press about travellers are couched in terms of the travellers being a nuisance, of illegal campsites and of leaving piles of rubbish behind when they decamp. (No mention is made that this may have something to do with the fact that the local police moved them on at 6 am!) The real motive underlying the antagonism may be economic. They fear that a travellers' site near their homes will devalue house prices, or in the case of pub landlords, that the presence of gypsies will deter customers.

The media covers 'negative' stories concerning travellers and not 'positive' ones. This is probably because ordinary members of the public rarely come into contact with travellers other than in a confrontational situation such as wanting a camp moved on. Both travellers and house dwellers lack good shared experiences of each other. Until this happens it is unlikely that unhelpful myths and legends will cease to be believed.

Dealing with bureaucracy

Travellers face many difficulties because they remain nomadic or semi-nomadic within a non-nomadic society. Our state institutions, most of them large, bureaucratic organizations, tend to function more efficiently when they are dealing with people who can be contacted at a fixed address! At the same time because such agencies have difficulty in contacting and working with travellers, so travellers experience a great deal of hardship coping with the requirements of these bureaucracies.

Helpful individuals exist in all state agencies, such as the police, health service and education departments, but it is usually the structure, rules and regulations of such bodies that cause problems in their relationships with travellers. Difficulties can arise around a whole range of complex issues, for example presenting traffic documents at a police station, registering with a GP, or placing their children in a particular school. Our social agencies are not particularly geared towards travellers' needs. Furthermore, the situation may be compounded by a low general level of literacy amongst travellers; forms have to be filled in!

A government committee of enquiry into the education of children from ethnic minority groups stated in its report (Swann report, 1985) that it was disturbed by the 'universal hostility and hatred' which was meted out to travellers. In the final section about other ethnic groups, the report stated that travellers' children were badly affected by 'racism and discrimination, myths, stereotyping and misinformation, and the inappropriateness and inflexibility of the education system'.

Local support groups provide an immeasurable amount of help to travellers. These are just some of the issues which one local support group assists travellers with on a day to day basis:

- advice on rights
- policing issues
- DSS regulations
- tax returns
- education
- creche facilities and under-five playgroups – while children are being cared for parents can seek assistance on other matters
- literacy help – writing a specific letter or filling in a form
- putting travellers in touch with legal assistance, liaising with police, solicitors or probation officers
- a mail collection and dissemination point – this acts as a permanent address when travellers are moving around the locality
- it acts as a 'neutral' meeting place for travellers liaising with health, education and welfare services e.g. social services, GPs, mental health services, education services or specific schools.

Other problems faced by travellers

'I will tell you my views about the local authority sites. Those that I've seen are fairly good. The only thing is, it's like the Indians in Canada and America, these reservations, the gypsies on them can't move.'

(Jimmy Penfold, traveller, in Sandford, J., *Gypsies*, Abacus/Sphere Books Ltd, 1975, p. 100)

Not all travellers want to settle; some prefer to be either permanently or intermittently on the move. The ability to earn a living can be limited, however, if the travellers are always on the move; they need to remain in one place for some period of time in order to earn some money. If travellers do want to settle for a time, they are faced with the difficult task of finding a site.

Sites for travellers vary in status. Some are publicly owned by local authorities while others are privately owned, in some cases by travellers themselves. Facilities differ from site to site; they are partly determined by whether or not they are authorized and whether they are permanent or temporary. Good facilities will include an electricity supply, fresh running water, hot piped water, a bath or shower room, a weekly refuse collection, flush lavatories and public lighting.

Of all the legislation regulating sites for travellers, the Caravan Sites Act (1968) is of key importance. Section 6 states 'it shall be the duty of every local authority (county council or London borough) so far as may be necessary, to provide adequate accommodation for gypsies residing in or resorting to their area'. Gypsies were defined in Section 16 of the Act as 'persons of nomadic habit of life, whatever their race or origin, but does not include members of an organized group of travelling showmen, or of persons engaged in travelling circuses, travelling together as such'.

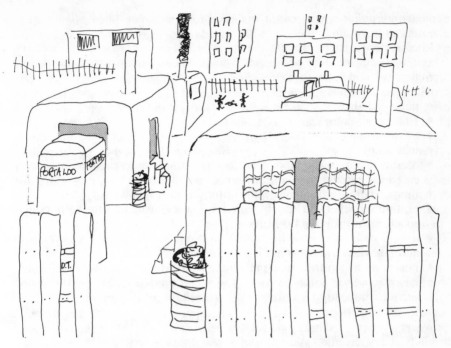

Most urban sites for travellers are far removed from the romanticized, traditional image.

The duty of local authorities to provide sites commenced from 1 April 1970, but since then there have been constant criticisms concerning both the quantity and quality of provision. The key terms in the act that are very much open to interpretation are 'so far as may be necessary' and 'adequate accommodation'. As a result there is a very wide diversity in the application of the act by local authorities. As far as quantity of caravans is concerned, a national count of caravans in 1988 indicated that there was a shortfall in provision of 33 per cent. Some commentators believe this is to be over optimistic. This is despite the fact that from 1978 local authorities received a 100 per cent capital grant for the provision of sites. There is no statutory guidance as far as the quality of provision is concerned and therefore the authorities have a free hand.

If site provision is good to start with, then travellers, as is usual with most residents, tend to take pride in their immediate environment. This in turn leads to travellers taking greater care of the site and its surroundings. It will also tend to have a further 'knock on' effect of facilitating greater integration and better relations with non-travellers in the vicinity. If site provision is not good all these positive aspects will be negated and conflicts and resentments will arise.

The management of sites is also a key factor in their success. Some private sites are run by the travellers who own them, but in the main travellers prefer sites to be managed by an independent authority rather than by travellers. Local authority managers have a variety of titles including 'gypsy site manager', 'warden', 'gypsy liaison officer' or 'travellers officer'. Diplomacy and administrative skills are essential attributes for a manager. She or he needs to consult and maintain a dialogue with the travellers in order to ascertain their needs and viewpoints.

At the end of a study of site provision in five London boroughs, Mavis Hyman concluded that 'more sites should be built rapidly, particularly by non-providing authorities. Eviction and designation (a local authority's power to evict those travellers not on "authorized" sites) could then cease to have any place in the scheme of travellers' lives' (p. 221).

If an eviction takes place, for whatever reason, it lays travellers open to much insecurity and vulnerability. They may be constantly moved on by the police, or be the subject of a number of vehicle or traffic offences. Moving on also creates problems with health and education, as it renders registering with a GP or finding a settled place for children in a school impossible. It may also involve, at times, what will be considered by many travellers to be the intrusive attention of Social Service Departments.

Travellers and social care

The many support groups around the country for travellers provide an invaluable source of advice and assistance. They have the further advantage of not 'stigmatizing' travellers. Contact with a social worker can in itself be a stigmatizing experience for anyone, but especially for a travelling family. However sensitive and informed social workers may be, they are settled house dwellers. They have no experience of a travelling life-style and they may well have subconscious negative feelings towards the quality of life experienced in a caravan on the move. With heightened awareness of 'child abuse' in Britain and occasional attacks of public paranoia about the responsibilities of parents towards children, some of it media-induced, it is little wonder that travellers tend to regard social workers with a certain amount of mistrust. The mothers among travellers are usually well aware of child care powers vested in social workers.

Travellers are a marginalized minority in our society and it is therefore crucial that those of us working in social care do not add to the traveller's sense of isolation. We must accept them and their life-styles on their terms and respect their history, traditions and culture. Wherever possible we should work through an intermediary, such as a support group, who will have a fuller knowledge and understanding of the special needs of travelling people.

5.7 Gays and lesbians

'. . . not only homosexuals, but also many heterosexuals, suffer from the unwillingness of society to allow them to act truthfully, in accordance with their diverse emotions. For such people, this denial of experience diminishes the prospect of a full and satisfying life.'

(The Gay Liberation Front)

Of all the groups mentioned in this book, gay women and men are perhaps the most consistently and blatantly discriminated against. They have a long history of oppression both in this country and throughout the world. The hostility towards homosexual women and men is so entrenched that many gay people do not feel it is safe to reveal their sexual orientation, and they therefore masquerade as heterosexual in public in order to keep their jobs, preserve public office or simply to keep discrimination at bay. As a result of this the true proportion of the population who are gay is not known but it is commonly estimated at between 10 and 20 per cent of the population. In the main homosexuality has been forced to be expressed in secret and it has given it a certain mystique which makes it appear a less common form of sexual orientation than it is, and this reinforces society's prejudice.

'. . . for after all, there are millions of gays in England – and not all dress designers and ballet dancers, but practical people like civil servants, hospital workers and school teachers.'

(Colin MacInnes, *New Society*, 23 October 1975)

One of the chief prejudices faced by gay people is that they are invariably seen solely in terms of their sexuality, for example, a gay social carer is seen first and foremost as being gay. All kinds of assumptions are then made about how this fact will affect her or his ability to perform the care task, and her or his other personal qualities and abilities will recede into the background.

Language

Homosexual is the word used to describe the relationship between people of the same sex. 'Homo' comes from the Greek language and means 'the same', and not from the Latin meaning 'man', and is therefore applicable to both women and men. *Homophobia* describes 'the fear and resulting contempt for homosexuals' expressed by *heterosexuals* (people who are attracted by people of the opposite sex). *Heterosexism* is used, like the words racism and sexism, to describe prejudicial attitudes and actions towards homosexuals. In recent times the term *gay* has been adopted by many homosexual women and men as a positive assertion of their identity and pride and is used instead of the more neutral word homosexual.

Legal discrimination

Until the passing of the Sexual Offences Act 1967, acts of homosexuality between men were illegal in England and Wales. This was later extended to both Northern Ireland and Scotland in 1983 following separate European Court rulings. Before this date engaging in homosexual acts was a crime punishable by imprisonment, even if it took place between consenting adults. Since 1967 homosexuality between men has been legal only in private and between men over the age of 21. (It should be pointed out that 'in private' is defined as a private house – a hotel room, a prison or a hostel are not private in terms of the law.) The age of consent for heterosexual sex in Britain is 16. Sex between consenting females over the age of 16 is only forbidden in the armed forces.

At 21 years, the age of consent for male homosexuality in Britain is the highest in Western Europe. In some countries, in East Germany for example, it is as low as 14 years. Further, the majority of European countries do not distinguish between the age of consent for homosexuality and heterosexuality.

Additional legal restriction on the lives of gay people was introduced under section 28, more popularly known as 'Clause 28', of the Local Government Act (1988). This act states that a local authority shall not 'intentionally promote homosexuality'. According to the National Association of Probation Officers' (NAPO) good practice guidelines produced in May 1980, 'To contravene the Act would require a deliberate attempt to increase the prevalence of homosexuality. No local authority or probation committee could introduce any measure which could change people's sexual orientation' (p. 5). The paper continues, 'Section 28 does not provide any legal basis for discrimination nor does it prohibit or restrict the supply of counselling, advice, support or information services to lesbians and gay men. Nonetheless, section 28 has inflamed prejudice and bigotry and encouraged further discrimination against lesbians and gay men in their family, working, social and personal lives' (ibid).

There is evidence that the application of discriminatory legislation causes a good deal of distress amongst homosexual men. In a letter to the *Guardian* (9 March 1990), Peter Tatchell, a former prospective Labour MP, points out that more gay men are prosecuted in this country than in any nation in Europe and that 'the number of gay men hauled before the courts is greater today than it was before the passage of the 1967 Sexual Offences Act which supposedly legalized male homosexuality'. He adds, 'In England and Wales during 1988, 23 men over the age of 21 were imprisoned for consenting and often loving relationships with other men aged 16 to 21 years'. Adding, that in the year earlier, '41 gay teenagers (sic) aged 16 to 21 years were prosecuted for consensual homosexual acts, with one of the youths being sentenced to 12 months custody'.

Much has been written about the possible 'causes' of homosexuality although the same question is rarely asked of heterosexuality. Heterosexuality is assumed to be the norm from which all other forms of sexuality deviate. Homosexuality is sometimes considered to be biologically determined but society has always considered it to be a sickness and has tried to treat it as such. However it is less common nowadays for psychiatrists and others to try to counsel gay people out of their orientation. Others take the view that homosexuality is culturally determined; that it is acquired through social influence, and society's solution this time is to try and limit the influence of gay culture or to apply behaviour modification techniques in order to enable a gay person to 'unlearn' her or his sexual orientation. Finally, gayness is seen as a choice made by individuals, and in this case society expects gay people to accept the consequences and tolerate society's antagonism. There has been no satisfactory explanation of why people are gay and in a sense the question is irrelevant, because it is merely one form of sexual orientation.

Gay people, and men in particular, have been strongly associated in the public eye with various forms of anti-social behaviour. Stereotyped views abound and are reinforced by the media which considers gay men and women as an easy target. For example, in May 1990, Garry Bushell of the Sun newspaper was reprimanded by the Press Council for using language offensive to gay people. In a retort printed in the same newspaper, he left out specifically offensive words but continued to employ invective and innuendo throughout his article. He stated that: 'homosexuals traditionally wanted society to leave them alone, but it didn't end there. When they achieved that, they demanded society's approval. They even demanded subsidies from the rates and got them. Now they want homosexuality to be thought of as being just as healthy as heterosexuality. They want our children to be taught that their perversion is normal.' He went on to state: 'The mass of people have no great sympathy or understanding for homosexuals. They accept that they exist and should be left alone. But most of all they want the homosexuals to leave them alone. Especially their children' (*Sun*, 18 May 1990).

Popular journalism, in particular articles of this nature, not only helps to create prejudicial attitudes, it feeds on and influences the homophobia already present in the readership. The idea, ambiguously alluded to in the last line of the article (that gay men will sexually exploit children) is a popular myth totally unsupported by any evidence. In fact it is acknowledged that the majority of child abuse and child sex abuse is perpetrated by heterosexual men. Gay men have been similarly negatively presented by the press on other social issues, notably the spread of the human immunodeficiency virus (HIV). As the epidemic nature of the disease became apparent in the mid 1980s, the popular press were quick to blame the gay community for its cause and spread, although the origin of the virus was not known and is yet to be scientifically established. Gay men were portrayed as being morally inferior, promiscuous and a threat to heterosexuals. It later became clear that HIV was both heterosexually and homosexually transmitted and that everyone, regardless of their sexual orientation, was at risk. Even so this fact is not popularly acknowledged and gay people continue to be over identified with the disease.

Marginalization

Discrimination against gay people takes many forms and is perpetuated both by individuals and institutions. On an individual level, gay people are subjected to a personal abuse ranging from the use of insulting and derogatory language and mimicry, to actual physical abuse and even murder. According to Outrage, a group formed in 1990 in response to the increased number of attacks on gay people, 32 gay men were murdered between 1986 and 1990 (*Guardian*, 11 August 1990). Outrage have called on the police to monitor attacks on gay men and lesbians in the same way that racially motivated crimes are recorded. The intolerance and hostility which surround gay people contributes to their isolation. This is particularly true for gay teenagers who because of their sexual orientation have additional anxieties over and above their heterosexual counterparts.

At the institutional level, gay people are discriminated against in the job market. Only within the organizations which operate an Equal Opportunities policy can gay people feel free to 'come out' and declare their sexual orientation. In other organizations gay people may run the risk of being dismissed if their sexual orientation becomes known. 'Clause 28' has helped create an environment in which local authority personnel, including teachers and social carers, are less likely to 'come out' than they were previously. For example, a woman nursery worker was dismissed because she was gay. Her appeal against unfair dismissal was disregarded on the grounds that the children's parents threatened to withdraw their children if she continued to work at the nursery. Thus public prejudice was upheld in this case. In actual fact gay people have no specific employment protection rights.

The phrase 'coming out' is used to describe the process by which homo-sexuals figuratively 'come out of the closet' and openly declare their sexual orientation and confront society's prejudice. 'Being out does not mean becoming flamboyant, funny, extra caring or changing one's personality. It means being positive about being gay; it means telling people; stopping people (generally men) from telling anti-gay jokes, and generally trying to educate people about what being gay means (*Community Care Supplement*, 25 June 1987).

This description of 'coming out' was made by an 'out' gay man working in a relatively safe environment. For other gay people 'coming out' can mean revealing one's sexual orientation to a few close friends only. There are therefore varying degrees of self-disclosure. The term 'outing' is used to describe a recent practice carried out in America, where gay groups deliberately expose a prominent person's hitherto undeclared gayness. This is done in order to lend credence to the homosexual community and to help break down the prevailing stereotypes. It is argued that the more gay men and women there are who come 'out' the more usual homosexuality will seem and as a result there will be more positive role models for young gays to identify with.

The Christian church continues to be unsympathetic towards gay men and women. It refuses to sanction 'marital' partnerships between members of the same sex and continues to outlaw homosexuality amongst the clergy. Elsewhere gay women and men in prominent social positions, for example within the judiciary or the civil service, are still susceptible to threats of blackmail and can be dismissed if their sexual orientation is exposed. Of course while homosexuality is considered abnormal, the vulnerability to blackmail will not recede.

The bestowal of a knighthood on Sir Ian McKellen (in 1991) marked an important breakthrough for gay people. He was the first 'out' gay person to have been granted such an honour. However, his acceptance of the knighthood was greeted with hostility among some gay people. Many were astounded that Sir Ian could accept an honour from a Government that had introduced anti-gay legislation, such as 'clause 28', and had contributed generally to the marginalization of gay people in society. Others supported and applauded Sir Ian's nomination and acceptance of his knighthood feeling that it was a step towards society's fuller acceptance of gay people and underlined the irrelevance of a person's sexual orientation when judging her or his talent.

Resistance

In June 1969 outside the Stonewall Inn in New York, a group of gay people finally retaliated against the abuse and victimization to which they had been subjected and made a stand against police intimidation. The action taken by lesbians and gay men led initially to a riot. It also marked the beginning of the Gay Liberation movement in America which has done much to improve the social standing of homosexuals in that country. Its influence has been felt in this country and the gay movement is now established. There are several gay organizations, clubs, magazines and newspapers. Some newsagents, however, continue to refuse to stock gay magazines including *Gay News*, which merely includes listings of events, news features, and other articles. The simple fact that standard gay periodicals are often not available locally to gay people serves

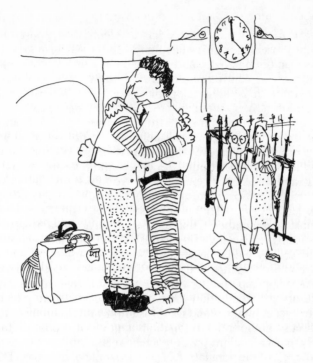

It is still considered unacceptable by many people for gay men to express their feelings openly.

further to marginalize them and in a small way contributes to the insecurity and low self-esteem experienced by young gay people in particular.

Social care

There is plenty of evidence of Social Service Departments discriminating against homosexuals. In particular, lesbian mothers have been considered unsuitable to look after children. For example, a contributor to a recent Women in Mind publication (1990), stated 'Losing custody of my child was the most devastating experience of my life so far. The Welfare Officer who made a report on us for the court, told me that my daughter was one of the sanest children he had ever met – which he said must be due to the way I had brought her up – yet he still recommended that she would be better off in a "normal family"' (p. 52). She added, 'He also said how tragic it was that the pain and stress of custody cases drives mothers to nervous breakdowns, so that the court is unable to give them custody even when it wants to.'

In some cases the children have been removed on the grounds of being in 'moral danger'. Similarly gay teenagers have been made the subject of care orders because of their sexuality. However, there is much more awareness about the needs of gay people today and some local authorities have developed sympathetic practices. Much of this progress is a result of pioneering work undertaken by community and voluntary organizations.

Help available

Nearly every town in the country has a telephone support system or gay helpline and most major cities have gay centres where people, particularly young gays, can obtain advice and support. Only one centre outside London, the Manchester gay centre, employs full time workers. The Manchester gay centre also offers a 24 hour telephone support service which is staffed by trained counsellors. Very often they receive 'silent' phone calls. These calls are thought to be either from 'cranks' or from genuinely troubled people who have plucked up enough courage to seek help but are not yet ready to be explicit about their problem. Whatever the circumstances a silent caller is respected. The counsellor will speak through the silence and reassure the caller that there is no hurry, and that she or he does not have to say anything. The counsellor may provide information about the centre and will give her or his name to the caller in order that the caller can request them should the caller want to ring again. It must be remembered that gay people have the same kind of problems as heterosexuals, especially teenagers, but their difficulties are often compounded by society's antagonism and the lack of appropriate help available.

A prime aim of the centre is to ensure that young people are able to join and meet with a peer group of other young gays. It is recognized that many young, gay people are isolated within their own immediate family or among their heterosexual acquaintances and that it is important that they have the opportunity to discuss, argue and develop their identity with people of their own age.

It is likely that a higher proportion of teenagers who are gay are received into care than the rest of the population of young people of their age. This is because in addition to other problems, so many have difficulties concerning their sexual orientation and disclosing it to those to whom they are close. Many parents react or are expected to react negatively to their daughter or son's disclosure in line with society in general. Consequently young people who grow up with the knowledge that they are gay may break away from the family at an early age and be more vulnerable to reception into care. The lack of a secure and accepting environment, isolation and or homelessness can also increase the likelihood that they become involved in crime.

It would be true to say that social care, whether provided by field social carers, hospital social workers, probation officers or residential workers, has done very little so far to eliminate the discrimination levelled at gay and lesbian members of our society. Only in recent years has significant attention been granted to their needs. Some local authority Social Services Departments are aware that lesbians and gay men have been denied social justice and have been marginalized by their policies. For example, the rights of gay people to adopt or foster children have now been acknowledged. It is especially realized that teenagers need positive role models and so young gays are now fostered with gay women or gay men.

What social carers can do

Sexuality is still very much a taboo issue within social care. Only recently, for example, has anything been done to acknowledge the sexual rights of all clients in residential settings. In some establishments attempts are being made to enable clients to express their sexuality in the same way as the rest of the population. This positive acceptance needs to apply to gay people also, so that they too can live full social and emotional lives. Peter Berry, a gay social worker, talks of how he regards his sexuality as a kind of 'hidden handicap'. He says, 'My biggest headache has been what is commonly called the corruption theory. This is that children should only have heterosexual models for fear that a gay social worker's homosexuality will unduly influence the child, especially as social workers are seen as models of acceptable behaviour and that a positive, adult homosexual model would be wrong. (*Community Care*, 25 June 1987). He feels that this stems from the popular misconception that gay men are more sexually attracted to children than their heterosexual counterparts. It is not only working with children that has its problems for gay men. Any client group in any social care setting 'where the client is deemed to be susceptible to undue influence is subject to particular scrutiny'. Peter Berry points out that 'gay social workers are no more likely to take advantage of clients than any other worker; rather, perhaps the opposite is true. We are aware that if we put a foot wrong, the system will come down on our heads with the weight of the public behind it.' (ibid.).

It is likely that many heterosexual social carers will not even consider the possibility of their client being gay since within their lives they have not come across any one who is openly gay. To act in this way is to flaunt basic social care principles and thus deny the client an integral part of themselves. It is not only important that young, gay clients have their sexual orientation acknowledged and accepted, but the same is true for adult clients. According to the London Charter for Gay and Lesbian Rights (1985) there are at least 50,000 elderly lesbians and gay men estimated to be living in London. The Charter points out that many of these elders 'are isolated, have kept their sexual orientation a secret or they may have been subjected to abuse from neighbours where it is known they are gay'. It is possible that the absence of children may add to an elder's feelings of isolation.

Social carers who are not gay themselves need to learn about lesbian and gay issues, their lifestyles and politics and to have a knowledge of the basic resources available. They need to become involved in creating or supporting others in creating initiatives which will make the social care service more appropriate to the needs of gay people. They need also to address all forms of discrimination, open or covert, personal or institutional, casual or entrenched. Finally, support should be given to colleagues and every effort should be made to create a safe environment in which both client and carer can reveal their sexual identity. Care should be taken not to burden one member of the team as the unpaid expert and sole spokesperson for gay issues. This is our joint responsibility. For as Colin MacInnes has pointed out, 'Sexual freedom, like social and racial freedom, is indivisible; by which I mean that heterosexuals can never be entirely free so long as homosexuals are not' (*New Society*, 23 October 1975, p. 224).

5.8 People with mental illness

What is meant by the term 'mental illness'?

It is very difficult to provide an exact definition of 'mental illness' because human behaviour varies so much from culture to culture; much depends on the dominant ethos of each individual society and the social setting in which so called 'normal' behaviour takes place. When it takes place must also be taken into consideration because perceptions and values change with time. Much too depends on the individual's natural personality. We all have certain characteristics in common, but we also possess characteristics that make us different from each other; indeed these are the very characteristics that make us 'individuals'. Just as an example, let us take a common physical characteristic; no two people have identical fingerprints. And so it is with the 'print' of our mental make up; no two people are exactly alike.

For exactly the same reasons outlined above it would be even more hazardous to even attempt to define 'normal behaviour'. It would be more useful, in attempting to understand the complex subject of mental illness, to provide some behavioural patterns that our society perceives to indicate mental illness.

We might say that someone is suffering from mental illness when a person's usual coping mechanism, for example with stress or anxiety, fails to be effective and consequently their day to day functioning suffers as a result; their behaviour is thought to be dangerous to her or his well-being, or that of others; their thoughts or emotions are clearly out of control; they are unable to maintain relationships with others because of severe emotional stress; they lose the ability to communicate effectively, or their behaviour is incongruous or inappropriate in, or to, their situation.

These behaviour patterns are not mutually exclusive; a person may exhibit several of them simultaneously. Any diagnosis of mental illness will be a process based on comparing an individual's usual, or normal, behaviour pattern with exhibited behaviour that is untypical. Thus there can be no absolute definitions of 'mental health' or 'mental illness' as such.

In short, one may say that a person who is mentally ill will manifest behavioural patterns that often differ in *degree* from that which is considered normal, rather than in *kind*. A mentally ill person tends to display an exaggeration of thoughts and/or feelings we *all* have, rather than different kinds of thoughts or feelings.

An illustration of this might be *depression* – we all feel 'down' from time to time or have bad moods. We may even say that we are 'depressed'. We are able, however, to continue to get on with our daily lives; in fact doing so may cause the feeling to pass. Depression as a serious mental illness (it is sometimes referred to as 'clinical' depression) will, on the other hand, profoundly interfere with our daily functioning to the point where someone may even contemplate or attempt suicide. The depression may totally dominate a person for a time, and throw her or his life 'out of balance'. It may prevent the person from taking effective care of herself or himself or from fulfilling her or his responsibilities towards others.

Mental 'illness' should not be confused with mental 'handicap' or 'learning difficulties' as it is now known. The first is usually not a permanent condition; it may be experienced over a very short period of time. A 'learning difficulty' is technically speaking 'permanent', but people born with the condition may be helped to cope effectively in spite of their handicap. Someone who has learning difficulties may also suffer from mental illness. Mental illness is more common than mental handicap. One person in every 100 is born mentally handicapped, whereas as many as one person in six will be affected by mental illness at some time in their lives.

A large number of medical, or psychiatric terms are used by doctors and psychiatrists to define specific types of mental illness. However, there is much professional disagreement regarding the use of such terms and the conditions which they describe. As social carers we should certainly treat these medical appellations with caution, question their relevance, and find out as much as we can about the meanings of such terms. Further complications exist concerning the diagnostic terms used by psychiatrists because certain mental illnesses have the same, or similar, symptoms and people may suffer from more than one mental illness at a time.

What are the causes of mental illness?

Explanations as to what causes mental illness have changed a great deal over the past century. In the nineteenth century, it was still believed that 'lunatics', as they were then called, were governed in their behaviour by the changing phases of the moon. Earlier, even more primitive views held sway. Some people suffering from mental illness were believed to be possessed by 'evil spirits'. Women in particular were from time to time burnt as 'witches'. Generally speaking people were labelled 'mad' or 'insane' simply because they were 'bad' or because it was believed they had been cursed.

Today we take a more enlightened approach but we are still a long way from fully understanding what causes mental illness and several theories exist. It has been agreed that in almost every case a number of varied causes work together to produce the illness. Some are intrinsic, others are external to the individual – in their family, their immediate environment or in wider society.

Our physical and mental health are closely intertwined, and therefore have a close effect on one another. For example a long physical illness can cause depression and a young person, worried about her or his weight and physical shape, may suffer from anorexia nervosa or other 'eating disorders'. Mental disturbance is also often manifested in physical symptoms – tension, increased heart-rate, sweating, dizziness and migraine.

A great debate has taken place about the contribution *biochemistry* makes to the cause of mental illness. Some researchers believe that it does cause some serious mental illness, which might be defined as 'schizophrenia'. Post-natal depression is another example where chemical changes in the body can have wider mental and emotional effects.

It is not thought that *heredity* plays a clear or definite part in causation but it is agreed that certain distorted family environments can have an adverse effect on those who grow up in them. The children of such families may suffer mental anxiety, confusion or disturbance as a result of poor parenting or destructive unharmonious relationships. Such distorted family patterns may be passed on and thus occur repeatedly through a number of generations. A poor physical and emotional environment in the early years may lead to a later predisposition towards mental illness.

Lifestyle and environment play very large parts in determining mental health. Both can create stress within individuals irrespective of their socio-economic positions. We live in an increasingly competitive and materialistic society in which the pace of life for many is accelerating. As a result people are subject to an ever increasing amount of stress and this is having a significant effect on the incidence of mental illness.

How many people experience mental illness?

Mental illness is far more common that is generally appreciated. As stated earlier, one person in six in Britain will be affected by mental illness at some time in their lives. The most common conditions – anxiety and depression, cause four million to five million people each year to consult their GP. About 30 million prescriptions for psychotropic (mind altering) drugs are written, on average, each year by doctors in England alone (*Guardian*, 14 March 1990).

As regards state provision, almost one pound in every ten spent by the NHS is allotted to mental health care. At any one time there are over 50 000 people in psychiatric hospital beds in England and this represent about 20 per cent of all NHS occupied beds. There are approximately 8000 psychiatric beds in Scotland. In addition there are almost 2 million psychiatric out-patient attendances each year in Britain.

As a result of recent community care policies and the closure of several large, Victorian-built, mental hospitals, fewer mentally ill patients are hospitalized today. At the beginning of this century, there were nearly 100 000 patients in asylums. The peak was reached in 1954, when the number of beds taken by psychiatric patients was 148 000, since when it has steadily declined (*British Medical Journal*, 21 April 1990).

Marginalization and mental illness

We may think we have come a long way since mental illness was thought to be devil possession or the work of evil spirits or the moon, but plenty of negative attitudes remain and are manifested in several different ways. In the eighteenth century, socially stigmatized asylums were sometimes visited by members of so called 'respectable society' as a form of entertainment. We have advanced but little; the social stigma attached to mental illness still exists although it tends to take more subtle or hidden forms today.

Although much mental illness is temporary, people who experience it are often regarded as if they never fully recover. Those around them may, as a result, become wary believing that the illness may return at any time. This will result in their not treating the person who has experienced a mental illness in an open and honest way.

Sadly, in our early years and throughout our school life we tend to pick up prejudicial attitudes towards mental illness. Words such as 'nutter', 'loony' and 'bonkers' are common terms of abuse used by children. However, these derogatory terms are also used in adult life and tabloid newspapers frequently feature such negative colloquial expressions in large headlines. The media generally sensationalizes a mental health issue; it will usually be a 'bad news' story and it is quite likely to have a 'criminal content'.

Horror films such as *Psycho* and *Dr Jekyll and Mr Hyde* help to fan prejudicial fears because they depict mentally ill characters who turn into dangerous monsters. In this way people's fears, suspicions and prejudices are inflamed while more enlightened and realistic attitudes are stifled.

Social stigma and prejudice can take serious practical forms. If someone who has had a mental illness applies for a job and truthfully fills in the section of an application form headed 'Any history of mental illness?' some employers may reject them for interview, especially in times of high unemployment when employers will have plenty of other applicants to choose from. Social stigma and prejudice can therefore negatively affect a person's job or career prospects and correspondingly her or his material quality of life.

The common response to a proposal for a hostel or group home for ex-psychiatric patients is 'anywhere but here'; this patently reflects social prejudice and stigma. Early in 1990, Bath Health Authority planned to house eight former residents of a psychiatric hospital on a private estate. The developers objected. Their objection, according to the comment column of the magazine *Community Care*, stemmed from 'a belief that mentally ill residents on an estate will lower property prices or diminish the supposed desirability of the estate. Thus those with a mental illness are not one of us, not citizens, but persons of secondary importance, with fewer rights about where they can live than others. It is a grubby little bit of home-grown apartheid' (3 May 1990).

Unequal treatment

Treatment for mental illness covers a wide range and includes 'talking treatments', either on an individual or group basis; drug therapy; a move into a therapeutic community; art, music or drama therapy; electro-convulsive therapy (ECT) and in rare cases, psychosurgery. Treatment will often consist of a combination of these. Fierce debates take place from time to time as to the efficiency or even the morality of different treatments especially ECT and brain surgery. Our knowledge of some treatments and how they work is still relatively primitive. Little is known, for example, about the longer term side effects of certain drugs, or how ECT actually works, and whether or not it has long-term damaging effects.

The incidence, diagnosis and treatment of mental illness varies a great deal depending on our position in society. They are affected by our class position, by our gender and by our race or colour. The social or environmental factors which lead to stress in people's lives tend to be more destructive at the lower end of the class system. Poverty, deprivation, unemployment, poor housing and impoverished local amenities are experienced more by the working class, and in recent years, amongst members of the emerging 'underclass'.

Inadequate material provision leads to a lack of power and control as well as a lack of choice. For example, council house tenants cannot usually choose *where* they live, they have to take what is offered.

Women in the working class or 'underclass' are particularly badly affected by stress. They make up the majority of single parents and bear the brunt of most child care responsibilities. They therefore are less able to take full time, well paid jobs than men and as a result they are more likely to experience poverty. Not surprisingly, women particularly working class women, experience a higher rate of anxiety and depression than men.

A research study in Camberwell, London, into depression in women (Brown *et al.*, 1975), discovered that 25 per cent of working class women living in the community, suffering from depression, were not receiving any psychiatric treatment. This compared to only 5 per cent of middle class women. The study defined various 'vulnerability factors', including loss of mother in childhood, having three or more children under 14 years living at home, and the absence of a close confiding relationship. All of these were found to be class related; they were experienced more by working class women.

In the same research, long-term mental illness amongst working class women had as its main causes, poor housing conditions, poverty, child care responsibilities and poor relationships in marriage, including violence and sexual abuse. Irene Starr came to a pessimistic conclusion after considering such research studies – 'for women, the alternative to chronic depression in an unhappy marriage is often poverty, a dead end job and the additional stress of child care responsibilities' (*Social Work Today*, 26 August 1985).

Working class people and poorer women cannot afford to buy psychiatric treatment privately. They are therefore dependent upon NHS services. This means, for example, that they cannot usually benefit from 'talking treatments' such as psychotherapy or psychoanalysis. They are far more likely to receive drugs as treatment, which may only affect the symptoms and not the cause of a psychiatric problem. The patient, therefore, will not gain the benefit of obtaining more insight or understanding of her or his condition.

Women also suffer from the gender stereotypes held by the men who make up the majority of doctors and psychiatrists. This is likely to result in more women receiving drug prescriptions than men and more being hospitalized for mental illness than men. A commonly held male prejudice is that women are less able to cope, less independent, more emotional and more obsessive about their emotions.

In recent years there has been a growing concern about the relationship between race and mental illness in this country. It has become increasingly clear that black people are not getting fair treatment for a variety of reasons. Much of this is thought to stem from cultural ignorance on the part of doctors and psychiatrists who, as a result of this lack of understanding, misread 'normal' behaviour and erroneously diagnose ordinary distressed people as mentally ill or sick. British psychiatric practice in general is culturally limited, it is too ethnocentric. Consequently some mistaken decisions are inevitable.

Particular fears have arisen about the diagnoses of 'schizophrenia', a serious psychotic illness. Approximately one person in every 100 suffers from one of the types of schizophrenia at some time in their lives. In Britain, Afro-Caribbeans are three times more likely to be diagnosed as schizophrenic than white people. Until a satisfactory psychiatric explanation for this discrepancy is provided, it is difficult to avoid the conclusion that racism is a principle factor.

Black people are also disadvantaged in general terms when we consider mental illness. Research has discovered that black people are more likely to be given major tranquilizers (e.g. Largactil and Stelazine), than white people; are more likely to see junior or unqualified psychiatrists; are more likely to be hospitalized than treated in the community or as an out-patient; are twice as likely to be the subject of a Mental Health Act 'Section' and so be held in a hospital involuntarily; are more likely to be sent from a prison on to a mental hospital and are more likely to be treated with ECT and to be given more 'shocks'.

Community care

In Britain the state began to get involved in the 'care' of the mentally ill with the 1808 County Asylum Act. This provided for the 'care and maintenance of lunatics' and gradually asylums were built throughout the country. They were usually very large, prison-like buildings, both in their external appearance and in their internal planning and organization. Their structures were so daunting and de-humanizing that Henry Maudsley said of them in 1871 – 'one effect of asylums is to make some permanent lunatics'.

The 1930 Mental Treatment Act replaced the term 'lunatic asylum' with 'mental hospital'. Gradually conditions in them improved, but as Andrew Scull (1984) said they were 'still a convenient way of getting rid of inconvenient people' (p. 128). Incarceration in a mental hospital, even if helpful in treating the illness, meant a break in usual social life, loss of family, home and employment, sometimes permanently, and being condemned to face social stigma upon returning to the community. Around the middle of this century, many argued that much mental illness was produced in society by social factors, and therefore it should be dealt with within the community rather than by shutting people away in an unreal environment where they may well experience a decline in their capabilities.

The programme to close the large Victorian mental hospitals began in the 1950s. It was assisted by the discovery of a number of psychotropic drugs, which could control people's behaviour without the need for physical restraint or confinement. This allowed them to remain in or be released into the community.

However, not all mentally ill people are able to live in the community – some are too disturbed or vulnerable, or even in a few cases dangerous. Total decarceration in any case is not desirable. The original meaning of the word 'asylum' was a 'place apart' a place of safety or refuge where someone can have time and space to recover (in this sense it is still used in terms of 'political asylum'). Some people experiencing mental illness will actually choose to have such a resource away from the stresses of the outside world.

Having said this, however, in medical and social care terms 'community care' will be most beneficial for most people if it allows them to live as full and 'normal' life as possible. Where this has been implemented, self-determination has been encouraged by giving clients more power and control over their own lives; self-advocacy projects have grown in number; independent living programmes and group homes have been established, and some Health Authorities and Social Services Departments have initiated 'Crisis Intervention Teams' in order to contain psychiatric problems within the community and without needing to resort to hospitalization. Such teams, based on good co-operative working practice, have seen psychiatrists, psychologists, community nurses, occupational therapists and social workers working more closely together.

Thus, artificial boundaries between different care disciplines may be broken down. Future developments may include the actual amalgamation of some areas of work: a prime example would be community psychiatric nursing and mental health social work. The aim of such closer co-operation must be that of dealing with mental illness in a more holistic and appropriate way, and not in separating medical from social problems. Accordingly, community care for the mentally ill has been defined by one writer, Chris Heginbotham, as 'a humanizing trend to reintegrate people into the community or enhance their already existing social networks' (*Social Work Today*, 1 November 1983, p. 8).

All is far from satisfactory with community care for the mentally ill however. One major criticism is that policy changes are still not matched by the financial resources. Some people seem to believe that the new policy approach was merely a cost-cutting exercise, resulting in a reduction in services, rather than a change in the pattern of service provision. Dr Jim Birley, President of the Royal College of Psychiatrists, points out that the amount of money for mental health has not increased in real terms since 1974. Between 80 to 90 per cent of this is still spent on hospital provision. He adds that 'provision in the community has to be on a large scale, and if it's not provided, the mental hospitals will have to stay open' (*Guardian*, 14 March 1990, p. 31).

Another major criticism is that hospital closures or bed reductions have taken place too quickly and in an unmonitored way. Trish Groves, writing in the *British Medical Journal* says 'Nearly 100,000 long stay patients have been discharged from Britain's mental hospitals in the past 35 years and fewer than 4000 places have been provided in local authority hostels' (21 April 1990, p. 1060). As to the discrepancy in numbers, she says 'the Department of Health does not know what has happened to that invisible cohort'. Many may have returned to families with inadequate support. The mother of a schizophrenic patient is quoted as saying, 'He was discharged into a community care system that turned out to be me' (*The Times*, 12 July 1989).

There is evidence that a growing number of mentally ill people, some of them discharged from hospitals, are destitute, homeless and 'getting by' on the streets. Many more appear to be in prison, in surroundings quite unsuitable and, in fact, actually damaging to them. Pressure has therefore grown to slow down hospital closures; the Government announced it was doing so at the end of 1989.

Some commentators do not believe that the real problem is closure of the hospitals, but one of a lack of general social provision. Dr Jim Birley is one who resents political pressure 'for the mental hospitals to stay open to keep the streets clean' (*Guardian*, 14 March 1990). Nicki Pope, writing in *The Guardian*, expands on the same theme: 'until society is able to help with their social

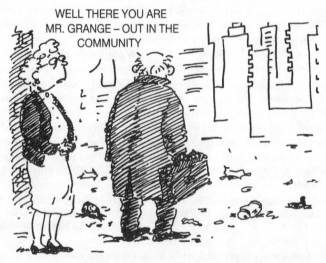

WELL THERE YOU ARE
MR. GRANGE – OUT IN THE
COMMUNITY

(Reproduced from *Care Weekly*, 31 May 1990 with the permission of Sophie Grillet.)

needs properly, psychiatric patients living in the community will be clamouring to get into hospital. It is better than being cold and hungry' (30 November 1988, p. 29).

5.9 People with physical disabilities

One of the most significant features of disablement is its diversity: it may affect a person's mobility to the extent that she or he may need a wheelchair in order to move around; it may be a sensory impairment of sight, hearing or speech; or it may be that a person suffers from either a subtle or complex neurological disorder as a result of a stroke, spinal cord injury or epilepsy. Not all disabilities are obvious; many will go unnoticed. The cause of disablement also varies a great deal. A condition may be inherited or it may be congenital (the disabled person is born with it, but it is not inherited). Accident, illness or disease may also cause a disability, and these can happen at any time in life. Ageing itself is a process that often brings with it disabled functioning as people slow down and experience a weakening of their powers.

Disability is spread fairly evenly in terms of class, gender and race, and it spans all ages. Not only do people with disabilities have to cope with the impairment itself, they also have to deal with able-bodied peoples' reactions to their condition. These can, of course, at best be helpful, sensitive and mature. At worst, they can be patronizing or prying; the latter often motivated by voyeuristic curiosity.

Some people object to the term 'able-bodied' because it is a myth which implies that all people are either able-bodied or disabled. In fact, human physical conditions comprise a wide continuum of differing abilities, so that a young person, for example, with a limp as a result of contracting poliomyelitis in her or his childhood, may be fitter and have a fuller range of mobility than an elderly person who is not classified as disabled.

Able-bodied people can be insensitive if they themselves are embarrassed: they may avoid the gaze of a person with a visible handicap, or talk over somebody in a wheelchair. The long running Radio 4 magazine programme for disabled people, *Does He Take Sugar?*, is so named because of this phenomenon. It may be that it is because people in wheelchairs occupy a distance above the ground roughly equivalent to the height of young children, they are treated thus. This is, of course, no excuse. Adults who wish to relate to young children squat on their haunches to do so, or sit down on the lowest chair. There also exists the fallacious correlation in peoples' minds between physical disability and mental impairment. Whatever the rationale, the effect of being by-passed or ignored is demoralizing and hurtful. Christy Brown, a writer who had cerebral palsy, describes his feelings on receiving 'looks of pity':

'They went right through me, those looks from people in the streets. My brothers didn't think I took any notice, but I did.'

(Brown, C., *My Left Foot*, p. 52)

Social stereotypes of people with disabilities are also unhelpful and dehumanizing. One of their characteristics is that they are usually extreme. Michael Oliver, himself disabled, refers to the stereotypes of disabled people as 'super-cripples' or 'pathetic victims'. Oliver (1990) has highlighted the existence of two major approaches to disability. He terms these, the *individual* and the *social* models of disability.

The older, traditional model is the 'individual' one. In his words, this 'sees the problems that disabled people experience as being a direct consequence of their disability'. Thus the onus is placed on the disabled person; she or he has to adapt to society, to make the best of a situation and to accept the imposed limitations it brings.

More recently, there has been an increasing acceptance of the 'social' model, in which, again in Oliver's words: 'adjustment . . . is a problem for society, not for disabled individuals' (p. 23). Here, the onus is on society to adapt to the needs of the disabled person and to cater for these needs as much as possible. This model promotes a view of disabled people as struggling positively, often in the face of society's non-co-operation, to overcome and surmount the limitations of their condition.

> 'In the cookery class 14 year-old Angie was putting the finishing touches to a salad. "You would have made someone a good wife," the teacher told her. "What do you mean – I would have?" the girl asked. "What I meant to say was that if you marry a disabled man, you would make him a good wife," the teacher explained carefully.'
> (Angie, who has cerebral palsy, in *Community Care*, 1 October 1984, p. 14)

How many disabled people are there?

A report from the Office of Population Consensus and Surveys (OPCS 1988b) surprised many people, including the Government, when it disclosed that one in ten people are disabled, either physically or with learning difficulties. This is approximately six million – over two thirds of the total (4.3 million) are over the age of 60.

Soon after the OPCS report, the Disability Alliance, which represents more than one hundred voluntary organizations, published its own material on the deprivation suffered by a large number of disabled people. It reported that some two thirds of disabled people (4 million people) were living at or below the poverty line. The report also stated that those people of working age are twice as likely to be living on or below the poverty line, than are their able-bodied counterparts. Thus, the hardship faced by most disabled people is two-fold: those practical difficulties which result from their physical conditions, and in addition, the related material hardship and deprivation (Disability Alliance, 1988).

The overwhelming dependence of people with disabilities upon state benefits, and the difficulties so many of them have in finding paid work, often leads to severe financial hardship. This is compounded by the expense associated with being disabled, e.g. aids to physical mobility, household adaptations, and special medical treatments and diets. Although there is some state support to meet such costs, they rarely cover them in full. Consider, for example, the cost of a new lightweight wheelchair for a teenager is between £400 to over £1000. Disabled people's experience of poverty leads to an over-representation of disabled people in the 'underclass'.

Mobility and access

Our society has come a long way in its treatment of people with disabilities. No longer are they treated as 'curiosities', or simply shut away in residential institutions, but there is still much further to go. The general public's awareness of the needs of people with disabilities has to be raised, and services need to be far more extensive. The concept of '*normalization*', which attempts to enable disabled people to live as 'normal' and as enriched a life as possible, has replaced the *institutionalization* of people with disabilities, and finds its practical expression in community care.

> 'A person can just as easily be handicapped by the lack of a lift as by the lack of a limb.'
>
> (*Guardian* 30 March 1990)

One of the chief obstacles to facilitating the ordinary community involvement of physically disabled people is that of 'access'. To many disabled people kerbs represent an effective barrier to everyday mobility. Although all new shops and offices must now be fully accessible, other buildings open to the public need only be accessible on the entrance floor. These may include cinemas, theatres, sports and leisure complexes. Many professional football grounds do not cater for visiting disabled supporters. Ninety five per cent of cashpoint machines are said to be inaccessible at the present time. In London, our largest city, only 38 per cent of museums and 20 per cent of cinemas are currently adapted for wheelchair use (*Guardian*, 2 September 1989). Almost all insist that a user has an 'able-bodied' companion with them.

> 'It's part of our culture that architects and developers are trained to build for an elite which is male, fit, and aged 18–45 . . . The further you are from the stereotype, the more difficulties you have.'
>
> (John Penton, architect, quoted in *Guardian* 2 September 1989)

Some transport systems such as the Tyne and Wear Metro in the north east of England and the Docklands Light Railway in London are fully accessible, but the majority, including the Glasgow and London underground systems, can present great difficulties. Taxis are mostly non-adapted, although the situation is improving, while buses remain largely inaccessible. To a large extent, disabled peoples' frustrations with regard to mobility and access is shared by parents with young children. Everyday activities such as shopping, recreation and travel are all made more difficult by high kerbs, heavy doors and the proliferation of steps and stairs.

Access is more than just a question of physical barriers. People with disabilities have long protested about their fundamental exclusion from many spheres of everyday life. Although there is more social awareness of the needs of disabled people, and a certain amount of real progress is being made in order to enable their fuller integration, disabled people are still marginalized and many feel angry.

In broadening the definition of 'access', Rachel Hurst, from the British Council of Organizations of Disabled People, highlighted the range of discrimination levelled at disabled people. Speaking at the 'Get Your Act Together' Conference on Disabled Persons (1986) she said,

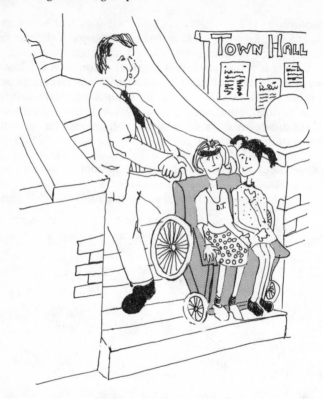

Not all public buildings are as yet accessible to all people

> 'The fact is that we don't have access to education as disabled children, the full education of able-bodied children. We don't have access to housing. We don't have access to employment. We don't have access to public facilities. We are not in fact members of the public – we don't have access to proper living standards and we don't have access to influence.'

Disability and sex

Much taboo and embarrassment exists around the issue of disability and sex, once again most of the embarrassment being felt by able-bodied people. In the book *Images of Ourselves*, Angie, who has cerebral palsy, recounts an interaction with a 'gas man' who found her alone at home: 'As he was leaving the flat he turned and asked if I was married. I told him I was. Then a funny look came into his eyes and he asked if I had sex. I was shocked at his question, and at first was stuck for words. Then I was angry and said the first thing that came into my head – 'Yes, do you?' He looked embarrassed and hurried away' (p. 14). The gas man clearly would not have thought of asking an 'able-bodied' woman the same question!

In a similar way the issue is seldom raised with regard to people with learning difficulties. Many who are not disabled in any way like to ignore the whole question of sex and sexuality, largely to quell their own feelings of awkwardness. As Michele Cheaney writes: 'Many social workers and parents deny that disabled people have sexual feelings and see no reason to promote such an idea since "no-one's going to fancy him or her anyway" (*Guardian* 27 March 1990).

However an integral part of normalization is to encourage people with disabilities to get in touch with and express their emotions. Sex will be a part of such an expression, and it is therefore important that disabled people should be encouraged to find helpful ways of fulfilling their needs for warmth, love, acceptance and sexual activity. Morgan Williams, director of SPOD (Association to Aid the Sexual and Personal Relationships of the Disabled) acknowledges that genital sexual intercourse may not be possible for some, but points out 'any part of the body can be an erogenous zone' (*Guardian* 27 March 1990). Plenty of aids and adaptations exist where physical intercourse is difficult.

Paid employment and disability

A common complaint from people with disabilities and those that speak on their behalf is that of the failure of legislation concerning services to disabled people. The 1970 Chronically Sick and Disabled Persons Act raised the profile of disabled people, but was not strong enough to force local authorities to provide certain services (i.e. it was *enabling* but not *mandatory* legislation). Sixteen years later, the 1986 Disabled Persons (Services, Consultation and Representation) Act, was brought in to strengthen the 1970 Act. It too, has received a great deal of criticism. Michael Oliver described it as 'relatively weak'. In fact some local authorities have not allocated funds for its operation. Sections 1 and 2 of the Act which enable a person with disabilities to have an authorized advocate and section 3 which puts a duty on local authorities to assess the needs of disabled people in their area, have not yet been implemented.

Also unsatisfactory is the legislation intended to provide paid employment for those with disabilities. As Greville Janner, a QC and Member of Parliament says: 'There are few statutes more honoured in the breach than the Disabled Persons (Employment) Acts 1944 and 1958. The requirements are equally ignored in the private and in the public sectors' (*Social Work Today* 11 January 1990). Section 9 of the 1944 Act states, 'It shall be the duty of a person who has a substantial number of employees to give employment to persons registered as handicapped by disablement for the number that is his or her quota'. 'Substantial' is defined in the Act as twenty people or upwards. As to the 'quota' there is a 'standard percentage' – 3 per cent at the present time, and a 'special percentage'. The latter means that an employer can employ more people with disabilities than the 'standard percentage', or more usually less, on application to the government.

An employer who is obliged to employ a quota of disabled people has to keep records of such people, and false records can lead to prosecution. However, although it is known that many employers breach the quota regulations very few prosecutions result. Gerry Kinsella, in a newspaper article states that 'not a single government department observes it' (*Guardian* 4 September 1989). Some disabled people object to the quota system on the grounds that it is patronizing and would rather people were employed on their merits regardless of handicap.

Media images of people with disabilities

Disabled people share a similar position with women and black people with regard to the mass media – they are rendered largely invisible, or if represented, are usually shown stereotypically. Despite the fact that disabled people represent as many as one in ten of the population, they are rarely featured in everyday settings on radio and television. The image that most people have of disability is one of pathetic helplessness. This image is often deliberately reinforced and exploited by advertising agents, because they know it will kindle sympathy and increase the financial support voluntary organizations need for their survival.

Able-bodied people dominate the media, whether it is reading the news, acting in drama or soap operas, or featuring in advertising. In theatre or films disabled people will mostly be played by able-bodied people. Overall, there is a dearth of *positive* images of disability. Furthermore, disability and sexuality receives virtually no representation, thereby contributing to the false notion that sex is unimportant for disabled people.

> 'In today's society we are constantly bombarded with the image of the body beautiful, and anyone who is even slightly overweight is made to feel totally undesirable. In such a climate, it is no wonder that disabled people are considered sexless.'
>
> (Michele Cheaney, *Guardian* 27 March 1990)

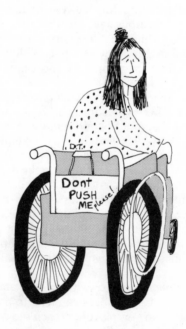

Social care and disability

Good practice in social care must include fully endorsing and utilizing the 'social model' of disability. As Gerry Kinsella says – 'It's time to stop trying to sell handicapped people to society. Society has a responsibility' (*Guardian* 4 September 1989). This model avoids *disablist* or *handicappist* language and terminology by using phrases like 'people with disabilities' or 'people who are physically challenged'. These are preferred to 'the disabled' or 'the handicapped'. Our language is important and will be reflected in more progressive attitudes. Good practice may also involve confronting and rejecting negative language and attitudes in others, sometimes our colleagues.

In working with people with disabilities we should always recognize and respect their individuality and reject stereotypes. We should encourage their striving for a 'normal' life-style, for independence and autonomy. This may include a full expression and fulfilment of their sexuality. This striving for a 'normal' life illustrates why *mobility* and *access* are of integral importance, not mere *tokens* or reflections of an attitude, because they mean disabled people can become *involved* in the mainstream of life and live it to the full.

Christy Brown, who had cerebral palsy and control and co-ordination only of his left foot, was reliant on his go-cart and brothers for participation in ordinary childhood activities. In his autobiography, he writes:

'Even in the space of a few weeks, since my old go-cart broke down, I had become as different in mind as I now knew I was in body. I had become more sensitive, more apprehensive to those I met outside my home. I looked on dumbly at my brothers and pals as they played around me, not even using my grunt now. I found no pleasure in their games. I had become a spectator now instead of one of the participants.'

(*My Left Foot*, Faber, 1989, p. 52)

Exercises

1. *A close friend comes to stay*

A close friend is coming to stay with you for the weekend. This friend is 'able-bodied'. Plan the weekend activities for the two of you. Now plan the weekend for yourself and your friend who is either:

i) severely visually disabled
ii) severely hearing disabled
iii) uses a wheelchair.

Consider the differences between the plans you make in each circumstance.

2. *Project on a minority group*

Select a minority group not dealt with in this book and produce a detailed project which gives information about the group and focuses on how its members are marginalized by society. For example you may choose to examine the social situation of people who are long-term unemployed; people who abuse drugs; people with alcohol-related problems; transvestites; transexuals or people with specific medical conditions such as myalgic encephalomyelitis (ME).

3. *Choices*

You have arrived at work or at college at the beginning of an average working day. This will mean that you have already made a number of choices. On a sheet of paper make a list of all the personal choices you have made so far. These might include what you have decided to wear, whether or not you chose to have breakfast or how you travelled to work or college.

After making a full list, imagine that you are a client in any of the following settings and make a list relevant to their situation:

  i) a hostel for people with learning difficulties
 ii) a day care centre for people with learning difficulties
iii) a person with learning difficulties living at home with your parents
 iv) a mentally ill person in an open hospital ward
  v) an elderly person in a residential establishment
 vi) a physically disabled person living at home with 24 hour social care support.

You may also apply this list of choices to any client in any other social care setting. Now compare the two lists you have made.

4. *Mental illness*

Study the following poems by Spike Milligan, comedian and author.

Oberon

The flowers in my garden
   grow down.
Their colour is pain
Their fragrance is sorrow.
Into my eyes grow their roots
   feeling for tears
To nourish the black
   hopeless rose
   within me.

Opus 1

This silent call you make
A silence so raging loud
I fear the world knows its
meaning
If you fill every corner of a room
Where can I look?
If I close my eyes
   the silence becomes louder!
There is no escape from you.
The only way out
   is in.
(S. Milligan, *Small Dreams of a
   Scorpion*, M. and J. Hobbs/
   Michael Joseph, 1972.)

Consider what insight the poems give into the experience of mental illness. Make notes of your thoughts and feelings and compare them with those of another member of your group. Discuss together any similarities or differences you may have.

5. *Media representation of minority groups*
With regard to one or more of any of the minority groups covered in this chapter, carry out a media survey on any one day or over a period of one week. Obtain copies of a number of newspapers or magazines and make sure you include at least one 'serious' national newspaper, one 'tabloid' newspaper and one local newspaper. Examine these papers for news, features and articles on your chosen group. In addition you may broaden your study by monitoring TV or a local radio programmes over the same period. Consider the following questions:

   i) Does the group have a high profile or do you feel its interests are marginalized or ignored?
  ii) Are members of this group depicted positively or negatively, seriously or disrespectfully?
 iii) To what extent have minority group members themselves been involved in the representation of the material produced in the media?

What conclusions can you draw about the media representation of your chosen minority group?

6. *Not in my backyard*
You have the task of informing a community about a proposed residential provision which is to be sighted within the neighbourhood for one of the following: people with learning difficulties, people with HIV, travellers or mentally ill people. At this stage you anticipate an adverse reaction from local residents and you want to present the group's interests as favourably and honestly as possible. It is important not to gloss over potential difficulties which might occur.

Draft a letter to local residents outlining what the practical consequences of the proposal might be. This situation could be taken further as a group discussion or role play, where individual roles of officials and local residents might be allotted.

Questions for essays or discussion
1. The use of the term 'learning difficulty' in preference to 'mental handicap' leads to a dilution of the condition and means that resources are not directed to those who need them.
2. Only heterosexual parents can ever give children a balanced upbringing because they provide appropriate role models.
3. Travellers represent such a threat to 'settled' society that society needs to erect so many barriers and blocks in order to effectively stop them living their chosen life style.
4. There is no such concept as 'able-bodied'.
5. Mental illness is a convenient way of labelling inconvenient behaviour.

6. We can expect older people to be prejudiced and need to tolerate to a certain extent racism and sexism in older people since we cannot hope to change them.
7. Every single parent would like to have a partner.
8. With reference to any client group consider the validity of the following statement: Residential establishments should encourage and enable all residents to express their sexuality.
9. 'But they are not normal are they?' This is a common reaction of parents of people with learning difficulties to attempts to normalize their lives.
10. All a carer working with people with HIV can do is to prepare and counsel them for death.
11. You arrive at a closed swing door at the same time as a person in a wheel chair. Do you automatically open the door for them? Give reasons for your answer.
12. Children of single parents are permanently damaged by the absence of the other parent.

Further reading

Academic sources

Acton, T., *Gypsy Politics and Social Change*. Routledge and Kegan Paul, 1974. An interesting academic text which includes a good deal of history, as well as more current developments among travellers.

Brearley, C.P., *Working in Residential Homes for Elderly People*, Routledge, 1990. A very concise and detailed book which describes what constitutes good quality care practice in residential homes for elders. Very readable and highly practical.

Burningham, S., *Not On Your Own – The MIND Guide to Mental Health*, Penguin, 1989. An accessible guide to mental health problems and the professional help available. It includes a section on self-help and sources of advice and information.

Gilbert, P., *Mental Handicap: A Practical Guide for Social Workers*, Business Press International Ltd, 1985. A 'practical primer' for social carers and social workers covering such topics as causes, assessment, communication, the law and community care.

Hicks, C., *Who Cares? Looking After People at Home*, Virago, 1988. A very detailed look at the lives of informal carers. Based on a study of 80 women and men, it outlines the frustrations, difficulties, stress and emotional turmoil experienced by those who care for disabled or elderly relatives at home.

Leighton, A., (ed.), *Mental Handicap in the Community*, Woodhead-Faulkner Ltd, 1988. A topical book which deals with a number of important issues such as the closing of institutions and the move towards community care, integration, education and work for people with learning difficulties.

McNeill-Taylor, E., *Bringing Up Children On Your Own*, Fontana, 1985. A practical guide to bringing up children as a single parent. The author, who has brought up her four children on her own, emphasizes the positive side of lone parenthood as well as outlining the difficulties with which many are faced.

Norman, A., *Triple Jeopardy: Growing Old in a Second Homeland*, Centre for Policy on Ageing, 1985. A book about the discrimination faced by ethnic minority elders in this country and the positive steps which can be taken to improve matters so that service provision is relevant and accessible to all sectors of society.

Oliver, M., *The Politics of Disablement*, Macmillan, 1990. An explanation of the 'social model' of disability which stresses the responsibility society owes to people with disabilities, as well as charting the rise of the 'disability movement'.

Stopford, V., *Understanding Disability – Causes, Characteristics and Coping*, Edward Arnold, 1987. A short useful handbook which provides a great deal of information and insight into a wide range of disabilities.

Tatchell, P., *AIDS: A Guide to Survival. A Radical Self-Help Manual for Understanding, Preventing and Fighting Back*, GMP, 1986. This book gives a clear and positive account of the major issues surrounding AIDS and HIV and suggests programmes for people with the virus aimed at strengthening the mind and body against the development of AIDS.

Sanderson, T., *How to be a Happy Homosexual. A Guide to Gay Men*, GMP, 1989.

Trenchard, L., *Being Lesbian*, GMP, 1989.

Both Sanderson and Trenchard offer advice and information across a wide range of relevant issues. Accessible and easy to read.

Other literary sources

Know Me As I Am: An Anthology of Prose, Poetry and Art by People with Learning Difficulties, Hodder and Stoughton, 1990.

Blythe, R., *The View in Winter*, Penguin, 1981.

Brown, C., *Down All the Days*, Secker and Warburg, 1983.

Dupoy, D., *Dare to Dream. The Story of the Famous People Players*, Key Porter Books, 1988.

Hall Carpenter Archives: Gay Men's Oral History Group, *Walking After Midnight. Gay Men's Life Stories*, Routledge, 1989.

Ireland, T., *Who Lies Inside*, GMP, 1984.

Mars-Jones, A. and White, E., *The Darker Proof*, Faber, London, 1987.

Nolan, C., *Under the Eye of the Clock*, Pan, 1988.

O'Rourke, R., *Jumping the Cracks*, Virago, 1987.

Reed, D., *Anna*, Secker and Warburg, 1976.

Sandford, J., *Gypsies*, Abacus/Sphere, 1975.

Sayer, P., *The Comforts of Madness*, Constable, 1988.

Films or plays

Aldrich, R., *The Killing of Sister George*, US, 1969.

Babenco, H., *Kiss of the Spider Woman*, US/Brazil, 1985.

Bogart, P., *Torch Song Trilogy*, US, 1989.

Cox, A., *Sid and Nancy*, UK, 1986.

Forman, M., *One Flew Over the Cuckoo's Nest*, US, 1975.

Ivory, J., *Maurice*, UK, 1987.
Loach, K., *Family Life*, UK, 1971.
Medak, P., *A Day in the Life of Joe Egg*, UK, 1971.
Parker, A., *Birdy*, US, 1984.
Sheridan, J., *My Left Foot*, Ireland, 1989.

6   Crime, policing and the penal system

Crime is deviant behaviour which society outlaws and labels *criminal*. What our society considers as deviant or criminal will change over time and will not necessarily coincide with other cultures. Much of what our criminal law outlaws is behaviour which causes harm to others. In so doing, the law lays down standards of acceptable behaviour which are necessary for social order.

Changing circumstances mean that society continually has to re-define crime. Advances in new technology bring new opportunities for criminal activity, for example, credit card and computer frauds.

The reasons why people commit crime are manifold and various. Apart from clearly negative motivations for committing crime, some people, particularly the young, will drift into criminal behaviour. Others may see crime as a legitimate way out of their deprived circumstances. Some may have a mental illness which may cause erratic and criminal behaviour. The motives for committing crime are not mutually exclusive. The truth may be a complex grouping of different factors and very hard to unravel. There is certainly no one unifying reason why people turn to crime.

Although the law defines what is and what is not criminal activity, there is much in other legitimate behaviour which does in fact have harmful and damaging effects. Some would regard as 'criminal' everyday business and professional practices. They might feel for example, that it is unfair for shop-keepers to raise the cost of their merchandise above the recommended retail price or for professional groups to charge excessive fees for necessary services. Because they are legitimate such practices are never officially condemned as being criminal.

How much crime?

For a large number of reasons we cannot be certain about just how much crime is committed. Every year the government publishes 'criminal statistics', but these merely inform us how much crime the police forces have actually *recorded*. This is clearly *not* the total amount *committed*. Social scientists refer to the concept of the 'dark figure of crime' as that which includes all the crime that actually occurs, regardless of whether or not it is recorded by the police.

Some commentators believe that the amount of crime recorded is more a reflection of how the police force operates within society rather than of criminal behaviour itself. Police tactics change from time to time, and they may, for example, choose to concentrate on certain types of crime, such as drinking and driving campaigns in the run-up to Christmas. Thus police activity will directly affect the amount and pattern of crime recorded.

An American writer, David Bayley (1983), calculates that there are nineteen factors which affect the relationship between the 'dark figure of crime' and the amount of crime that actually shows up in criminal statistics. These are:

1. Public ignorance of the law.
2. The accustomization of people to crime.
3. Crimes without specific victims (e.g. breaking the speed limit in a car, vandalism, graffiti).
4. The embarrassment of the victims of crime.
5. The fear of retaliation.
6. The physical inconvenience of reporting a crime to the police.
7. The anticipation of an unpleasant involvement with the police, if a crime is reported.
8. Peoples' perception of police ineffectiveness.
9. The desire of witnesses of a crime to be uninvolved.
10. Police uncertainty in classifying offences.
11. Interpersonal dynamics between the victim of a crime and the police.
12. The consequences to the police of recording an offence which may reflect badly on them and their 'clear-up rate'.
13. Bribery.
14. The organizational emphasis in policing.
15. The wilful repression of crime by the police.
16. Statistical errors.
17. A lack of standardization in reporting different crimes.
18. The size of a police force and the actual number of police working on the beat at any one time.
19. The attentiveness of the police.

This list may not be exhaustive.

Obviously a great deal of crime occurs without anybody being aware of its occurrence except the perpetrator; it is carried out in secret. Prominent criminologists who have undertaken a number of research projects on crime patterns and the victims of crime state that 'what is in little doubt is that the actual figures of crime are double the figures known to the police'. They add further that, 'the dark figure varies by type of crime, so that for instance, "taking and driving away" figures are extremely accurate'. This is because car insurance terms require car owners to report car thefts to the police.

On the other hand, 'crimes of violence probably reflect only one third of the total'. Figures for murder are the *most* reliable of all official crime statistics reported, whilst the crime of rape is grossly under reported for a variety of reasons, including the insensitive treatment victims receive from the authorities.

The amount of recorded crime has continued to rise each year for a very long time, with a few exceptions. For example, from 1952 to 1954 there was actually a reduction in 'notifiable offences recorded by the police per 100 000 population' in England and Wales. In 1966 and 1983, there was no change over the previous years' crime rate – it remained stable. There are also from time to time reductions in particular crimes e.g. there was a reduction in theft and handling stolen goods in 1983, compared with the previous year. However, the overall trend seems to be an inexorable rise in the crime rate, no matter what complexion of government is in power.

Who are the victims of crime?

An encouraging recent trend both among academics who study crime and in society generally, has been the increasing attention paid to the victims of crime. Politicians have also added their voice to those who want our society to show more concern for the victims of crime. Crime may emanate from social or personal factors, or both, but whatever conclusions are drawn as to the causes, we must take crime and its consequences seriously – the victims certainly do.

Victim support schemes

From small scale beginnings, Victim Support Schemes are now organized on a national basis. The Home Office spends a large amount of money on their running and paid co-ordinators exist for most local schemes. Volunteers provide support of various kinds to the victims of crime. Some local schemes have widened their brief to include special projects on particular forms of crime or specific issues, for example domestic violence or racial harassment.

Areas with higher crime rates tend to be those which already suffer a good deal of deprivation and lack adequate community resources. People living in these areas are more likely to be unemployed and in receipt of state benefits. One of the reasons for this is that people in areas of higher affluence tend to take more precautions against crime because they can afford to do so. They fit burglar alarms more frequently and are able to purchase more effective security devices for their houses.

Neighbourhood Watch schemes (where local people watch for suspicious behaviour or activity which might be criminal in their area) tend to be more active in middle class rather than in poorer areas. There is a danger that people living in areas with a very high level of crime will become 'de-sensitized' – as Bayley says, they become 'accustomed' to crime and so fail to report criminal activity. This soon becomes a 'vicious circle'. Crime, therefore, tends to escalate in such areas.

Some researchers assert that women are more likely to be the victims of crime than men. In their Islington 'victimization' study, Jones *et al.* (1986) found a 'considerably higher rate of female victimization'. They believe there are three main reasons for this:

1. The victims of sexual assaults are almost exclusively female.
2. The same is true of domestic violence, of which it is thought only a small proportion comes to the notice of the police as it is so easily hidden.
3. Street robbery against women is greater than it is against men.

They cite the example of 'non-sexual assault' and say that women are 40 per cent more likely to be attacked than men. This was especially disturbing as women took more precautions than men against crime. The women they interviewed were, for example, 'five times more likely to never go out after dark than men, three times more likely always to avoid certain types of people or streets, and . . . six times more likely always to go out with someone else instead of alone' (ibid., p. 15).

Another writer on gender and crime, Frances Heidensohn (1985), speaks of 'a great deal of crime which is carefully hidden from the police, from families, friends and neighbours' (p. 52). She is referring to domestic violence, abuse of children, incest and marital rape. (Rape in marriage has only recently been acknowledged as a criminal offence.) The overwhelming majority of this domestic crime is perpetrated by men.

Finally, not only are women more often victimized than men, but women who are less well off fare worse than those more affluent. This means that *working class women* are particularly vulnerable.

Agencies of social control

The police force is the agency in our society most directly associated with dealing with and controlling crime. There is no denying that such a job is an extremely difficult one. The police will have to get involved in many situations which are threatening, and situations that involve hostility, aggression, violence and in extreme cases, danger to life. Many incidents to which the police will be called will involve them trying to hold a 'balance' between hostile factions in extremely difficult confrontations.

We can describe the police, therefore, as agents of 'formal social control'. There are other agents, for example, the courts, the Magistrature and Judiciary, the Probation Service and the Prison Service.

Although we tend to think of social workers primarily as delivering care, we must recognize that a great deal of their work also involves an element of control. Social workers will act to modify certain kinds of behaviour which may be regarded as anti-social or damaging to the actual perpetrators of that behaviour. For example, social workers may be called upon to remove children from their parents, compulsorily admit mentally ill people to hospitals, and take neglected elderly people into residential accommodation. Because of this controlling role, social workers have sometimes been referred to as 'policemen in plain clothes'. Having said this, the police remain the agency to which we turn when a crime is discovered.

The police

Within the police force there are a number of different groupings and units with specific ways of operating. Apart from the general uniformed section of the force, there are plain-clothed sections such as the CID (Criminal Investigation Department), the 'traffic division', and specialist teams like the mounted police and dog handlers, usually used in the control of large crowds.

There are also a range of tactics which the police can deploy. They will police different areas in different ways. Decisions as to policing methods will often be affected by the level and type of crime in any particular area. There is, therefore, a spectrum of police behaviour ranging from the 'soft' end of 'community policing' and the 'bobby on the beat', through conventional policing, to the 'hard' end, where the police operate with paramilitary manoeuvres with units like the Territorial or Divisional Support Groups. These may include a full range of 'riot equipment', such as shields, batons, tear gas and, in Northern Ireland, rubber bullets. Whilst we associate the 'soft' end with conventional or 'street' crime, we associate the 'hard' end of policing with public disorder and large crowds in the streets of our cities.

The gender and racial make-up of the police

The majority of the police in the United Kingdom are white males. Just 8.5 per cent (almost *one in twelve*) are *women*. This percentage varies among the counties of the UK. It is highest in England – 9.3 per cent and lowest in Scotland (5.4 per cent).

The number of police who are drawn from ethnic minorities is even more disproportionate than the number of women. At the beginning of 1985, in England and Wales there were only 680 black officers, 253 of whom were in the largest force, the Metropolitan Police, which serves most of London. Eighty-seven were in the West Midlands force; this left very few indeed across the remaining forces in the country.

In 1981, following the urban disturbances in Brixton, South London, a report written by Lord Scarman recommended that many more ethnic minority members be recruited into the police. In the London area, as elsewhere, this has not been successful. In 1987, 114 ethnic minority officers joined the Metropolitan Police Force as new recruits. The following year, the number was just 66. In 1989, almost as many ethnic minority members left the police force as were recruited; some, as a result of racially-based hostility (*Observer*, 3 December 1989, p. 4).

In order to reflect the proportion of ethnic minority members in London, the 426 black police officers in the London force in 1988 would have to be increased ten-fold. In common with other areas of employment, people from ethnic minorities are over represented in the lowest grade of the service. In 1988, 90 per cent were constables.

The main barrier to more recruitment of ethnic minority members is believed to be the racism within the police force. Recent official reports have repeatedly highlighted this problem. In 1983, the independent Policy Studies Institute (PSI) published a report entitled *Police and People in London*. This research, initiated by the Commissioner of the Metropolitan Police two years earlier, was the most detailed ever conducted into the relationship between the police and the public. One of its major findings was that racist language and attitudes were prominent and pervasive in the police (*Observer*, 20 November 1983).

In December 1989, Walter Easey, policing adviser to the Association of London Authorities stated, 'The problem is in the force; it's a matter of cleaning up the Met. and eliminating racism in the canteen culture' (*Observer*, 3 December 1989, p. 4).

The nature of 'cop culture'

Obviously the managerial directives given to the police and the tactics and operational methods decided upon by managers in the police are extremely important. We must take them into account in studying the activities of the force. However, what actually happens face to face on the streets between members of the police and members of the public may have little to do with activity at managerial levels. Directives from above may, for example, outlaw racist language and behaviour, but individual police officers have a great deal of discretion about how they actually behave towards those they come into contact with in their working lives. As Francis Salandy says, 'I can meet the Chief Constable and have a friendly, intellectual conversation about policing. But he's just the Chief. He's not in the forefront' (*New Society*, 18 February 1982).

What they do on the streets in their dealings with the public is largely determined by their own culture or 'cop culture' as it is sometimes referred to. Studies such as the PSI research portray a police force which is largely isolated from the rest of society, especially in terms of social and leisure activities. It *is* a demanding job, and this tends to lead members of the police force to retain close ties with one another in the face of what they might regard as a rather 'hostile' public. A prominent writer on the police, Robert Reiner, sums this up by referring to 'the marked internal solidarity, coupled with social isolation of police officers' (Reiner, 1985, p. 92).

Other aspects of police culture are largely determined by the fact that the majority of the force are *white* and *male*. With so many white males working in such close proximity to each other, facing a good deal of danger, public hostility, and most of them wearing a common uniform, it is not surprising that research portrays a body of people which is conservative, both morally and politically. Another factor of crucial importance borne out by research is that there is a strong masculine ethos in the force that promotes machismo. An over emphasis on masculinity can lead to the predominance of physical resolutions to problems at the expense of appropriate sensitivity.

Such qualities will, of course, affect how the police force deals with women and black people in our society. Women may frequently be treated in a patronizing way (a hangover of old 'chivalrous' attitudes) or may bear the brunt of generally sexist attitudes. The PSI report (1983) stated that 'the dominant values of the force are still in many ways those of an all man institution such as a rugby-club or boys' school' (p. 372). These values will show themselves in a hostility towards homosexuals (a 'heterosexist' attitude) and in a good deal of 'sexual boasting and horseplay' (pp. 91–7), often for the 'benefit' of female colleagues.

> 'If *all* people experienced "policing" the way especially black people, peace women, the miners, young people and the politically active do, an unstoppable head of steam for change would build up.'
> (Jefferson, T., Smith, I., *Critical Social Policy* No. 13, p. 132)

Much criticism was levelled at the police in the past for the insensitive ways in which they dealt with rape victims and the victims of other kinds of sexual assault. However, improvements have been made in recent years. They have often set up specialist teams of female officers who work hard at putting victims at their ease while at the same time reassuring them that they should in no way feel responsible for the traumatic things that have happened to them.

We live in a racist society and we cannot expect one of its major institutions, i.e. the police force, to be otherwise. Robert Reiner (1985) sums up many research findings by saying that police officers are racially prejudiced, 'but only slightly more so than the community as a whole' (p. 100). He goes on to quote two American researchers, who write – 'Policemen reflect the dominant attitudes of the majority people towards minorities'.

It is dangerous to assume that *attitudes* of racial prejudice within the police will automatically be translated into *racist behaviour*. The PSI report (1983) found plenty of evidence to suggest that this is not so. 'Our first impression after being attached to groups of police officers was that racialist language and racial prejudice were prominent and pervasive . . . on accompanying these officers as they went about their work we found that their relations with black and brown people were often relaxed or friendly' (p. 109).

Other writers however, do not agree; they say that the police are more likely to stop young black people (mostly male) than their white counterparts. A Home Office report (Stevens and Willis, 1979) showed that the police were far more likely to 'stop and search' young black men rather than young white men under the 1824 Vagrancy Act, in a section known colloquially as the 'Sus' law. The same research showed that black people were 14 or 15 times more likely to be arrested than whites who have been stopped and questioned.

> I walk in-a Brixtan markit,
> believin I a respectable man,
> you know. An wha happn?
>
> Policeman come straight up
> an search mi bag!
> Man – straight to mi.
> like them did a-wait fi mi.
> Come search mi bag, man.
>
> Fi mi bag!
> An wha them si in deh?
> Two piece a yam, a dasheen,
> a han a banana, a piece a pork
> an mi lates Bob Marley.
>
> Man all a suddn I feel
> mi head nah fi mi. This yah now
> is when man kill somody, nah!
>
> 'Tony,' I sey, 'hol on. Hol on,
> Tony. Dohn shove. Dohn shove.
> Dohn move neidda fis, tongue
> nor emotion. Battn down, Tony.
> Battn down.' An, man, Tony win.
>> (James Berry, *In-a Brixtan Markit* in *News*
>> *from Babylon – The Chatto Book of West*
>> *Indian – British Poetry*, Chatto and
>> Windus, 1984, p. 191, with permission)

The 'sus' law has now been repealed, but there are fears by the black community, especially in London, that the police have begun to use a new tactic in order to harass black people. In October 1989, the Joint Council for the Welfare of Immigrants (JCWI) stated that hundreds of black people are stopped and detained every month while the police check their 'immigration status'. Alison Stanley of the JCWI said 'It is the experience of many lawyers, advisers and community groups that in certain areas of London a new 'sus' law is effectively being operated, in which black people are regularly stopped on the pretext of minor road traffic infringements and then asked to produce passports' (*Observer*, 15 October 1989). She summed up the situation as she saw it. 'It amounts to harassment of young black men' (ibid.). She claimed that many were held overnight in police custody, and some even for two days.

What of black people who join the police force? As stated earlier, why do so few appear to remain in the force for very long? It is suggested that their situation is made very difficult because they suffer from a 'double marginality'. This means that they are treated as 'outsiders', both in their professional world (by their white colleagues) and in their social world (by their white colleagues, and also by fellow black people who consider they have joined a 'racist' institution). The ostracism suffered becomes too great and they quit the force through a kind of 'loneliness'.

How well do the police do their job?
The police fulfil a large number of tasks: they answer distress calls of all kinds; they direct traffic and have the onerous task of usually being first on the scene at accidents; they control large crowds of people; they provide advice, assistance and information on a number of subjects and, of course, they detect crime. Many would consider the latter to be by far their most important role. Statistical evidence shows that the police force, though an essential service, is in fact inefficient and expensive with regard to clearing up crime.

In addition to the *criminal statistics* published each year by the Home Office, a British Crime Survey is now regularly produced by the same source. This gives a great deal more detail about crime in this country including rates at which crime is cleared up. These surveys clearly illustrate that the police rely heavily on the general public for information concerning serious crime. This was found to be true in over 90 per cent of cases. In inner-city areas it rose to 95 per cent (Hough and Mayhew, 1985).

From 1945 until the early 1970s the overall clear-up rate for all crime remained around the level of 45 per cent. Since the early 1970s however, it has steadily declined. By 1979 it was 41 per cent. This had fallen to 32 per cent by 1986.

The actual clear-up rate for specific crimes varies a great deal. Murder has the highest rate of 92 per cent, whereas burglary is only 25 per cent (in England and Wales). In the Metropolitan Police District the clear-up rate for burglary in 1986 was as low as 9 per cent. In fact the Metropolitan Police has the lowest overall clear-up rate of any force in Britain (in 1986 it was 16 per cent). This has declined more than any other force.

In general, crimes that require a good deal of police detective work tend to have low clear-up rates. In referring to these very low rates of detection, some authors (e.g. Lea *et al.*, 1987) speak of a 'crisis' in crime control. 'Detection rates have declined below the level that would have even a marginal deterrent effect: this is the extent of the crisis in the control of crime' (p. 34).

'We are losing control of the streets. It sometimes takes ten men in a van to deal with a problem which the absence of one man has produced . . . and we are starting to lose public support.'

(Robert Birch, Chief Constable of Sussex, *Observer*, 9 October 1988)

We must remember that although the police force is the agency most closely associated with crime control, all of us have a responsibility to prevent crime, where possible, and to report what criminal behaviour comes to our notice. Crime cannot be left to the police force alone. Given that 90 per cent of serious crime in Britain is reported by the public to the police, this flow of information is crucial to the police. Without public support the police officer's job would be largely unworkable. The policing of crime is achieved by the police *plus* the community.

Police accountability

In recent years a mounting concern has been expressed about the public accountability of the police. The exposure of a number of instances of corruption within the force, as well as examples of brutal treatment of individuals or groups of people in public demonstrations, and a number of deaths in custody, have combined to create a sense of public unease.

A tripartite system of accountability has traditionally existed: to the law, through the principle of the individual legal accountability of the constable; to the Home Secretary, through the Chief Constable; and to the police committees of the local authorities, of which two thirds are elected councillors and one third are magistrates. But despite the existence of this machinery, it is felt that there is no true accountability. Also in existence are new procedures under the Police and Criminal Evidence Act 1984, implemented in 1986, which provide for liaison between the police and the public. These Police Liaison Committees are too new as yet to be meaningfully assessed.

The Police Complaints Authority, which receives complaints from the public about the police, is not fully independent, and this factor gives rise to some concern about its effectiveness. It may well be that a radically different system of police accountability needs to be introduced. As Simon Holdaway (1983), now an academic, but once a member of the Metropolitan Police, says: 'Public accountability is . . . of the essence, in policing a democratic society' (p. 175).

The penal system – class, gender and race issues

Until the last few years, gender and race have largely been ignored in the study of crime. More work has been done on the relationship between *social class* and crime.

Social class and crime

As mentioned at the beginning of this chapter, society and its penal system generally have a distorted image of crime. This lopsided view results in the misplaced concentration in our society on young, working class men as the perpetrators of crime. As the authors of *Crime and Penal Policy* (Smith and Fowles, 1986) state

'Criminal justice is overwhelmingly concerned with what is sometimes called "street crime": the visible, obvious, almost universally condemned, but mostly petty crimes which are the characteristic offences of the young and the poor. Most of these offences, even when they are relatively serious, are not planned, calculated affairs. The professional criminal of popular imagery is not a myth, but he is extremely rare.'

(p. 22)

Other writers refer to 'street crime' as 'conventional crime' (Box, 1987, p. 35).

Every year in England and Wales, one half of all known offenders committing indictable offences (those dealt with in the Crown Court) are aged under 21 years and about one third are under 17 years. Generally, therefore, the greatest proportion of offences are committed by the young. For certain specific offences, the proportion of young offenders is even higher than shown in these general statistics. Seven out of ten burglaries are committed by those under 21. The 'peak age' for shoplifting is 14 to 16, and that of assault, damage to property and drug-related offences are between 17 and 20 years of age. The tailing-off of their involvement in criminal activity illustrates the fact that most young offenders grow out of crime as they mature and take on more commitments and responsibilities (Rutherford, 1986).

There is no research evidence that absolute deprivation (e.g. poor housing, poverty, unemployment) leads *directly* to crime. Criminologists will, for example, point to the relatively *low* crime rate in the 1930s, when Britain was in a profound economic slump and there was high unemployment. What *is* clear is that such deprivation ultimately increases the tendency to commit crimes of the kinds that have been mentioned.

In order to correct the imbalance of this concentration on 'conventional' crime, it is necessary to examine crime committed largely by those at the other end of the social class scale. Such crime is usually referred to as 'white-collar crime', less commonly as the 'crimes of the powerful'.

The kinds of crimes referred to are often work-related and are committed by people who generally have well-paid jobs, for example, income tax fraud, or income tax evasion, embezzlement and using property or equipment that belongs to one's employers for oneself.

A section of 'white-collar' crime is 'corporate crime', that which is committed by large businesses or corporations, for example, the underclaiming of profits, failure to pay National Insurance contributions, price-fixing, illegal pollution, selling unsafe or untested products and ignoring health and safety regulations.

> 'They hang the man and flog the woman who steals the goose from off the common, but let the greater criminal loose, who steals the common from the goose'.
> (Common saying at the time of the 'enclosure' of land in Britain, in the 1700s)

Often, it is fairly easy to disguise the fact that such offences are being committed because they occur in the private or 'closed' realm of work. Often they are not reported to the police because employers are keen to retain their 'good name'. They dispense 'private justice' instead, and thus deal with the matter internally. To pursue an employee through the courts would involve time, energy, money and possibly adverse publicity.

Another factor which acts as a barrier to the prosecution of offenders is the sheer complexity of many fraud or tax evasion cases. Such cases can take several years to investigate and cost a great deal of money.

People who commit such crime do not fit the public stereotype of an 'offender' because they have a 'white-collar' job and an outwardly respectable life-style. Such people do not strike fear into the general public because they do not pose a direct threat to them.

The public remain largely ignorant of the existence of much of this crime. In fact, a good deal of so-called 'sharp practice', which is not strictly illegal but borders on it, is actually admired. It is often portrayed in the media as astute and competitive behaviour and reported as an example of 'enterprise'. There is often a very thin dividing line between the legal and the illegal!

'You put the small thief in prison but the big thief lives in a palace'.
(Graham Greene, *Stamboul Train*)

It is extremely hard to assess the damage which such white-collar criminality does to both the national economy and to the well-being of people in society. A recent government estimate put the amount withheld by businesses for National Insurance contributions for their employees at £365 million a year or £1 million a day (*Observer*, 25 February 1990). The London Business School puts the cost of crime to United Kingdom companies at £3 billion per year, more than half of it due to cheque card fraud (*Observer*, 11 March 1990).

In 1986 there were 14 000 prosecutions for welfare benefit fraud, the cost of which was said to be £500 million. In the same year there were a mere 20 prosecutions for tax fraud (most importantly, submitting false tax returns or making false claims for personal allowances). The estimated total cost of *all* tax fraud was said to be £5000 million (*Observer*, 23 October 1988). This is a considerable cost to society, and it is significant that for each person prosecuted for tax fraud, 700 were prosecuted for benefit fraud.

The Observer carried an account of this unequal situation and stated why it believed the two offences appeared to be so differently treated by officialdom: it said it believed that in government circles, illegally taking money *from* the state is a greater crime than illegally withholding money *owed* to the state (*Observer*, 23 October 1988). An example such as this may give credence to the view that there is 'one law for the rich and another law for the poor'.

'When a youthful nobleman steals jewellery, we call the act kleptomania, speak of it with a philosophical smile, and never think of his being sent to the house of correction, as if he were a ragged boy who has stolen turnips.'
(George Eliot, *Middlemarch*)

The 'underclass' and the criminal justice system

The recent emergence of a so-called 'underclass' in Britain has raised concern about law and order and policing issues. Many members of the 'underclass' suffer unemployment for long periods, if not permanently. They frequently experience other related deprivations, such as poverty and poor housing conditions, and they are often over represented in run down areas of the inner cities. Owing to their exclusion from the workforce, they are sometimes referred to as a 'surplus population'.

Disaffected, and with no way of legitimately improving their situation other than by the unlikely solution of finding full-time, well paid employment, many will turn to crime and thus an involvement in criminal activity can develop. When represented in large numbers in confined geographical areas such as the inner cities, this so called 'surplus population' is often seen by formal social control agencies, most notably the police, as a 'control problem'. Rather than deal with the economic, political and social factors which have led to the creation and the continuance of such an 'underclass', we all too often merely hear cries for more 'law and order' and for tougher ways of controlling and dealing with offenders. This situation leads many to feel that the urban disturbances of the 1980s will not merely be a thing of the past.

> 'I'm not a sociologist, but if you have a society which is disturbed because of unemployment, bad housing etc., resentment is turned inwards on that society, and the police who are easily identifiable, reap a bad harvest.'
>   (Brian Fairbairn, Policeman, on the Brixton disturbances, 1981,
>   from *We Want to Riot, Not to Work, The 1981 Brixton Uprisings*.
>   Riot Not Work Collective, 1982, p. 160)

Social class and the penal system

We have already mentioned that the majority of people who appear before the courts are from working class backgrounds. When they are in court they are dealt with by people who are, in the main, from more affluent and privileged social class backgrounds. It has been estimated that around 80 per cent of magistrates are drawn from classes I and II of the Registrar-General's classification (NACRO, 1989a). Very few indeed are drawn from the unskilled working class. This is a reflection of the selection procedure of magistrates; they are not legally qualified and are chosen because of their perceived standing within the community.

In carrying out research for a book entitled *The Politics of the Judiciary* (1985), Griffith discovered that judges were drawn from an even more privileged background. About 70 per cent of them had attended a prestigious 'public' school, followed by either Oxford or Cambridge University.

It would be spurious to assume that there is therefore a class bias in sentencing in our courts, but it does lead to a questioning of how well the magistracy and judiciary will understand the kind of social class background of the majority of offenders who come before them. 'Equality before the law' is the central tenet of our legal system, and some people would argue that it is compromised by the existence of such social class differentials.

Gender and crime

We have already stated that some researchers believe that women are more likely to be the *victims* of crime. We noted that they suffer especially from the large proportion of undisclosed crime that remains a 'secret' of their domestic situation.

As far as the *perpetrators* of crime are concerned, not only are the majority of them *young*, but they are mainly *male*. Only around 12 per cent of all offences processed by the courts each year are committed by females (Hart *New Society*, 30 August 1985). For the most serious crimes, e.g. murder, causing death by reckless driving, wounding and robbery, the percentage of women who commit these crimes is as low as between three to five per cent. In this country the only serious crime for which more women are found guilty than men is cruelty to children, which does not include sexual abuse. This is partially explained by the fact that women generally spend much more of their time with children than men do.

Women commit fewer crimes than men. This is true in all countries, for all periods of recorded history, and for all age groups. In this country, the percentage of women in prison has never exceeded three to four per cent. In 1970, the Home Office stated its intention to have *no* female prisoners by the year 2000 (Blackstone, 1990). But the fact is, the numbers have risen.

However, although the prison population is predominantly male, women are still greatly affected. Many prisoners leave wives, girlfriends and children in the community. These female partners and relatives of those in prison are left to cope while their men are 'inside'. In a very real way they are punished because they have to struggle with new difficulties. These can include financial problems, especially if the prisoner was the only wage earner; housing difficulties, which may relate to their financial security, and social stigma as a result of their predicament. Visiting and keeping in touch with their partner in prison can be inconvenient and time consuming. In addition, they have to cope with their own emotional distress at separation from their partner. Also, mothers have to cope with their children's response to a father's sudden and prolonged absence.

Women and the penal system

One of the social effects on a woman who has committed a crime and is brought before the court is that she tends to be the subject of more social stigma than a man. Obviously the key reason is that women are a substantial minority coming before the court and therefore their appearance is considered more remarkable. Local press reporters may well pick up on a case which they would otherwise ignore, if it involves a woman.

There is evidence that courts treat women as 'doubly-deviant'. Firstly, women suffer as a result of their rule-breaking or 'criminality' as do *all* offenders. Added to this, however, is a second stigma. Women have acted out of their role as women, or as 'unfeminine', in committing that which is usually done by men. As a result, the consequences for them are harder than for men, especially if they are sent to prison.

Women workers in the penal system are to a great extent '*marginalized*'. Of the 27 500 magistrates in England and Wales, 11 500 are females. In the Crown Court, the situation is more starkly unbalanced. In March 1987, of the 79 High Court Judges, only 3 were women; of the 393 Circuit Judges, only 16 were women; of the 534 Recorders, only 23 were women; and of the 467 Assistant Recorders, only 28 were women (NACRO, 1989a). This situation is still essentially the same and applies to Scotland as well, although the criminal justice system is quite different there.

Within the legal profession, women are again under represented. In Britain as a whole, only 12 per cent of solicitors and 17 per cent of barristers are female. Although the proportion of female Probation Officers in the Probation Service is more healthily balanced at the basic grade, the differential becomes marked at senior level and above. Only 5 of the 56 Chief Probation Officers are women. The Probation Service only exists in England and Wales. It ceased to exist in Scotland after 1969 and its duties were taken over by the Social Work Departments.

In conclusion, women may well form the majority of victims of crime. At the same time, they are under represented as people in positions of authority within the penal system, particularly in the more senior positions. This corresponds to their inferior position in the majority of our society's institutions.

Black people and crime

Despite legislation such as the 1976 Race Relations Act, there is still plenty of evidence that ethnic minority groups experience racism and disadvantage in the criminal justice system. An important report called, *Black People and the Criminal Justice System* (NACRO, 1986), concluded that 'measures to ensure the provision of fair and non-discriminatory treatment to black offenders and victims of crime are a low priority for most of the responsible organization' (para 8.2).

Racial stereotypes linking black people with crime are firmly established within our society at all levels. In a speech to the Carlton Club in June 1986, Douglas Hurd, who was then Home Secretary, said on the subject of crime in Britain

> 'The heart of the problem, as I see it, is the existence in a number of our cities of a hard core of perhaps no more than 200 youths in each, many of them black, who have become completely detached from their society. They are hostile because every influence in their lives has been discouraging. They turn easily to crime because too many people have filled their minds with an exaggerated despair.'
>
> (cited in Mathews, 1988, p. 43)

Similar sentiments were present in a manifesto published by the National Front for the 1983 General Election. 'The streets of our larger towns and cities – once safe for all, the old, the weak, and the infirm – have become jungles plagued by gangs of vicious – predominantly, though not exclusively, black – muggers who hunt down our old folk for pitiful sums of money' (*The Times Guide to the House of Commons*, 1983, p. 352).

A good deal of research has examined the way in which society, or some sections of it, have used certain groups of people as scapegoats, making them appear exclusively responsible for certain crimes, and thereby distorting reality. This is the case with black, male youths and the crime of 'mugging'. This is not a legal technical term, but a rather emotive one that was in the main invented and canvassed by the media. Although the word was not used in crime reporting in this country until August 1972, the crime it referred to was not itself new. It was 'robbery with violence' which has certainly been around for a very long time.

The most important media distortion was not the discovery of a new type of crime, but more sinisterly, the almost exclusive reference to young blacks as perpetrators of the crime. This was done despite the fact there was no way of knowing the ethnic origin of offenders at the time as the Home Office did not then collect ethnic-specific data on those committing crimes. The media was able to generate strong feelings amongst sections of the general public based on a distorted over exposure of a handful of cases involving black offenders. This may have had a detrimental influence on magistrates and judges when sentencing black offenders, especially on charges of, or those akin to, 'mugging'.

Black people and the penal system

Racism is again evident in the disproportionate number of black people (especially Afro-Caribbeans) in prison serving sentences. According to Prison Reform Trust statistics issued in August 1989, Afro-Caribbeans are imprisoned seven to eight times more than white people. The figures were 775 out of every 100 000 for the former compared to an overall rate of 98.2 per 100 000 for the latter.

Prison Department figures for black people in custody also shows that black people tend to serve longer sentences on average than white people. Eighteen per cent of those serving four or more years were black compared with under 8 per cent of those serving less than 18 months (NACRO, 1986). Other figures show an estimate that in some prisons in the south east of England over 20 per cent of inmates are from ethnic minorities, while in some juvenile institutions it is as high as 60 per cent (Lea *et al.*, 1987). The authors conclude that 'Since offenders from ethnic minorities receive generally longer sentences overall than white offenders, it seems certain that the prisons will become increasingly filled with black prisoners' (ibid., p. 47). Based on 1985 figures for the 17–20 age group, the 2250 male Afro-Caribbean offenders sent to prison that year represented 1 in 20 of all (some 40 000) Afro-Caribbeans in that age group.

One of the reasons why so many black people are being sent to prison may be contained in the findings of a NACRO report, entitled *Black People and the Criminal Justice System*, published in 1986. They discovered that Probation Officers made fewer recommendations in 'social enquiry reports' for the courts for supervision in the community, 'because they lack the confidence to carry this out successfully' (p. 16). Consequently, black offenders are often pushed higher up the 'tariff' of sentencing options more quickly than their white counterparts.

Turning to those prisoners who have not yet been sentenced, it can be seen that the proportion of black people *remanded in custody* has also been growing. In December 1989, the National Association of Probation Officers (NAPO) issued a briefing paper which showed that black people represented 20 per cent of the remand population in prisons in England and Wales: in London this figure was 38 per cent. It needs to be borne in mind when considering these figures that black people comprise less than 5 per cent of the general population. Since the monitoring of ethnic minority numbers in the prison system began, the proportion of them remanded in custody has steadily risen.

This gross over representation in the prison population contrasts with the under representation of black people in positions of authority within the criminal justice system. In 1989 only 500 of the 27 500 magistrates in England and Wales were from ethnic minorities, i.e. less than 2 per cent. In the same year there were only two black recorders, two black assistant recorders and one black circuit judge (NACRO, 1989b). In 1988, the Probation Service began ethnic monitoring of its workforce. Black people now make up less than 2 per cent of all probation staff. There are no black Chief Probation Officers, only one Assistant Chief, and four Senior officers throughout the service (England and Wales).

Prisons

Tessa Blackstone (1990) sums up the current state of our prisons: 'Britain's prisons are institutions of which we should be ashamed. They are absurdly expensive, yet scandalously inhumane.' Many are old, Victorian buildings intended for far fewer inmates than they now hold. Over-crowded, insanitary and undignified conditions contribute to the de-humanization of prisoners. Any claim that prisons reform or rehabilitate have receded and all but disappeared. Their primary function would now seem merely to contain. The stresses endemic to the prison system which erupt from time to time were most dramatically manifested in a number of penal establishments in April 1990. The siege at Strangeways Prison, Manchester, which began on April 1st and lasted for 25 days, was the longest and most serious in modern times. Amongst other things, these events illustrated the pent-up frustration and anger that found expression in violence and destruction.

> 'The top could blow off these penal dustbins at any moment.'
> (Lea *et al.*, *Law and Order – 5 years on*, 1987)

At the present time, there are 129 penal establishments in England and Wales – 117 for males and just 12 for females. Officially they have places for approximately 45 000 people, but are actually holding over 50 000 (NACRO, 1990). Over the last few years the prison population has steadily risen and there appears no sign of this trend changing in the foreseeable future. In fact the

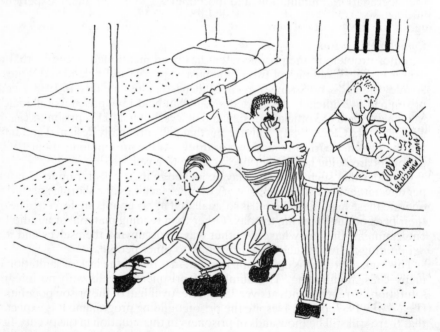

Prison cells are often overcrowded, unstimulating, dehumanizing and occupied for most of the day.

government has embarked on a very large prison building programme, and recent history suggests that spare places will quickly be filled.

In 1988 the United Kingdom had the highest prison population of the 21 countries which make up the *Council of Europe*. This is both in terms of absolute numbers and also in relation to its overall population. There are approximately 48 200 males and 1800 females in prison.

As well as the moral argument for keeping more people out of prison there is an economic argument. It is established that many people currently in our prisons need not be there because their crimes do not pose a serious threat to the community. Furthermore, it is argued that incarceration only serves to foster criminality. It can breed contempt and harden anti-social attitudes, as well as effectively damage people's chances of leading an ordinary life after release. The huge expense incurred by the prison system is a further argument in favour of reducing the prison population.

In the financial year 1988–9, the average cost of keeping someone in prison was £288 per week (NACRO, 1990). The cost varies according to the type of penal establishment; from a lowest figure of £199 per week in an *adult open prison*, to a highest figure of £541 per week in a *dispersal prison* (these are *maximum security* prisons holding the most serious types of offenders).

Some people argue that it is necessary to deprive offenders of their liberty, and that this in itself is a sufficient punishment when meted out by a 'developed society'. Others argue that conditions should be sparse in order to discourage people from abusing the system and seeking 'asylum' in prison. However, it would be hard to produce a moral argument for subjecting our prisoners to the degradation, humiliation and boredom so many of them experience 'inside'.

Conditions in prison

A major problem in the prison system has been mentioned already – that of *overcrowding*. Examples of two of the busiest prisons in England and Wales – Armley in Leeds and Strangeways in Manchester illustrate this. In 1988, Leeds prison had 642 officially designated places, but held 1347 prisoners (all male); Manchester had 653 officially designated places, but held 1132 prisoners (again all male) (NACRO, 1988). This means that cells originally designed and built for one prisoner currently hold two or three. At the present time about 19 000 prisoners are being held either two or three to a cell.

Consider that such prisoners may be locked in their cells for up to 23 hours per day, either because of lack of work or other facilities or a shortage of staff to operate these facilities. The cell is so small that its occupants are forced to lie on their beds or bunks during the day. Other than reading material or a radio for entertaiment, they may have no other way of occupying themselves and it is debilitating to live at such close proximity to other people.

This lack of privacy is dehumanizing and, in terms of the lack of sanitation in many cells, humiliating. The number of prisoners in cells with no integral sanitation currently stands at over 25 000, i.e. over half of the prison population (Lea *et al.*, 1987, p. 45). Despite the prison building programme it is expected that there will still be thousands of prisoners in this situation in the twenty-first century. The lack of sanitation results in what is called 'slopping out', described by the Chief Inspector of Prisons in a 1984 report.

'When the time for slopping out comes the prisoners queue up with their pots for the few toilets on the landing. The stench of urine and excrement pervades the prison. So awful is this procedure that many prisoners become constipated – others prefer to use their pants, hurling them and their contents out of the window when morning comes.'

(p. 45)

Prisons have the benefit of 'Crown immunity', which means that standards of health and hygiene cannot be legally enforced. This means that even if conditions resulted in the illness, injury or even death of a prisoner court proceedings could not be instigated against those responsible.

In many ways the regime in prison is harsh and restrictive. Female prisoners are allowed to wear their own clothes (and to have three changes) but only male *remand* prisoners are allowed this. All sentenced male prisoners have to wear prison issue clothing and baths or showers are restricted. Prisoners serving a sentence can only send out one letter a week which is paid for by the prison, others they have to pay for themselves. There is widespread official reading of both incoming and outgoing mail, except in *open* prisons where it is not read. Only those in open prisons have access to a telephone.

The point is frequently made that it is actually the wives and families of prisoners who may suffer more during a relatives' term of imprisonment. Prisons are often located in isolated rural areas making transport difficult for visitors. Commonly, a prisoner is sent to a prison far from her or his home, which makes it not only difficult and time consuming but also expensive to visit loved ones, although some expenses may be reclaimed.

The frequency and duration of visits is strictly limited, and this puts a further strain on family relationships. Prisons vary in their visiting arrangements, but minimum requirements for all are laid down. Sentenced adult prisoners are allowed just a half-hour visit every 28 days. Added up over a year, this constitutes 6½ hours for those over 21 and 13 hours for those under 21. Given that visits take place in the very public surroundings of a large visitors hall this puts considerable pressure on both offenders and visitors. Is it any wonder that many relationships do not survive a prison term?

Does prison work?
Rule one of the Prison rules states that the purpose of prison is to encourage prisoners to lead a 'good and useful life' on release. Prison certainly punishes those sent there, most especially by depriving them of their liberty, but whether it *reforms* and deters offenders from crime is very doubtful. Prison has been described as 'criminogenic' because many offenders have gone on to commit more serious crimes on release, following their initial experience of prison.

The 'odds' are often stacked against prisoners on their release. Many marital and familial relationships will have foundered whilst they have been away. It is estimated that owing to this, as well as other reasons, a quarter to a half of prisoners are homeless on release. These women and men will only have a small release grant to help them. Without an address, problems over claiming benefits and finding work in order to settle and stay out of trouble are extreme. The difficulty of finding work is compounded by the attitudes of many employers: it is often awkward to try to explain away a prison record. The temptation to re-offend may be hard to resist in the face of such difficulties. It is estimated that petty offenders who were homeless on release had a rate of re-conviction almost 3 times that of those who were not homeless.

There remains the further question of whether prison itself has a constructive effect on the prisoner. Despite work facilities in prison, especially the more well equipped, prisoners remain too idle for too long. The plight of 'remand' prisoners is especially severe; they are often locked in cells for 23 hours a day with nothing to do except wile away their time as best they can.

Only one prison establishment in England and Wales (Grendon Under-wood) is designated as a 'psychiatric prison'. Here, and in specific units within other prisons, a good deal of therapy takes place, much of it in the form of group-work. In most prisons, however, little or nothing is done to help prisoners to modify their behaviour during their incarceration and after release. This is particularly true of sex offenders who may seek protection under 'Rule 43' which guarantees their isolation. There is little therapeutic intervention for such people in prisons.

Stanley Cohen, a sociologist, refers to prisons as 'human warehouses'. Given that the mental condition of violent men and women and those who have perpetrated sexual attacks on women or children may well have actually deteriorated whilst 'inside', the prison establishments may be releasing people into society who are more dangerous than they were at the time of being sentenced.

'Prison life is the dependency culture at its most extreme.'
(Douglas Hurd, Ex Home Secretary, *Independent*, 15 October 1988)

Media images of crime

In several ways the image the media creates of crime is misleading, unhelpful, and even actually damaging. Some of the key factors concerning the media representation of crime are listed below.

1. The media, which understandably has to be selective in order to function, frequently focuses on what is sensational. Horrific crimes, often of a very violent or sexual nature, will receive a great deal of detailed attention. Minor crimes will only be featured when they are committed by well known person-alities like film or pop stars, or politicians. In both cases, the media obscures the generally petty and unsensational nature of crime.

2. Linked to this first point, the type of media reporting that sensationalizes crime often adds unnecessarily to the public *fear of crime*. The original *British Crime Survey* (NACRO, 1982) stated in reference to the media, '. . . some people are able to recognize and discount exaggerations when they occur: others are less likely to do so, and these may well include groups who are most fearful of crime – the isolated and the elderly among them'.

3. We have already mentioned the part the media played in creating a false picture of 'mugging' as an exclusively black crime. Not only was this sen-sational, it was largely untrue and very misleading. Again, if we turn to the 1982 British Crime Survey, it specifically referred to this bias and to the need for

accurate information on crime. The true picture of 'mugging' was that it was rare (although in some inner city areas it occurred much more frequently than elsewhere), that it did not usually result in injury, and that elderly women were seldom victims.

4. The lack of an accurate and balanced portrayal of crime in the media also stifles open and honest debate on criminal and penal policy. Tessa Blackstone (1990) states that 'The right-wing tabloid press frequently screams for tougher penalties for convicted criminals, described as "monsters" and "beasts", who should be put away for the rest of their lives. Believing that these newspapers reflect their readers' views, as well as moulding them, ministers respond accordingly' (pp. 23–4).

5. The sensational and alarmist reporting of the tabloid press creates what sociologists have called 'moral panics'. Stanley Cohen made a study of such phenomenon which he observed as being generated initially by the identification of what he called a 'folk devil' – a figure to terrify and alarm the general public. Although his original study focused on the early 1960s 'battles' between groups of 'mods' and 'rockers' on various seaside beaches, the process continues today. The 'black mugger' mentioned previously is a good example. The stereotyping of a racial nature meant that media reports of black people frequently had a very negative, criminal connotation. Such stereotyped images of black people also resurfaced during the media reportage of the urban disturbances of the 1980s.

The future

Crime is a serious social problem. The police and the official social care agencies, such as the Probation Service, cannot be left to deal with it alone, although, of course, they have a crucial contribution to make. Crime should concern us all, and our informed caring should embrace both offenders and the victims of crime.

Predictions as to the general level of crime in the near future vary; some expect it to increase, and along with it the prison population. Others predict a decrease owing to demographic changes which mean there are, and will be for some time, less young people around the age when the commission of crime is at its peak.

There are many calls for more 'law and order', for tougher sentences and more control. These are made despite all the evidence concerning the ineffectiveness of imprisonment. Calls for tougher sentences tend to only deal with crime as an illegal act and ignore the fact that it is but a symptom which has its roots in deeper social tensions and problems. The latter, which include poverty, unemployment, inequality and homelessness, may not directly lead to crime, but they all contribute to a more desperate social climate in which crime is more likely to flourish. This is especially true when those who are unable to legitimately afford material goods are constantly bombarded by a media and advertising industry that tempts people to spend at an ever increasing level. The implications of non-ownership of a whole range of desirable material possessions are incomplete social membership and individual failure.

The present plans to introduce and extend more control in the community (i.e. non-custodial measures such as 'tracking' and the 'electronic tagging' of offenders) will have a limited success if basic inequalities not only go unchecked but actually increase in the years to come. We will never eradicate crime in our society. It is a 'fact of life' we know we have to live with. Should we therefore concentrate on limiting its worse effects, but meanwhile take as many sensible preventive precautions as we see fit?

Exercises

1. Spend some time in the public gallery of your local Magistrates or Crown Court. What can you deduce about the class, gender and race of:

    The defendant
    Magistrates, Judges or Sherriffs (Scottish Courts)
    Social Workers
    Solicitors
    Barristers (Advocates in Scotland)
    Victims of crime
    Probation Officers (England and Wales only)

What conclusions can you draw?

2. *Media study*
Select a number of local and national newspapers, preferably a range from 'light' to 'heavy'. Measure how much space each devotes to the reporting of crime. What type of crime is it? 'Blue' or 'white-collar'? How is it reported and what language is used? Is it sensationalized or treated seriously? Select some individual words or phrases which you think indicate a particular papers' crime reporting.

3. Given that women may represent the majority of the victims of crime, most especially violent and sexual assault, find out what support, assistance and advice exists for them in your local community.

4. You are a member of staff working in a probation hostel for male and female offenders between the ages of 17 and 21. As a team member you have been asked to deliver a talk (of about twenty minutes duration) to a small group of visiting Magistrates who are all new to the 'bench'. Your brief is to outline the *social* factors that contribute to criminal activity.
Stage 1
Use the material contained in this chapter and the suggestions for further reading. In small groups of 3 or 4, develop the main points of your presentation, substantiating, where possible, with relevant statistics. This task may require more than one class session.
Stage 2
Each group of 3 or 4 will in turn make their presentation to the rest of the whole group, who will be 'acting' as the visiting Magistrates. The Magistrates will be given an opportunity at the end of the presentation to ask questions.

5. Contact your county police headquarters. Find out what practical steps they are taking to recruit more black people to the Force. What success have they had? Can you obtain figures on how many have joined and how long they have remained? What inhibiting factors do the Police feel exist around the recruitment of black people?

Questions for essays or discussion

1. Crime statistics tell us no more than how active the police are and where they are concentrating their resources.
2. Probation officers and qualified social carers are merely 'police officers in plain clothes'.
3. Were the urban disturbances of the 1980s simply criminal activity, or were they the symptoms of deeper social problems?
4. 'There are all those things like not getting jobs and people leading miserable, bleak lives, so that crime becomes the only avenue.' (Commander Jenny Hilton, Metropolitan Police, quoted in the *Observer* 30 September 1990).

   'It does not surprise me that some poor people are driven to drugs or violence or immorality. What else have they to do?' (Dr John Vincent, President of the Methodist Conference, quoted in the *Independent* 21 October 1989).

   In your opinion what validity do these statements have?
5. Prison merely contains and in no way reforms.
6. Why do women commit far less crime than men?

Further reading

Academic sources

Downes, D., Rock, P., *Understanding Deviance*, Clarendon, 1988. A very thorough account of the main sociological theories of deviance and crime, which interestingly presents them in the historical order in which they originally appeared.

Moore, S., *Investigating Deviance*, Unwin Hyman, 1988. An accessible and up-to-date discussion of the major ideological approaches to crime and deviance, including sections on gender, ethnic minorities, the 'contemporary left' and the 'New Right'.

Heidensohn, F., *Women and Crime*, Macmillan, 1985. A radical critique of past and present sociological writings on women and crime and a review of current debates in feminist criminology.

NACRO, *Race and Criminal Justice*, NACRO, 1988. A report examining the experience of black people in the criminal justice system in Britain.

Reiner, R., *The Politics of the Police*, Wheatsheaf, 1985. A comprehensive study of the British police which, as well as sections on the history and the politics of the police, also examines the sociology of 'cop culture'.

Simey, M., *Democracy Rediscovered. A Study in Police Accountability*, Pluto, 1988. From 1981–6 Margaret Simey was Chairperson of the Merseyside

Police Authority. A study of police accountability in Liverpool during a period which included the Toxteth disturbances.

Blackstone, T., *Prisons and Penal Reform*, Chatto and Windus, 1990. A brief, outspoken account of the current state of our prisons and possibilities for penal reform.

Stern, V., *Bricks of Shame*, Penguin, 1987. A critical view of the state of our prisons which questions why we sentence so many to custodial institutions at such great expense.

Other literary sources

Behan, B., *Borstal Boy*, Arena, 1990.

Boyle, J., *The Pain of Confinement*, Pan, 1985.

Dostoyevsky, F., *Crime and Punishment*, Penguin, 1951.

Greene, G., *Brighton Rock*, Penguin 1970.

Hill, P., with Bennett, R., *Stolen Years – Before and After Guildford*, Doubleday, 1990.

Pearson, J., *The Profession of Violence*, third edition, Granada, 1984.

Films or plays

Cox, A., *Repo Man*, US, 1984.

Hart, H., *Fortune and Men's Eyes*, US, 1971.

Parker, A., *Midnight Express*, UK, 1978.

Roeg, N., Cammell, D., *Performance*, UK, 1970.

7   The media in a democratic society

'To me a free society and a free media are inseparable'
(Margaret Thatcher, 1984 cited in Hennessy, P.,
What the Papers Never Said, Portcullis Press, 1985, p. 160)

We live in a so-called 'free' and 'democratic' society. One of the freedoms we are supposed to have is freedom of *speech*. This principle not only applies to public speaking, but also to our media. In this chapter, we will examine how far this is true. We will discuss the 'mass media' – which includes television, film and video, radio, records, books, journals and newspapers. We will concentrate on television, radio and newspapers because they are the most popularly used forms with the most up-to-date, immediate and direct impact.

If we want to learn what is going on in our society and in the wider world, we have to turn to such forms of media – they are the only resources we have. We cannot travel to all the locations where a 'news story' is unfolding and see for ourselves. This is why the media is in a powerful position, although its precise influence is difficult to determine.

As informed and effective carers we need to know what is going on in our society. We need an understanding of the 'climate of public opinion', of social problems and their development, of changes in the law and local government, all of which may directly affect our work. Most importantly, we need to see our clients in their social setting. So we turn to the media.

What we find will be limited in two important ways. Firstly, there are a restricted number of organizations and companies involved in media production, news and current affairs. In Britain we have four main television channels plus satellite and cable TV companies, although more are planned. There is only one national radio company (BBC) plus an increasing number of local and independent ones. There are now only a dozen high circulation national daily and Sunday newspapers, a much lower figure than in the first half of this century (Table 7.1). The second limitation is that the media is, and has to be, *selective*. It cannot report *all* that happens in our society, let alone the wider world. Therefore, *what* it selects, *how* it selects it, and *why* it selects it, are extremely significant questions.

A further general point is that the way the media is produced and presented creates the impression that news coverage is unbiased – that it represents the balanced truth. Small wonder then that we tend to believe what we see, hear and read in the media. We do not find ourselves disbelieving or questioning the very news reports themselves – we assume their basic truthfulness in a generally unquestioning way.

Table 7.1   The decline in the number of newspapers published 1900–1987.

	1900	1921	1947	1987
National dailies	21	12	9	11
Provincial morning	70	41	28	16
Provincial evening	101	89	75	64
National/Provincial Sundays		21	16	13

(Reproduced from Negrine, R. (1989), *Politics and the Mass Media in Britain*, Routledge.)

It needs to be pointed out that the quality of all the different kinds of media varies considerably. The contrast between a so called 'quality' or 'serious' (or 'heavy') newspaper and a popular 'tabloid' size (or 'light') newspaper is very stark. Whereas the first will concentrate on reporting news stories and providing serious comment, the second will go more for what are called 'human interest' stories, 'society gossip' or accounts of the goings on in TV 'soap operas'.

The tone of news bulletins on the various radio stations we can tune into will vary enormously – the important 'lead' story on one may not even be mentioned by another. The same is true of television, where much of what is broadcast varies depending on the time of day or night it is shown. This will often be determined by the TV company's estimation of what kind of audience is viewing at any particular time.

We must beware, therefore, of believing that the quality of our media is of a standard and consistent kind. Some of those involved in media production have responded positively to what they believe are the genuinely expressed feelings of its audience, including those of minorities. The picture is therefore a mix of progressive elements and more traditional ones which tend to continue delivering the same kind of product.

'Good' and 'bad' news

The actual content of what is called 'news' is mostly 'bad'. Deaths, disasters, accidents and crises appear to have more 'newsworthy appeal' to television, radio and newspaper editors. Frequently, the only lighthearted or humorous item in a television or radio news bulletin will be the final one – acting as a 'sweetener' before the end, with the intention of retaining the viewer/listener. In a similar way the 'sensational' news item is given prominent and lengthy coverage, especially in 'tabloid' newspapers. These popular papers are dependent on very large circulations for their survival and so they are frequently drawn to the more outrageous news items. Such pressures clearly distort the coverage of news stories that such papers provide.

In addition to news the mass media also presents factual documentaries, drama, entertainment, sport, political and 'strip' cartoons amidst a great deal of other material. Underlying a large amount of the total material presented are a range of 'messages' to the consumer – in the form of values, attitudes, beliefs and political ideology. These 'messages', not surprisingly, reflect the views of those who own, edit and produce the various media forms and who are largely white, middle class men. It is less common for minority views to be aired.

> 'The *Sun* prefers the working class to be tucked safely away in their front rooms
> watching *Eastenders*, and then once every five years going out to vote Tory.'
> (Murphy, A., *The Heavy Stuff*, no. 1, London Class War 1987, p. 9)

The media and advertising

The media has a very close relationship with advertising. All newspapers and the independent radio stations and TV channels carry advertising. Most newspapers derive well over half their income from this source. Without it many would simply not survive, so advertising revenue is very important to them. It is small wonder that newspapers tend to have a 'conservative' nature; they are at pains not to offend the sources of so much finance!

The independent radio stations, of which there are some 50 in the UK, and the 15 regionally based television companies rely on advertisers for their income. Advertisements are presented either between programmes or in a break during the running of a programme. Only the BBC is funded from licence fees.

It is important to consider the kinds of images they present; for example, the picture of family and social life is usually an extremely conventional one, made up of well-groomed members of nuclear families, so-called 'attractive' people, who are most likely to be white, middle class and 'well spoken'. Although we shall deal with this in more detail below, it is worth pointing out that working class people, black people, women (other than as sex objects or housewives), gay people, the elderly and those with disabilities, very rarely feature in advertising, whether in the press or on radio and TV.

What effect does the media have?

A great deal of research into the effect of the media, especially on the portrayal of violence, crime and sex on TV, has proved disappointingly inconclusive. It seems when the media is studied more questions than answers come to light. Certain cases of individuals committing serious crime as a result of being influenced by TV have come to notice, but the more general effect on the population at large is much harder to assess. Many feel that rather than mould us, change us, or directly influence us, the media is more likely to merely reinforce our already existing views, value systems and political ideology. In fact, they believe that we tend to seek out the newspaper, radio or TV programme which will fit in with our values and feelings.

It is so difficult to assess media effect because there are so many complex, interacting factors which we have to take into account. If we take a television programme, relevant factors include; the time it is broadcast, its length, content, its likely audience and the age, class, gender and racial make-up of that audience. This shows that any simplistic statements about the media having a direct effect, which has been called the 'hypodermic syringe model', are mistaken.

One of the negative effects the media certainly appears to have is that of *de-*

sensitization. This especially takes effect if images, items and stories are repeatedly presented over a long period. Thus photographs or films-clips of famine and starving children, urban unrest and war would seem to create less and less response in people the more they are subjected to them. The audience mentally and emotionally 'switches off' – we take little notice of another bomb explosion in Belfast or a fresh food shortage in a developing country. If such news items are to continue to evoke a response, perhaps their presentation should be more selective or intermittent. Events in the world come so quickly into our homes via the mass media that as an audience we tend to be less affected, less moved, less shocked, in total less *sensitive*.

'In the emergence of the yob, the *Sun* bears a far greater share of responsibility, than all the lager in the land.'

(Richard Ingrams, *Observer*, 23 April 1989, p. 14)

Another process that is used by the media is manipulation especially in news coverage, by the very *ordering of items*. This process which may be unconscious or deliberate, works by presenting a news item against which there may be strong public feeling. This item is immediately followed by one which may be *associated* with it in the public mind, and the association will taint the second item. For example:

1 { Item 1   The Russian Chernobyl nuclear power station explosion.
    Item 2   Safety at Sellafield nuclear power station, Cumbria.

2 { Item 1   A terrorist attack on an aeroplane.
    Item 2   IRA activity in Northern Ireland.

3 { Item 1   A child in the care of the local authority is killed by a parent.
    Item 2   A pay rise claim by local authority social workers.

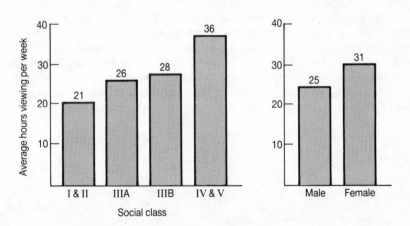

Fig. 7.1 Who watches TV? (Reproduced from *Social Trends*, 1988, with permission.) It is perhaps not surprising that women watch more TV than men as they spend more time in the home. Members of lower social classes (Registrar General's classification) use TV as a cheap form of entertainment.

It is not difficult to see how such association can work – and also to see how negative it can be. These items might not be related in any way, and yet one will colour the other simply because of the ordering. The working of this can be clearly seen in the case of TV and radio, but the same is also true for the press. Newspaper stories can be run side by side where their close proximity can easily spark association. Not everyone will be aware of this process, therefore they will be oblivious of its working and subtle effect.

Personalizing issues

It appears that an increasing trend in the media generally is to personalize issues. This was noticed very markedly during the year long miner's strike of 1984–5. The original cause of the dispute was the threatened or planned closure of certain pits. However, for the media it soon became a struggle between the personalities of Ian Macgregor, the National Coal Board (now British Coal) Chairman, and Arthur Scargill, the President of the National Union of Miners. It is easy to see how tempting it is to do this, for it provides more of what the media call 'human interest' input and it might fulfil the need for new 'angles' on the dispute. Having said this, many observers commented on how the issues got lost beneath the more trivial coverage of individuals' personal and private lives.

The personalizing of issues probably accounts for the popularity of stories of the Royal Family and of the growing number of soap operas on the radio, and especially television. They are both very much focused on people and the details of their lives, rather on issues or arguments.

In conclusion it has to be said that we cannot make very definite statements about what effect the media has. However, as it is often our *only* way of learning about what is happening in our society and the wider world, it obviously has some effect on what we call *public opinion*, and this effect is important. Public opinion is a very difficult term to define because there is such a diversity of opinion on such a wide range of issues. There is, however, a certain amount of broad agreement. The way in which money pours in for such charitable causes as famine relief (e.g. the annual 'live' Telethons) or disaster funds, proves how effectively the public can be mobilized through media coverage. However, many question marks over media effect do remain.

The following diagram illustrates how the intervention of the media can affect the events it is reporting.

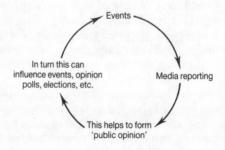

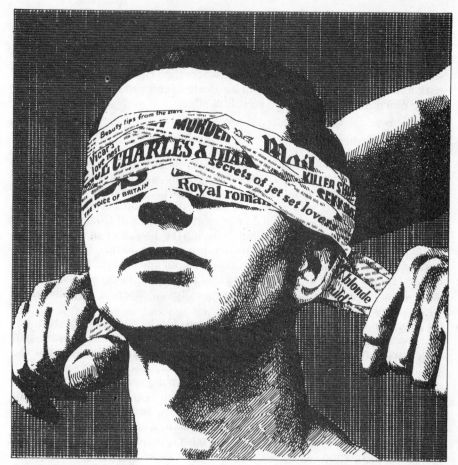

Fig. 7.2 Blinded by trivia – what effect does the press have on us? By Ingram Pinn. (Reproduced with permission from Campaign for Press Freedom and Leeds Postcards.)

A very clear example of the effect of the media was provided by the Strangeways Prison Siege in Manchester in April 1990. The fact that the prisoners involved broke through onto the roof of the jail meant that they could be directly observed from outside the walls by television cameras and press photographers. What could have remained an internal prison-system problem became a 'media event'. The prison was, in a very real sense, 'opened up' to public scrutiny. This had a clear effect on the prisoners involved in the siege who then 'played to the gallery' of waiting and watching media people. The final five prisoners even orchestrated their eventual descent from the roof, in a mechanical hoist, in full view of the world's media.

Media attention also brought relatives and a large number of the public to the scene. Some of those present cheered as the hoist was lowered and the five men were returned to custody at the conclusion of the siege – 6.22 pm on 25 April. The timing actually meant the event was covered 'live' by national television and radio broadcasts. Malcolm Pithers, writing the following day in the *Independent* said: 'The siege also raises questions about constant media coverage of the riot. Some officials believe that allowing the inmates to "play" to a television audience may have prolonged the siege' (26 April 1990, p. 2).

What images do the mass media present?

Those who do not fit neatly into the conventional nuclear family structure and whose lives do not have a nine to five full-time working routine are often portrayed very negatively by the mass media. It is easy to detect prejudice, bias and stereotyping when news stories involve such groups of people. Black people, some women's groups, gay men and lesbians, gypsies and 'travelling families', and so-called 'hippy' groups such as the 'peace convoy', can all suffer from media *distortion*.

The majority of newspaper editors and radio or television producers do not share the way of life of such groups or understand their values and attitudes, so we repeatedly find them 'putting such people down' and representing them in a very trivialized and negative way.

One newspaper reported the eviction of a number of so-called 'hippies', who formed part of the 'peace convoy', from land in the New Forest (*Daily Telegraph*, 10 June 1986, p. 1). Not only was the tone 'negative' throughout, but the article was also notable for the 'militaristic' language of the reporting. It was as if a war was being fought between the 'hippy convoy' and the police.

Under headlines 'Bedraggled Hippies Dispersed' (the police had woken the camp members at 4 am!) and 'Dawn Swoop Catches Hippy Camp Napping', it referred to a 'meticulously executed operation' (by the police). It referred to 'the defeated and bedraggled hippy army', as being 'decommissioned' by the police. The Chief Constable, John Duke, in charge of 'Operation Daybreak' said that the 'invasion' of the hippies was 'neutralized' by the police. The language and style of reporting created an image of the convoy as being 'alien' to, and set apart from, wider 'conventional', 'normal' and 'decent' society.

In 1986, 29.8 million people (i.e. adults aged over 15) read a daily national newspaper, while even more, 32.8 million, read one on Sunday. The impact of the press is potentially very powerful, and such negative images of women, black people, or people with unconventional life styles, go into a very large number of homes and are 'consumed' by a large proportion of the public.

Three specific examples of how negative portrayal works against women, black people and disabled people are listed below.

Women

The media has a gender stereotyped image of women. Elements of this may be that women are obsessed by their appearance and want to look attractive to men; that they have certain characteristics which include caring, nurturing, servicing others and lacking ambition and drive! This will be reflected in the media representation of the jobs they do. Women will be shown as employed in nursing, social care, secretarial work, catering and housework. Women's interests, as perceived by most of the media, tend to be very narrow – e.g. fashion, cosmetics, cooking, or generally looking after their men! This trivializes women and ignores the more serious issues with which they are concerned.

'People tend to see women's topics as either militant lesbianism or how to make a dress out of a lampshade!' (Roma Feltein, Controller of Women's Programmes and Commissioning Editor, British Satellite Broadcasting, *Guardian* 6 March 1990, p. 38).

Women's marginality is also evident when their role as radio and television presenters is considered. They are less numerous than men and they are more likely to be restricted to magazine-style women's programmes. The more serious and important programmes are 'fronted' by men. Furthermore, women are generally expected to be 'attractive', and are usually under 50 years of age. Men are not similarly restricted.

The media has also created its own specific images of women, the best example of which is probably the 'Page 3 girl', presented by the *Sun* newspaper and copied by others. Today many national daily and Sunday newspapers carry pictures of naked, semi-naked or scantily-clad women in the knowledge that these pictures will sell papers.

> '. . . this paper's boring mindless mean
> full of pornography the kind that's clean
> where william hickey meets michael caine
> again and again and again and again
> i've seen millionaires on the dhss
> but i've never seen a nipple in the *daily express*
> (Cooper Clarke, J., you've never seen a nipple
> in the *daily express*. Reproduced from *10 years*
> *in an open necked shirt*, Hutchinson, 1983,
> p. 108, with permission)

In addition, the media also compounds negative stereotypes found in wider society, e.g. the 'nagging housewife', 'difficult mother-in-law', 'dumb blonde', 'sexy secretary'. All this adds up to a portrayal of women which is unfair, untruthful, and does not accurately reflect the diversity of their interests, roles and occupations.

Black people

One of the most important 'messages' which our media sends black people in Britain is that their life-styles should conform to white society. There is very little representation of black peoples' cultural identity in the main-stream media. Black people are largely 'invisible' in advertising and in news coverage. If they *are* featured in news items it is often because a disturbance has occurred, for example, during the annual Notting Hill Carnival in West London. Rarely is such coverage balanced by positive representation.

> 'When we win races, we're British, but when we mug, we're black.'
> (Lorna Lee, Kilburn College Student, 1989)

Although a very small number of black people have appeared on TV screens to read news bulletins, generally the news is delivered by white readers with 'classic Oxford' or 'received' English. Even regional accents or dialects are hard to find amongst white presenters. The message to black people is that they are *marginal* to mainstream culture. If a programme is specifically designed for a minority, ethnic audience it will often go out at an unusual viewing time, perhaps very late at night or in the early morning, although some TV channels and radio stations are rectifying this situation.

Some time ago, there were several 'stories' circulating in the press that attacked Labour Party controlled local authorities in London and represented black people in a negative way. Haringey council was supposed to have banned black dustbin liners as being 'racist'; Hackney, Islington and Brent councils were said to have banned the nursery rhyme 'Baa Baa Black Sheep' in their schools; and Haringey was supposed to be teaching West Indian dialect in schools. Several other accounts trivialized women or gay people's issues. When the Goldsmiths' College Media Research Group (1987), a part of London University, investigated the background to these items, they found that 'not one of these stories is accurate' (p. 1). Some significant details were wrong, or misleading, others were complete inventions. The research appears to contain serious implications about the integrity of the press.

Disabled people
As we have seen representations of people in the mass media tend to be white, often middle class and very conventionally placed within their nuclear families. They also tend to be able-bodied. There are extremely few disabled people, whether physically or mentally impaired, represented in the media generally especially in commercial advertising, yet one in seven people has a disability. Although it is not always possible to tell that someone is disabled from seeing them, hearing their voice, or reading what they write, people with a disability have been largely rendered invisible. Just as it does with women and black people, the media again fails to portray life in our society in a realistic and accurate way. Often a *token* disabled person will appear in a documentary, or a series or soap opera, but they are rarely centrally placed. In addition, very limited air-time or column inches are devoted specifically to the special needs and interests of disabled people.

Comment
An examination of the images the mass media presents of women, black people, disabled people and a variety of 'minority groups', reveals a partial, one-sided and distorted picture. We find *sexism*, *racism* and *handicappism* reinforced. We do not recognize the society in which we live – it is an image 'edited' by those who make programmes and who own and edit newspapers.

Who owns the media?

Rupert Murdoch owns the largest media enterprise in the world. Britain is only one of several countries in which he has an interest. Apart from Sky TV, the first satellite company in this country, he owns three national daily papers, the *Sun*, *Today* and *The Times*, and two national Sunday papers, the *News of the World* and *Sunday Times*. Profits for his News International company were £175 million in the year 1988–9, which was a £25 millions rise above the previous year. The other chief media magnate in this country is Robert Maxwell who owns one daily and two Sunday national newspapers, the *Daily Mirror*, *Sunday Mirror* and *The People*. Together, they account for about 75

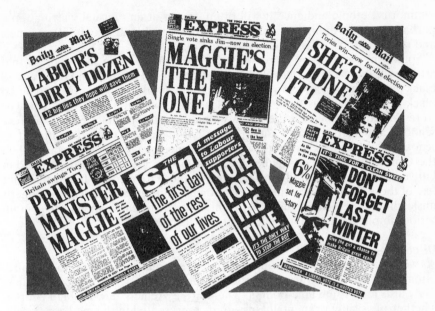

A selection of national newspaper front pages at the time of the 1979 general election by George Brown. (Reproduced from Campaign for Press Freedom and Leeds Postcards.)

per cent of all national daily papers sold and 85 per cent of Sunday nationals. Murdoch's papers are read by a total readership of 30 million adults – 13.7 million during the week and 16.3 million on Sundays. Maxwell's papers are read by 8.9 million in the week and 17.7 million on Sundays.

As we can see, the power of the press is concentrated in very few hands and this process has been going on for at least 50 years. Newspapers are increasingly owned, if not by 'press barons', then by conglomerates – companies which have a wide variety of interests in a number of different activities; these might include leisure and sports activities, hotels, manufacturing and banking.

> 'I run the paper purely for the purpose of making propaganda, and with no other motive.'
> (Lord Beaverbrook, owner of the *Daily Express*, in 1948. Cited in Royal Commission on the Press 1947–9, para 87 p. 25 HMSO, 1949. Command 7700)

Over the past few years the national press have gained a substantial interest in the shrinking number of regional daily newspapers. Choice has become more limited as titles have merged or disappeared, and some would say that this is detrimental in a democratic, pluralistic society.

Large proportions of other areas of the media are also owned by a few companies. Since the 1940s a duopoly has owned all the cinema 'chains' in this country. The only present alternatives to this are a few small, locally run, independent 'arts' or civic cinemas. In television, just four channels exist at

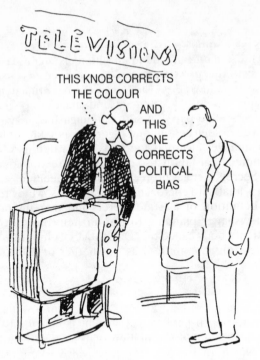

TELEVISIONS)

THIS KNOB CORRECTS
THE COLOUR

AND
THIS
ONE
CORRECTS
POLITICAL
BIAS

(Reproduced with permission of Colin Wheeler.)

present, apart from cable and satellite: two from the BBC and two run by the 15 independent companies. The government is currently in the process of 'deregulating' television and radio, but it is uncertain at the present time what *real* changes, if any, this will bring about.

Owners of newspapers can have a great deal of control, if they so choose, over what material is published. It is, however, very difficult to be accurate about what control exists. It can be hidden and subtle – one may need to actually be inside the organization in order to gain a true picture.

What is easier to judge is the political complexion of the product. With the demise of the *Daily Herald* – a Labour Party supporting paper in 1964, and *News Chronicle*, a Liberal Party supporting paper in 1960, our national newspapers are almost all of a conservative nature and are broadly in sympathy with the Conservative Party's policies, values and opinions. This means that more liberal and left-wing political views are not as fully aired as conservative attitudes. The views of the Labour movement, the Trade Unions, and a variety of minority groups' interests are unlikely to be accurately or fully represented in the mass media, especially in our national daily newspapers. To a certain extent minorities have found expression of their views by publishing their own newspapers for example *The Voice, Asian Times, Daily Jang* and the *Irish Times*.

Is our media free?

There has always been some kind of restriction on the freedom of the press and media. The libel laws enable an individual who feels slighted to seek redress in the courts. Access to this process, however, is limited because it can be very expensive! Newspapers have therefore always to bear this in mind when they consider publishing. Recently huge financial damages of over £1 million have been awarded to a libelled party. A satirical magazine such as *Private Eye* is continually involved in such actions and regards it as a 'fact of life', although at times the size of damages awarded continue to threaten its very existence.

Certain government legislation also restricts the freedom of the press. Since 1911 the Official Secrets Act has protected what are deemed 'state secrets'; this means the media is unable to encroach in certain areas. Many feel the Act is far too wide in its definition of a 'state secret' and that limitation should be introduced. A newspaper planning to run an item on an aspect of official secrecy is advised by a body called the 'D – Notices Committee' (The Defence, Press and Broadcasting Committee) as to whether or not to go ahead with publication. This voluntary system appears to have worked well as far as the press is concerned.

In 1988, the government introduced a Local Government Act, in which Section 28 outlawed the 'promotion of homosexuality by local authorities'. Later, on 19th October 1988, the government introduced new legislation which restricted 'live' media presentation of statements made by outlawed organizations in Northern Ireland. The practical working of the law would seem to be rather ridiculous – for example, an actor can read the words spoken on television, but the actual speaker cannot be shown speaking.

In fact Northern Ireland has become a special case in terms of the freedom of the press. For example, under Section II of the Prevention of Terrorism Act 1984, the BBC in Belfast were forced, in March 1988, to hand over to the Royal Ulster Constabulary film footage they had made of an IRA funeral at which people were killed. The film was to be used by the police to identify the people present. After protest, the film was duly handed over. The same thing happened in Trafalgar Square, London, in April 1990, following a demonstration against the introduction of the 'Poll Tax'. Photographs were requested from newspapers by the Police.

So far, we have looked at *official* external controls over the media. There also exists a number of consumer organizations or pressure groups which provide some kind of grass roots reflection of public opinion. These *can* act as an external control and bring about greater media accountability. The best known is probably the organization formed by Mary Whitehouse, for a long time a media campaigner, called the *National Listeners and Viewers Association*. They have concentrated on the portrayal of sex and violence, especially on TV, and are concerned about the detrimental effect such material can have on the consumer, particularly younger people and children.

In 1979 the Campaign for Press and Broadcasting Freedom was launched. It states as a central aim 'that *everyone* should have the right to information, news and opinion, and the right of access to the printed word and to the airwaves, so long as such rights are not abused to incite violence, race hatred or sexual discrimination'. They have a London office, salaried staff, and conduct research and publish a range of material. A National Council, as well as regional groups, has specialist sections represented on it – dealing with black, gay, women's and disability issues. A large number of organizations, including Trade Unions and academic institutions, are affiliated and many well known people act as sponsors. In August 1987, the CPBF organized a public reading from the book *Spycatcher*, by Peter Wright (which was banned at that time) at Speakers' Corner, Hyde Park, London.

Apart from *external* bodies and controls, there exist *internal* watchdog organizations. The press council receives and investigates complaints made about the press. The BBC, set up in 1926, and the Independent Broadcasting Authority, set up as the Independent Television Authority in 1954, oversee the content of the programmes presented by each of the respective sectors.

The Advertising Standards Authority acts as a control on commercial advertising. They investigate complaints and will uphold a complaint if they believe it causes 'grave and widespread offence'. This could include the portrayal of overt racism or violence towards women. However, much material it does approve of may be considered objectionable because it is exploitive and distasteful.

The media and social care

'They (the press) create a poor public image of social workers and morale in the profession suffers to the extent where some authorities now face difficulties in recruiting staff.'
(Bob Franklin and Gerry Lavery, *Community Care*, 23 March 1989, p. 26)

Amongst the millions of news items every year on radio, TV and in the press, only a very small proportion will actually report on the work of social carers, and it will almost always be when something has gone drastically wrong. The media is not interested in reporting all the many examples of good, positive practice and fine achievement that follows hard and thoughtful work. It is the death of a child of a family with whom the Social Services Department of the local authority are working, or the sexual assault of a boy in a community home, or abuse of elderly people in residential care that will be deemed 'newsworthy' because it is the kind of 'bad news' which most of our mass media relishes.

Representations of carers in the media

'Social workers do a job . . . which requires rare devotion and commitment . . . If the media were to hail success as often as we hunt failure we would serve both truth and our fellow citizens to greater effect than we do at the moment.'
(Jonathan Dimbleby, 'Witness', in *Social Work Today* (Supplement) 1988, p. 2)

As with women, black people and people with disabilities, we find that the representations of carers in the media are often stereotypical. Today, the traditional image of 'Lady Bountiful' – a rich, white, middle class woman with spare time on her hands has been replaced by the 'do-gooder', sometimes represented as 'interfering'.

'Social workers have a simple answer to the stress, over-work and violent abuse they face in their job. They should quit. These well-meaning do-gooders provide a crutch which stops people helping themselves.'

(Reproduced from the *Daily Mirror*, 30 May 1989, p. 24)

More recently, this has given way to the image of the young male or female radical who enters social care as a career and who seeks good prospects and a good salary. We find variations on these themes – from 'meddlers' (*Daily Express*, 18 November 1987) through 'hysterical, powerful personalities' (*Sunday Telegraph*, 10 July 1987) to 'authoritarian bureaucrats' (*The Times*, 17 June 1987) and 'abusers of authority, hysterical and malignant callous youngsters who absorb moral-free marxoid (sic) sociological theories' (*Daily Mail*, 7 July 1988).

All these comments were made about social workers in the Cleveland child abuse case (cited in *Community Care*, 23 March 1989, p. 27) and portray the conservative press in strident mood! None implies that these particular writers have great confidence in, or admiration of, social carers. One important question must be, do the targets of these statements take them seriously, or will they be dismissive of them?

'He hated the press as he hated advertising and television, he hated mass media, the relentless persuasion of the twentieth century.'

(John Le Carré, *Call For The Dead*)

Conclusion

We have discovered that our mass media does not always reflect truthfully and accurately what goes on in our society. A true, full and accurate account does not appear because it is distorted by a range of factors including limited ownership, profit seeking and advertising. The cultural attitudes and values of the media, partly a product of this, lead to certain prejudices and stereotyping, most especially of the more marginal, least powerful groups in our society. It is such groups, black people, women, travellers, gays and lesbians, and those leading unconventional life-styles, who are the victim of a 'labelling process' which often stigmatizes them. It is also noted that such groups have very little, if any, right of reply.

In one way, the media reflects society – both are constantly changing. Some sections of the media *are* making real efforts to change in a progressive way, to address sexism and racism; to be more aware of the needs and public image of women, black people, the elderly and people with disabilities. This is partly in response to public criticism, and it is encouraging. As consumers we should certainly applaud such efforts. For example, the BBC has committed itself to staffing levels which accurately reflect the composition of society by the year 2000. This policy will apply at all levels, and in all departments.

Finally, we should remind ourselves that we have a responsibility, both to ourselves and others, to develop a critical sense towards what we see, hear and read in the media. In the end, *we* have to decide what is and what is not factual, accurate and truthful. If we succeed in this, we will be more able to deliver a more effective service to those for whom we care.

Both read the Bible day and night, but thou read'st black where I read white.

William Blake (1757–1827)

Exercises

1. The following article appeared in the *Sun* newspaper on 22 July 1990 in response to the announcement of a delay in government implementation of new community care proposals.

'*How to waste £820m*
The Government is under fire for delaying for two years reforms of community care.

This would put local councils in charge of an £820 million budget designed to help the elderly, mentally ill and disabled.

If Ministers have any sense they will scrap the plans altogether.

Once councils get their hands on that kind of cash, we all know what will happen.

First, a Director of Community affairs will be appointed on fifty grand a year. Then three assistants and deputies will be recruited. They will all need company cars, secretaries and public relations advisers.

Legion
Hundreds of community care outreach co-ordinators will be hired, along with a legion of outreach co-ordinator co-ordinators.

Then there will have to be dozens of race and gay advisers to ensure there is no discrimination in the provision of care. They will need to be housed in a giant new office block, costing millions and probably named after Bishop Tutu.

Then someone will realize that there is no money left for old people's homes and meals on wheels. There will be 'cuts'. And the Government will get the blame.'

(p. 6)

Comment on the validity of the argument.

2. Select 10 TV advertisements at random and consider the message they convey about the roles of women and men. Examine, for example, such things as who does the talking? Who is in the background? What style of clothing are the people wearing? Who has the key roles? What relevance do such factors have to the product being advertised?

3. With regard to the following social groups:

- the working class
- women
- black people
- people with disabilities
- travellers
- gay people
- the elderly
- people with a mental illness
- people with learning difficulties

consider how they are represented in one or more of the following media areas: news, documentaries and current affairs programmes, 'soap operas' and TV documentaries, and children's programmes.

4. *Women in the press*
Select two newspapers or magazines. Note what kinds of subjects or topics are dealt with and consider what this implies about public perceptions of women in society.
5. Do you consider that minority groups should have separate media representation in newspapers, magazines or on radio or television? Consider this with specific relation to the following groups:

- gays and lesbians
- members of ethnic minorities
- people with disabilities
- elderly people.

Questions for essays or discussion

1. How can disabled people and members of other minority groups in our society present themselves more positively in the media?
2. Is it acceptable for a private individual to own a number of national newspapers?
3. The portrayal of social care events in the media is generally negative and is frequently sensationalized. Considering the large number of people engaged as either informal or paid carers, how do you account for their low profile within the media?
4. How are black people represented in the media?
5. As members of a democratic society we have a right to know what is going on. Should the police or other powerful social agency be allowed to withhold information from us?
6. Does the mass media have a direct effect on people or events?

Further reading

Academic sources

Curran, J., *et al.* (eds). *Bending Reality – the State of the Media*, Pluto Press, 1986. Describes how certain groups in our society e.g. women, ethnic minorities, trade unionists, peace campaigners and gays are consistently misrepresented by our media. It attempts to answer the question – what can be done about this?

Glasgow University Media Group, *Bad News* (Routledge, 1976), *More Bad News* (Routledge, 1980) and *Really Bad News* (Writers and Readers Publishing Co-operative, 1982). Studies how TV in Britain 'shapes' the news. The group, established in 1974, recorded news programmes over a six month period, focusing particularly on industry and the economy. News as the 'manufactured production of ideology'.

Goldsmiths College Media Research Group, *Media Coverage of Local Government in London*, Methuen, 1987. A research study of several cases of distorted media coverage concerning a number of Labour controlled London boroughs and race issues.

Hall, S., *et al.* – *Policing the Crisis – Mugging, the State, Law and Order*, Macmillan, 1978. An academic study of how the media (along with other state agencies such as the police) introduced 'mugging' as being exclusively a 'black crime'. It charts the process, and considers the implications.

Hennessy, P., *What the Papers Never Said*, Portcullis Press, 1985. A study of the 'Westminster Lobby' and three case studies of past news items which, with hindsight, are seen to have been reported in very incomplete and unsatisfactory ways.

Tunstall, J., *The Media in Britain*, Constable, 1983. Very comprehensive coverage of all aspects of the media, including a history since 1945. A great deal of facts and figures.

Other literary sources

Benn, T., *Arguments for Socialism*, Penguin, 1980.

Gould, T., *Inside Outsider – The Life and Times of Colin MacInnes*, Penguin, 1986.

Green, J., *Days in the Life – Voices from the English Underground 1961–1971*, Heinemann, 1988.

Pilger, J., *Heroes*, Pan, 1989.

Tatchell, P., *The Battle for Bermondsey*, Heretic Press, 1983.

Thompson, E. P., *The Heavy Dancers*, Merlin Press, 1985.

Films or plays

Kazan, E., *The Last Tycoon*, US, 1976.

Lumet, S., *Network*, US, 1976.

Pakula, A.J., *All The President's Men*, US, 1976.

Welles, O., *Citizen Kane*, US, 1941.

8 Social change, welfare and community care

Social care does not take place within a vacuum. It is therefore important that social carers are informed in their work by an understanding of wider social and political issues. Whether a carer is tending to the needs of a dependent relative, or she or he is employed as a paid carer by a statutory, voluntary or private organization, she or he needs to be aware of the relationship between the client and society in general. Additionally, carers need to acknowledge their own relationship with the wider society and the dynamic relationship between themselves and those for whom they care, so that their own positions and that of their clients can be seen within the same social context.

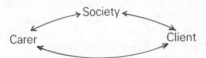

The above figure stresses the *relationship* between the carer and wider society. Notice the direction of the arrows indicating a two way process.

Most people who choose to enter the field of social care or social work may do so for two main reasons. Primarily they may be motivated by a sense of compassion, which may spring from deep-seated spiritual, moral or cultural grounds or may simply be an expression of their desire to 'work with people' or 'to do something worthwhile'. The other main concern felt by many entrants to the field of social care is to be able to become involved in purposeful social change and to be able to help create a more just society.

Change occurs within society all the time; some of these changes are gradual whilst others take place more quickly. The effect of some changes are minimal but others have a huge and lasting impact. Social carers, by the very nature of their work, are inextricably involved in the process of social change.

Consider for example a situation where a carer is preparing a physically disabled man for bed. By attending to his physical needs and ensuring that his cultural needs are met and that the client's dignity and self respect are maintained, the carer automatically becomes involved, however minimally, in the process of purposeful social change. The intervention itself has an immediate effect on the client's well-being, not least because his physical comfort may allow him now to obtain the rest his body needs. If care has been carried out positively it may well have the effect of increasing the client's confidence and independence and contribute to reducing his reliance on other people. The carer's involvement with the client may thus affect the lives of other people – perhaps those neighbours, relatives or other carers who would otherwise be responsible for the man's care.

Similarly, but on a larger scale, the impact of, for example, the introduction of a group living scheme in an elderly person's home which gives residents more autonomy, opportunities to take risks, to make decisions and to do more things for themselves, can be seen as a clearer more dramatic example of social change. The ramifications of such a move may spread beyond the walls of the home; the ensuing increased interaction and the greater satisfaction felt amongst residents who are significantly more involved in their own lives may coincide with an increase in staff morale and a growing sense of purpose within the establishment. Further, the effects of this might be felt by all visitors to the establishment and those who share the lives of the workers in the home.

Greater social change clearly occurs following the introduction of new or amendments to existing legislation and social policy. Whilst these changes are formally introduced by the government, instigation for change may well have occurred outside. Agitation by consumers, practitioners, professional associations and trades unions, the success of good practice and research, can all directly affect changes in policy.

A carer's understanding of wider society needs to go beyond the general impression created by much of the media and official organizations. The image projected is often of a stable, balanced society that rewards best those who are talented or hard working, and ascribes failure either to individual pathology or misfortune. In other words the individual is considered responsible for her or his circumstances. It is rarely admitted that hardship is often structurally determined. Instead the impression of social justice is fostered and notions of equality of opportunity and equal rights are taken for granted and considered to be the very basis upon which our society operates.

Anything other than a superficial examination of society will show this picture to be a false one. Throughout this book we have looked at the divisions within society and at the structural inequalities which affect people's lives and their ability to fulfil themselves. In particular we have noted the damaging effects of prejudice, discrimination and bias delivered by individuals and organizations from a position of power.

Structural inequality

Many people would now argue, judging by the evidence of their own circumstances and personal observation, that society has greatly prospered over the past decade. They would refer to the greater numbers of people who now own their own homes, the increased participation in share ownership and the general increase in consumer consumption. This new level of affluence is assumed to be shared by all members including those who are poor who have at least benefited from the 'trickle-down' effect of economic growth.

Whilst it is true to say that living standards for the majority of the population rose through the 1980s, not all society's members benefited from economic prosperity. In fact a substantial proportion of the poor became relatively poorer and divisions within society widened during the period. Observers have pointed to the growing polarization which exists within society between the increasingly well off sectors and those people who are poor. The very existence of the recently recognized emerging 'underclass' bears witness to this polarization. As we have seen the trapped and fixed nature of the 'underclass' severely restricts its members lives. Many are totally dependent on state benefits, the real value of which has been threatened by a number of factors.

Since 1987, a higher than expected inflation rate has meant that the levels of benefits have not been fully realized. Carey Oppenheim of the Child Poverty Action Group, noted other factors which have affected those people who are poor, when she stated that 'The safety net has many more holes – the burden of paying Social Fund loans and paying the poll tax and water rates, means hidden losses for many claimants' (*Social Work Today*, 7 June 1990, p. 4). The greatly increased draw on charities in Britain is further testimony to the worsening financial situation of this group of people. (See the FWA figures on p. 194.) However, it is not only those who belong to the so-called 'underclass' whose lives are restricted and who are therefore unable to share fully society's rewards. Others include those in low paid work; those suffering from ill health or a disability; some single parent families; some of those who are in retirement, especially those who had low paid jobs or who had breaks in regular employment. All of these groups experience a restricted involvement in society. What such people have in common amounts to a reduced citizenship and a marginalized existence.

The widespread nature of degradation amid prosperity has brought comment from various organizations, including the church. In December 1989 an all denominational group, Church Action on Poverty (CAP), condemned government policies and public apathy towards poverty. Their manifesto put forward a new 'penitential rite' which they wanted added to church communion services all over the country. Among recommendations were that the priest or minister taking the service should say 'it cannot be right' before each paragraph:

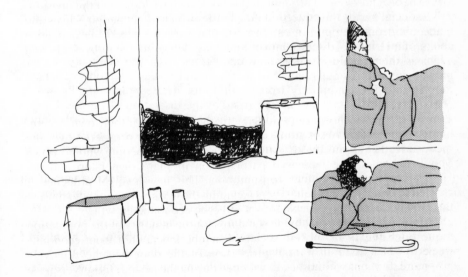

'It cannot be right that young people are living in cardboard boxes.' Church Action on Poverty, 1989.

'It cannot be right that some have to survive on less than £60 per week while others receive pay rises of £3000 per week.'
'It cannot be right that young people are living in cardboard boxes.'
'It cannot be right to cut taxes as an incentive to the rich, but to reduce incomes to spur on the poor.'

Other topics covered in the incantation include benefit levels, racism, hospital closures, teacher shortages, long term unemployment and short term job schemes.

Social policy changes

Social policy changes, particularly those related to welfare benefits, can be seen to have contributed to the disadvantage felt by those people who are poor. The attack on benefits and the 'dependency culture' has been aimed at reducing the number of people who are financially dependent on state aid. Whilst this directive recognizes the debilitating effect that dependency can have on those who receive benefit, the policy does not acknowledge that people receiving benefit do not always do so from choice. Claimants are unable to find an alternative source of income owing to a variety of reasons including poor health or disability, lack of appropriate employment opportunities, and the need to remain at home in order to care for a dependent relative or to look after young children. Social security changes, most notably the introduction of the *Social Fund*, the various restrictions on availability of housing benefit for young people, as well as general reductions in the real value of many other benefits, have caused the relative poverty of those people who are on benefits to become intensified.

The Social Fund, introduced in April 1988, replaced single payment grants made to income support recipients for essential household items such as cookers and fridges. Instead claimants may now apply for a discretionary 'loan' which is then repaid by automatic deductions from the claimants weekly income support. A small number of grants are still available but only to persons moving into the community from institutions. These grants are known as community care grants and are awarded at the discretion of the local social security office which operates within a fixed budget. In other words only a limited number of loans or grants can be made. It is estimated that two thirds of the social fund's applicants are sent away 'empty handed' (*Community Care*, 10 May 1990, p. 4).

As a consequence increasing numbers of people are seeking help from charitable organizations. Charities however have not got the resources to meet the growing demand. For example according to the Family Welfare Association (FWA), 'In 1981/2, the Association had sufficient funds available to meet requests for help in all but two weeks of the year, but by 1985/6, the number of weeks in which no funds were available had risen to 20, and in 1988 it stood at 39 – more than nine months of the year in which no money could be allocated' (*Community Care*, 10 May 1990, p. 1). The changes in the board and lodging arrangements have meant many young people without a permanent address have not been able to claim benefit. This factor combined with the growing shortage of cheap, accessible accommodation, especially in our major towns and cities, has seen a rise in the number of young people who are homeless, and a corresponding rise in the number of people who are begging on the streets. (Over 3000 people are annually prosecuted under the 1824 Vagrancy Act in London alone.)

The sight of young people begging; of people sleeping rough in shop doorways or in cardboard boxes; of women and men with alcohol-related problems, many of whom are in need of proper medical attention, sitting in our parks or city centres; and the alarming number of distressed adults who are clearly mentally ill, who are left to wander and shuffle against the back drop of conspicuous affluence, stands as an indictment to a so-called 'developed society' and provides evidence of the gross inequality which has been created.

Dr Bob Holman, a community worker, who works and lives in Easterhouse, Glasgow observed 'I have spent over 25 years in the world of welfare. At no time has the gap between the poorest and the rest of society been greater than now. At no time have I seen so many families without goods which others take for granted. At no other time have I witnessed parents having to cut down on their already inadequate food intake for the sake of their children (*Social Work Today*, 22 February 1990, p. 21).

Social policy and social services provision

The end of the 1980s saw the beginning of a period of fundamental change in social policy and social services provision which is expected to continue

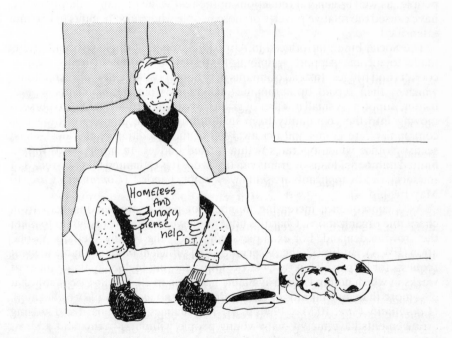

A common sight in many cities.

throughout the 1990s. During this period the policy of *community care*, albeit not new, came into prominence. It had been operating since the mid 1960s with the transfer from hospital of long stay mentally ill adults and people with learning difficulties back into the community.

The idea of community care has been debated for many years and was first recommended by the Percy Commission in 1957 which reported on mental health to the government and preceded the Mental Health Act (1959). The Act chose to ignore the recommendation that some patients may be better cared for in the community than in large scale institutions. Over the years other reports ensued, most notably, *Better Services for the Mentally Handicapped* (1971), and the Audit Commission (1986) *Making a Reality of Community Care*. Finally in December 1986, Sir Roy Griffiths was asked by the Secretary of State for Social Services, 'to review the way in which public funds are used to support community care policy and to advise on options which improve the use of these funds as a contribution to more effective community care'. His report entitled *Community Care: Agenda for Action*, was published in 1988. The focus of the report was not solely the care of those people returning to the community from institutional settings, rather it was concerned with the care already being carried out in the community by carers for dependent relatives. The report, (echoing the Barclay Report ten years earlier) acknowledged:

'Families, friends, neighbours and other local people provide the majority of care in response to needs which they are uniquely well placed to identify and respond to. This will continue to be the primary means by which people are enabled to live normal lives in community settings.'

(Griffiths Report, 1988, p. 5)

The level of funding was not written into the remit so therefore there was no attempt to assess the adequacy of current funding.

The principle of community care has an appeal to a wide range of political ideologies: to some politicians it represents a more humane service delivery and to others it is conceived of as being a potentially cheaper way of providing services. With regard to the actual costs, all welfare groups would argue that community care should never be considered as a cheap alternative to institutional care. Care within the community, if it is to be provided appropriately, has its equivalent costs. They go on to say that without proper funding community care policies will not meet needs.

Consider, for example, the cost of setting up a four person group home in an ordinary house with full time social work support for adults with learning difficulties who are being rehabilitated into the community. Disregarding the cost of the building, the staffing costs alone would need to be based on the cost of employing five full-time equivalent social care workers (after taking account of average training needs, sick leave, holiday entitlement and shift rotas).

In its response to the Griffiths Report, the Equal Opportunities Commission was concerned, 'that the emphasis on community care policies will increase the domestic burden on women and restrict their opportunities for paid employment and their personal prospects' (1988, p. 1) The Commission also felt that 'the Health and Social Service provision allocated to a household with a disabled member should be based on the needs of that person, and regardless of the sex of the carer'. This is a result of the research findings by the EOC, that women constitute the majority of carers and that generally they receive less health and social services support than male carers.

The Race Equality Unit (REU) of the National Institute for Social Work (NISW) pointed out that the Griffiths Report contained only one paragraph about multi-racial perspectives. According to the REU this was significant since 'the concept of community care is not a new one in the black communities. The problem has been the abuse of this by white organizations which, in the absence of appropriate services to certain black user groups, have expected black families, community and voluntary organizations to provide care in the community however appropriate or inappropriate that has been' (1989, p. 1). The REU recommended improved recognition and communication with the black community and voluntary care groups before the implementation of any community care legislation.

Residential care

Within the residential sector great changes have recently been made and will continue to be made throughout the 1990s. The Wagner Report, *Residential Care – A Positive Choice* (1988) sought to separate residential provision from its traditional negative image. Instead, residential care should be seen to be a purposeful resource; a 'positive choice' for consumers of social care. For Wagner, residential care should no longer be a dumping ground or a last resort for clients unable to be cared for in any other setting. Rather it should be seen as an integral part of community care. It is not seen as different in kind from other types of provision but as a pattern of care provided with accommodation. It is described as a form of 'supported housing' or 'accommodation plus support'. Wagner includes as a result; sheltered housing, group living, cluster homes and even boarding out (fostering) as forms of residential care. The report was keen to break down the artificial distinction between residential and community care which has the undesirable effect of separating residential care from the rest of the community.

'Choice' is the central theme of the report with the emphasis being on the client's right to exercise personal preferences between genuine alternatives. The clients involvement in the decision making process is acknowledged at all times, as is her or his right to full dignity and respect for cultural preference.

Community care

On 16 November 1989, the government published a White Paper on Community care entitled *Caring for People – Community Care: The Next Decade and Beyond*. It followed a long period of uncertainty after publication of the Griffiths report on community care. Many feared that responsibility for community care would be taken from local authorities and be given to health authorities and that widespread privatization and dismantling of public services would accompany this shift.

In fact a major transfer of responsibility did not happen. Local authorities retained responsibility for community care, but were required to work more closely with the private and voluntary sectors. The White Paper said in effect

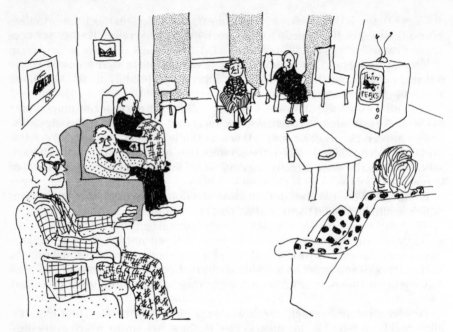

The traditional image of residential care – a thing of the past?

that local authorities will actually own residential provision and deliver services to a lesser extent than before. Instead they will become increasingly 'enablers' of service provision, making assessments and managing care, and become co-ordinators of facilities owned by others.

In what amounts to a definition of community care, the White Paper states 'Community care means providing the services and support which people who are affected by problems of ageing, mental illness, mental handicap or physical or sensory disability need to be able to live as independently as possible in their own homes or in homely settings within the community'. This policy should help such people to 'achieve their full potential'.

In the new proposals two important functions should be highlighted. First, local authorities are to be responsible for *assessment* of an individual's needs. This should be done in collaboration with any other relevant agencies, e.g. medical or nursing. 'Care packages' should then be designed in order to deliver services which will meet each individual's assessed needs. Assessments should always take account of the clients own perceptions and expressed wishes and needs.

Second, once assessment is complete a *care manager* will be nominated. This may or may not be the assessor. She or he may be employed by a Social Services Department, a Health Authority, a private or voluntary organization or may even be a carer, in many cases a relative. In the words of the White Paper, the care manager will 'take responsibility for ensuring that individuals needs are regularly reviewed, resources are managed effectively and that each service user has a single point of contact' (p. 21).

Client choice is of paramount importance, and no longer must the emphasis be on fitting a client's needs to an already existing service. Rather services should cater for individual needs, even if this means devising a new form of service delivery. This principle will hopefully mean that amongst other advantages services should be geared more appropriately to the neglected needs of ethnic minority communities.

Other duties of local authorities entail publishing three year community care plans and establishing procedures for receiving comments and complaints. Information is clearly of key importance and authorities are required to publish and disseminate clear details of the services they offer. Social Services Departments will also be more directly responsible for financial budgeting in respect of services to clients.

In July 1990 the government announced a departure from its original plans which would have seen the introduction of the White Paper proposals in April 1991. Apart from provisions which relate to mental health and new complaints procedures, full implementation has been delayed until 1993. This sudden announcement caused widespread anger and disappointment throughout the caring services and amongst individual carers. Local authorities who had been busy gearing themselves up to meet the original deadlines were especially outraged.

Amongst informal carers there was huge disappointment. Their expectations had been raised by the prospects of the new Act, under which every local authority was obliged to seek out those needing help, assess their need and draw up a plan for their care. The delay prompted Polly Toynbee to state 'Yet again, as with so many previous governments, the old and the disabled were relegated to the bottom of the waiting lists.' (*Observer*, 22 July 1990, p. 11).

As to be expected, criticism of the Health and Community Care Act proposals has been mixed. On the positive side overall administration of care remains with local authorities, who most believe are best placed for this task. It is good that care packages or programmes are to be individually based and that client choice and the wishes of clients are to be central to the whole exercise. Also good care practice should be enhanced through more rigorous assessment and care management procedures. Perhaps the major deficiencies centre around the future role of the Social Services Departments and the financing of such public services.

Sir Roy Griffiths said, shortly after the publication of the White Paper, 'I had provided a purposeful, effective and economic four wheel vehicle but the white paper has redesigned it as a three wheeler, leaving out the fourth wheel of ring-fenced funding' (*British Medical Journal*, **300**, p. 1187). Without guaranteed funding local authorities will struggle to improve community care policies.

The future plans for community care will continue to stimulate private and voluntary sectors alongside a correspondingly shrinking public sector. The government wants local authorities to retain some 'capacity, skills and experience', but only in a residual sense. Otherwise private or voluntary agencies will either directly provide services or be 'contracted out' by local authorities to do so. The public sector is likely to be left with 'people with high levels of dependency, or particularly challenging patterns of behaviour'. These will be those whom no other agency wants to take on. Harriet Harman, an opposition spokesperson, has said, 'It is clear that Social Services Departments will dwindle away until all that is left is a rump providing services for people private business cannot make money out of' (*Observer*, 10 November 1989).

It was thought in the past that community care was always a cheaper option than residential provision. This is far from the truth although occasionally it may occur. It is estimated, for example, that in the Oxford Regional Health Authority it will cost £30 000 per year to keep one person with learning difficulties in the community. This is almost twice the cost of keeping such a person in one of the local specialist teaching hospitals. Edward Pilkington has written, 'The fashion for community care has begun to wane as the costs add up. Mentally handicapped people are slipping down the list of priorities again, returning to their old marginalized position' (*Guardian*, 23 May 1990).

Bob Rhodes, head of mental handicap services in West Berkshire, stated, 'We are in a double bind. We haven't got the money to make the hospital service acceptable . . . We are convinced resources would be better spent in the community but we haven't got enough to do that either. So we have to choose between the devil and the deep blue sea' (*Guardian*, 23 May 1990, p. 33).

It is fine to have new proposals for more effective and innovative care in the community, but resources, financial and otherwise, must be there to facilitate their implimentation. Many social services administrators believe that local authorities have been 'set up to fail' with regard to the new care proposals because of a lack of funds. Falling government funding and rising costs have led to predictions from social service administrators of a financial shortfall of 100 million pounds by 1992 and half a billion pounds by 1994 (*Community Care*, 12 April 1990).

The community charge

The last few years have been difficult ones for local authorities and have been characterized by a great deal of upheaval. This has affected both their duties, powers and responsibilities, and also the way in which local authority services are paid for. After several years of financial cut backs in local authority services, the *community charge*, more commonly known as the *poll tax*, has replaced the traditional *rating* system as a means of raising money for services. People rather than premises are now being taxed in order to pay for revenue.

Since the Second World War local authorities have lost a good deal of control over a range of services. Health Services are now regionally organized and central government control over housing, the Police Service and the Probation Service has grown. These developments mean that the two largest remaining areas of local government expenditure and influence are education and social services. Social services usually make up the second largest slice of the budget after education.

Each local authority has had to set an annual rate at a level at which poll tax will be paid in the area from April 1990 in England and Wales, and April 1989 in Scotland. Levels of the tax have varied a great deal around the country according to a combination of local needs and the political persuasion of the local authority. The lowest poll tax fixed in the year of its inception was in Wandsworth Borough Council – £148. The highest was £538 in Lambeth. Central Government determines what levels will be fixed and in fact it decided to 'cap' 21 local authorities. This forced those authorities to set a lower rate of poll tax. It had the effect therefore of limiting the amount of money the local authorities could spend on Social Services. Over a third of Social Services Departments in England and Wales have had to reduce their services or cancel new developments as a result of the poll tax.

The disturbing effect of the poll tax is, therefore, to reduce public spending on Social Services, and to force local authorities to continually seek cheaper services. This is proving a severe restraint when, under the new government proposals for community care, local authorities are required to take on new and wider responsibilities.

The present government's intention is to diminish the public sector and to stimulate growth in the private and voluntary sectors. As the recently published White Paper *Caring for People* states 'Social Services should be "enabling" agencies. It will be their responsibility to make maximum possible use of private and voluntary providers' (p. 5). It remains the government's wish that local authority Social Service Departments will sell off residential provision to the private or voluntary sectors and will become instead administrators of care which will actually be provided by others.

The reduction of the influence and authority of state run Social Services Departments can be seen as part of a larger attack on the welfare state. The Post Second World War consensus on the desirability of a comprehensive welfare state to protect those who are in need and those who are vulnerable, has been broken in recent years. In some ways critics of welfare state services have been proved correct – services were often large scale bureaucratic affairs, delivered in very impersonal ways to their recipients. However, the application of free market forces to service delivery can mean a lack of over-seeing regulation, thus some of the poorest, deprived and most vulnerable members of our society may suffer or in extreme cases may not survive. As the Labour MP Frank Field has said 'There is no "hidden hand" to protect the poorest in our community unless voters and government decide to do so' (*Independent*, 10 May 1990, p. 2).

The uncertainty surrounding the poll tax, in particular the uncertainty over exactly how much money will be raised, makes the planning of social service provision extremely hazardous. The difficulties are further compounded at the present time when new community care arrangements are soon to come into operation. Planning cannot be performed when it is not known how much revenue will be available for services.

The poll tax is proving a very difficult tax to collect. Many people are opposed to it on moral grounds believing it to be unfair that all are taxed at the same rate, regardless of ability to pay or the amount of wealth, property or land held. There are those therefore who are refusing to pay. One such person, Dr Nigel Mason, told the Magistrate's court that he was refusing to pay his £379 poll tax bill on a point of Christian principle. 'In the Old and New Testaments it is quite clear that justice, as far as God is concerned, is important. Poll tax is an unjust act. It would be condemned by the Old Testament prophets and the Lord Jesus because he condemned an attitude which said stuff everybody else, I am alright' (The *Oxford Times*, 20 July 1990).

By July 1990 (i.e. four months after the tax was introduced in England and Wales) many local authority collection rates were only 50 per cent (*Observer*,

24 June 1990). After a full year of operation in Scotland, Strathclyde council had only an 80 per cent collection rate (ibid.).

Furthermore, some people may be tempted not to enrol on the electoral register in an attempt to avoid paying the poll tax and to avoid investigation. This has profound implications for the democratic right to vote and to undertake jury service. This point has been made by Peter Esam and Carey Oppenheim:

> 'Because the poor are hit harder by the poll tax and may, in many cases, be driven to desperation by the tax, it is they who are more likely to be tempted to give up their right to vote in the hope of evading the tax.'
>
> (1989, p. 114)

At local government elections those authorities who set a very low rate of poll tax can obviously present themselves in a very favourable light. What is sometimes forgotten is that needs vary greatly in different areas and that a low poll tax is achieved at the expense of public services. Those areas, including many of the inner cities which have a larger number of poorer or dependent people, whether elderly or with disabilities, will tend to require more services and will consequently have to set a higher rate of poll tax. Such areas may also have the added handicap of a larger proportion of poorer people within their boundaries who are unable to pay the tax in the first place.

Cuts in welfare

Wandsworth council has a deliberate policy of keeping its poll tax as low as possible and in 1990 it was the lowest in England (£148 per year). This meant services have had to be cut. Proposals to cut its social services bill have included: ceasing to do generic and non-statutory social work; transferring elderly residential provision away from the council; integrating under-five's daycare with nursery education and a re-examining of the policy of charging for Social Services. If funding remains as it is, it is certain that many if not all Social Services Departments will have to consider the same kind of measures.

What services will look like in a few years time is impossible to predict owing to all the many uncertainties. Cutbacks appear, however, to have already had severe repercussions. An official inquiry, chaired by Professor Olive Stevenson, into the murder of a three-year-old, Stephanie Fox, by her father, concluded that cutbacks in nursery provision in Wandsworth were a direct cause of her death. The inquiry stated that finding a day nursery place for Stephanie was a crucial part of her 'protection plan', and condemned the length of time it took (*Guardian* 21 June 1990). At the time Wandsworth's cutbacks meant that only two out of five day nursery staff posts were filled. Consequently, one third of places for children were not offered. Further to this over 10 children on the 'at risk' register in Wandsworth had no social worker owing to the staff shortages.

Charity

Hand in hand with the cuts in welfare is a drive to encourage charitable giving. The money raised can then be distributed to those in need. At root level, this is based on pure ideology: an objection not to raising money but to how it is raised. People in our society are urged to give charitably rather than to pay taxes which can fund public services. The main danger in this arrangement is its unpredictability. As Robert Morley of The Family Welfare Association has said, 'By its nature charitable giving is capricious, often spontaneous and rarely the object of careful thought about the needs of poor people and how those needs ought to be met' (*Independent*, 18 May 1990, p. 21).

Many people also feel that charity carries a stigma. David Blunkett, MP, has said, 'You cannot have dignity and self respect if you have to rattle a tin in the high street to raise money for the very basics of life'. He goes on, 'The very act of portraying an individual or group of individuals as a deserving cause belittles them and separates them out from the rest of the community because it plays on people's sympathy' (*Sheffield Star*, 12 October 1988).

It is patently false to believe that affluent people will want to give more. Some causes will be more popular than others; for example, those relating to children are likely to receive more public sympathy than say the single homeless. Ruth Lister has said, 'The unfashionable, the unnoticed, and the "undeserving" are unlikely to do well in the charity stakes' (*Independent*, 18 May 1990, p. 21).

'Piss on pity'

Every year the independent television company ITV organizes a charity fund raising event known as Telethon. It raises a huge amount of money – £23 million in 1989. A proportion of this money assists disabled people. Each year however a growing number of protesters make themselves heard at the event, many of them with disabilities. Their pressure group, the Campaign to Stop Patronage, accused the event of 'tokenism, patronage and portraying a negative image of people with disabilities' (*Guardian*, 28 May 1990). One banner at the event read 'Piss on pity' and Mike Higgins, one of the protesters, said the event 'just salves consciences and boosts flagging careers for stars' (ibid.). Mave Kennedy, writing in the *Guardian*, summed up the protesters views of the event as 'undermining their own efforts to obtain the help they need as of right paid for by Government' (ibid.). Ruth Lister echoes this view when she says 'Charity has an important place in our society but not as a substitute for legally based welfare right' (*Independent*, 18 May 1990, p. 21).

The active citizen

Closely allied to the drive for charitable giving is the concept of the 'active citizen'. The government set up an all party *Commission on Citizenship* under the patronage of the Speaker of the House of Commons in January 1989. It is partly funded by private industry. Membership is wide ranging and includes trade union representatives, MPs from all parties, educational institution representatives and some from professional bodies. Its aim is to promote the development of the active citizen.

In a report published in early 1990, the Commission on Citizenship stated that it wanted more recognition for the 'involvement of the citizen, or groups of citizens in the community'. The report defined the active citizen as 'the citizen acting in a voluntary capacity'. The Commission's first important aim is to introduce civic education to the National Curriculum in order to develop pupils' personal and social education'. Francis Morrell, Secretary to the Commission says, 'One part of that is the ability to understand they are part of a wider society. That they do have entitlements and responsibilities. That they can play a role in society. The aim is to instil into young people a sense of "obligation" to our society, a sense of "public spirit"' (*Social Work Today*, 4 January 1990, p. 16).

Morrell quite rightly says that when a young person leaves school and applies for work, too much stress is placed solely on educational achievement. Other abilities, sensitivities and achievements should be taken into account. One writer on the Commission interprets this view in saying 'employers and colleges should put out signals that a stint of volunteering in some form is a passport to a better job, education and career opportunities' (ibid.).

One of the problems with this theory is that it could profoundly distort the spirit of altruism, of doing something for nothing, of giving and not expecting a reward. A further problem is that it tends to be young people from more privileged homes and backgrounds who find it easier to sacrifice a few weeks or months for volunteer work. It can also be seen as a patronizing approach to social and community action which can divert attention from genuine grass roots activity, often of a spontaneous nature.

In considering the dismantling of the welfare state, the spread of market forces ideology into welfare services, and the concomitant push for charitable giving and increased volunteering, Ruth Lister feels that social justice and the rights of each of us as citizens are at risk. She states 'Ministers have conjured up the active citizen like the genie in the lamp, to paint a caring gloss over divisive polices which are corroding these rights. Obligations are being shifted from the public sphere of tax-financed benefits and services to the private sphere of charity and voluntary service' (*Independent*, 18 May 1990, p. 21).

Equal opportunities

Following on from legislation enacted in the mid 1970s, the CRE and EOC issued codes of practice which came into force in 1984 and 1985 respectively. Since this time many employers have declared themselves as equal opportunity employers, although follow-up studies have revealed an alarming lack of commitment to acompany the expressed sentiments. A survey carried out in 1988 involving all 514 local authorities in England, Wales and Scotland found that 206 of the 446 authorities who responded to the survey questionaire had no equal opportunities policy. Furthermore, 18 of those without a policy nevertheless described themselves as equal opportunity employers in their job advertisements. Whilst some employers are genuinely concerned to provide equal opportunities, it would seem that others may show a commitment only as an exercise in 'image management': their need or desire, according to Owusu-Bempath, 'to present a socially desirable or acceptable image of themselves and their organizations, which has the effect of a conspiracy to exploit the credulity of the public' (*Community Care*, 14 September 1989). He goes on to state, 'Image management by employers is a reaffirmation of racism in British institutions and society at large. It is a new institutional racism used by employers and service providers, large and small, to present an "acceptable face of racism"' (ibid.).

A similar criticism is levelled at social work organizations by Josie Durrant, director of Focus (a consultancy). She claims that social work organizations have recruited black people only to 'act as a buffer between the consumer and a white structure that does not seek change' (*Community Care*, November 1989). It is undoubtably true that progress towards equality of opportunity has been slow considering the length of time since the initial legislation, although some organizations have made inroads. But as Josie Durrant points out 'in order to measure progress we need not to look at the situation of the few but the circumstances of the many' (*Social Work Today*, Job Forum, 1989).

In November 1989, David Divine, an Assistant Director of CCETSW, was very critical of social work education and training. Along with many others he felt that often anti-racism was little more than rhetoric and that social work courses were unable to implement it practically. At the time he felt that social work education and training was undergoing a crisis. However, he felt there was cause for optimism. He cited the National Vocational Qualification which he felt would not discriminate on the basis of previous experience and would 'begin to tackle the existing elitist structures of so many of our caring agencies'. Furthermore he noted that the new social work training course, the Dip. SW, would have built into it 'all aspects of anti-racism and transcultural understanding'.

National Vocational Qualification (NVQ) or Scottish Vocational Qualifications (SVQ)

It is too early to comment on the impact that the new NVQ proposals will have on social care. This will depend once again on how well these initiatives are backed up financially by the government. The potential exists, however, to create a fully trained workforce across the field of social and health care within local authority, voluntary, private and health care settings, where each individual carer has the opportunity of being tested and accredited for their skills, or to be trained as far as they wish. At the beginning of 1990, it was estimated that over 1 million people were working in the UK's health and social services without any formal qualifications (*Community Care*, 8 February 1990, p. 17). They range from care assistants/officers to medical secretaries, and fulfil a vital role in supporting social workers and nurses and others with professional qualifications in the care field.

Education and training – working together

The establishment of NVQ followed on from a Government White Paper *Education and Training – Working Together* (1986). The aim was to produce a better qualified workforce in all industries throughout the country. The application of NVQ to certain trades and industries, such as engineering or catering, was relatively straightforward, since many of the components of the work could quite easily be dissected and broken down into separate units or competences. The reduction of tasks and duties carried out by workers within the care sector was more problematic because of the degree of human interaction involved: all care takes place within a dynamic personal relationship and the effectiveness of a worker is correspondingly harder to measure than say a caterer producing a cake which in itself is objective evidence of competence. Testing for competence, however, is not simply a question of 'the proof of the pudding is in the eating'.

Even within the catering industry it would not be possible to test a cook's level of competence by sampling what has been produced. 'Without observing the cook actually at work you could never tell whether they were using the rules of hygiene. You certainly could not tell whether they were wasteful in their use of materials. Assessment by results, therefore, is clearly not good enough' (*Care Sector Consortium Newsletter*, August 1990). In other words it is the *process* which is being tested.

The Care Sector Consortium was formed in 1988 and is made up of representatives from all the major caring organizations, local authorities, health authorities, the Council of Professions Supplementary to Medicine, voluntary organizations, the Probation Service, private bodies, trade unions and professional and educational organizations such as CCETSW and NHSTA. Their job is to set and maintain standards and to produce criteria for competences.

The notion of NVQ (or SVQ in Scotland) was not new. It had been in operation in France and Germany and other European countries. Not only does NVQ establish *levels of qualifications* but it also provides members of the workforce with an opportunity of *career progression*. Once a worker has achieved competence at one of the prescribed levels, then she or he is eligible to be considered for competence testing at the next, higher level. Within the field of social care for example, achievement at level 2 (basic competence) would qualify the worker to progress to level 3 – the level at which the new Certificate in Social Care (CSC) is set. Successful completion of the CSC would make the candidate eligible for full professional social work training (Dip.SW), although many workers may not wish to qualify further but instead remain at level 3.

The impact of NVQ within social and health care is yet to be seen, but it has generally been welcomed by employers, unions and professional organizations alike. Properly implemented and resourced it would lead to a better trained workforce and ultimately to improved service delivery.

Some of the advantages of NVQ are listed below:

1. It acknowledges the skills that many care workers exhibit in their everyday practice. As the National Institute for Social Work/Social Care Association have stated in *Making National Vocational Qualifications Work for Social Care*, 'NVQ should provide opportunities to the mass of social carers to receive formal recognition of their abilities and of their worth'. It continues, 'opportunities, which as the Wagner Report and others have frequently pointed out, have consistently been denied to this large and important workforce of people, the majority of whom are female, many of whom come from minority ethnic groups, and many work part-time; but without whose efforts the bulk of services would simply collapse'.

2. The emphasis is no longer solely on academic qualifications as before. Instead, a person's ability to do the job well is being tested irrespective of formal qualifications. Of course in order to perform a caring task effectively

one needs to be informed by an understanding of caring skills, social issues and a knowledge of what constitutes good practice, but essentially it is the ability to do the job which is being tested.

3. A worker's previous qualifications, life and work experience will be formally recognized and taken into consideration before she or he embarks on any training programme. It is expected that once the NVQ structure is fully in place candidates will be able to put themselves forward for Accreditation of Prior Learning (APL), and so possibly reduce the number of units on which they have to be assessed.

4. Workers are able to progress. Having achieved competence at one level the worker is in a position to prepare for future assessment at the next higher level.

5. There should be an opportunity for carers to achieve some *horizontal interchange* where this is sought. In other words, many of the core competences are common to a wide range of jobs within the caring services, so that, for example, a person training within a health setting may acquire similar competences to a person working within a social care setting and vice versa. Under NVQ it should be possible then for a person working in a hospital setting, for example with mentally ill adults, to eventually be able to work in a social services day centre with elderly people or in a nursery working with young children, having acquired the additional necessary competences on top of the *core* competences already achieved.

The success of NVQ will be greatly determined by how well it is funded. The cost of training a largely untrained workforce is going to require substantial resources, not least in order to provide for the initial establishment and training of work place assessors. It is to be hoped that training departments, through lack of resources, do not abuse the spirit of NVQ by channelling their resources on assessing carers only for their current level of performance. All workers should have the right to be tested to the level of their potential or at least as far as they wish to progress. It is hoped further that training resources are not directed towards the basic levels of competence at the expense of professional training.

The NVQ competences drawn up by the various caring bodies for the Care Sector Consortium have given issues of race, gender and disability a high profile and this is to be welcomed. The service user's right to respect and dignity and individuality is enshrined in the core units and core performance criteria and is required to be evident in the carer's approach to all caring tasks and duties.

Project 2000

Closely related to, but separate from, the arrangements for NVQ are the developments in nurse training known as Project 2000 (CCNMHV, 1986). This approach is about a new pattern of preparation of nurse education and sees a movement away from apprenticeship training towards one where the trainee nurse will have full student status. Much of the training will still take place in health care settings but the Project 2000 practitioner will be supernumary to staffing establishment throughout her or his training. The new three year training programme will emphasize health promotion and primary health care and prepare the nurse to work in both community and health care settings. Essentially 'The Project 2000 practitioner should be a "knowledgeable doer" competent to assess the need for care, provide care, monitor and evaluate and do this in institutional and non institutional settings.' The academic standard of nurse training is expected to improve and the successful Project 2000 practitioner will be awarded a Diploma in Higher Education in Nursing as well as a Registered Nurse Qualification.

The Project 2000 practitioner would be helped and advised by specialist practitioners who would assist in either a teaching or managerial role. They would also be supported by the new health care support workers who would undertake many of the tasks and duties previously undertaken by the traditional trainee nurse. The health support workers would be eligible for training under NVQ. By September 1990, three NVQ qualifications in health care were proposed by the Care Sector Consortium: Assisting Client in Personal Care – level 1 NVQ, Direct Personal Care – level 2 NVQ, Enablement Care – level 3 NVQ.

Some initial criticisms and difficulties

Despite the promise generated by the idea of NVQ, its actual implementation will not necessarily be as simple as it would seem. In order to ensure that accurate assessment is carried out and that workers are treated fairly in this process, certain precautions need to be taken. By September 1990, the organization Black Perspectives in Care had drawn up a set of questions that addressed issues of anti-discriminatory practice. Amongst some of the questions they have asked employers to consider are: 'Are the competences presented in a way that does not discriminate against individuals or groups of candidates? e.g. literary, sensory or physical impairment'. 'What positive steps are to be taken to prepare the candidates to undertake a set of competences?' 'What positive steps are to be taken to ensure fair representation of black assessors, verifiers etc.?' and 'What recourse do candidates have when they are considered "not yet competent"?' (*Newsletter no. 6*, September 1990, Association for Social Care Training). The complete list of 14 questions is available in an appendix to this chapter.

Inequality and the individual

Throughout the book we have noted the existence of structural inequality and the harmful effect this has on individuals who are denied full and equal participation in our society. We have stressed the need for carers to comprehend the influence of social structures on themselves and the persons they care for: the client should be seen within her or his social setting.

There is widespread understanding of the integral relationship between structural inequality and individual problems. This has always been acknowledged by social reformers and was articulated again over 20 years ago by the late Lord Seebohm, who chaired the committee which heralded the introduction of the Social Services Departments in 1971. He estimated that about 60 per cent of cases dealt with by social workers were caused by poverty and poor housing. As we have continually highlighted, inequality within our society is still marked. In some ways the divisions in society are more profound today than they were at the time of the introduction of the generic Social Services Departments.

We have observed too, that the very framework within which professional caring takes place, i.e. in local authority, health authority, voluntary or private settings, is undergoing enormous change and is surrounded by uncertainty. It is likely that the public sector will continue to diminish whilst the voluntary and private sectors expand.

Outside the formal network, the position of informal carers who look after dependent relatives has been acknowledged, yet very little has been done to assist the plight of such people of whom there is an estimated 6 million. Some are under considerable stress and very few receive official support. According to Jill Pitkeathly, director of the Carers' National Association, '80 per cent of carers get no help at all' (*Guardian*, 16/17 June 1990, pp. 24–5.). Whilst professionals like district nurses and social workers can offer carers advice they still need other services like day care facilities, home care aids and flexible respite care so that they can have occasional time off. Catherine Sadler points out, 'most of all, carers need Government recognition. The Carers' National Association estimates that each year the saving to the state is £24 billion, yet the Invalid Care Allowance is still a paltry £28.20 per week' (ibid).

The ICA (Invalid Care Allowance) is currently paid to those carers who would otherwise be available for fulltime paid work. Pensioners are therefore not eligible for the allowance.

Gay people

With regard to gay people, we have seen that although clause 28 of the 1988 Local Government Act provides no legal basis for further discrimination, the threat of being considered to be intentionally promoting homosexuality has made people cautious, or at least self-conscious, about offering support to gay people within the public sector. The current intolerant climate contributes to the anxiety and continued marginalization of gay people, particularly the younger gay people.

> 'And then, of course, there is clause 28. I wish I had had a teacher at school who had passed a few words of comfort and hope down to me, sitting edgily at the back of the class. To be told by a teacher – or a priest – that being homosexual wasn't the end of the world might have saved me a lot of suffering, made me stronger and more courageous now, a time when courage is called for. Clause 28 has locked teacher's mouths. Once again, the subject dare not speak it's name. The children are the losers.'
>
> (Michael Carson, *Weekend Guardian*, 17/18 March 1990, p. 12).

Britain in Europe

1992 sees the introduction of the *single European market*. This largely applies to economic and trading activities between the 12 countries involved but it may well also have social implications. Some fear that it will merely be a 'businessmans' bonanza' and deregulation of trade barriers and restrictions which will see multinational corporations and international banking and finance doing very well at the expense of individual nations. The European Community has laid out its intentions in a 300 point plan for a so called 'internal market'.

Wider issues are involved, however. Fears that the planned changes may result in what has come to be termed 'social dumping' i.e. the relocating of business from high to low wage areas, has led to a political response from the European Commission. Led by its President, Jacques Delors, it has developed the so called *Social Charter* or to give it its full name – The Community Charter of Fundamental Social Rights. This provides a framework of principles relating to employment and Trade Union rights, including the employment of children and young people. Given that individuals will theoretically have free movement within Europe, it also sets out to safeguard certain rights in terms of housing, childcare, social welfare and equality of gender, race and disability. The latter may relate to pay and benefit levels. Since Britain lags behind Europe in many areas of social provision, notably childcare services, it may be that this country will benefit from being drawn into line by the European Community.

As the law now stands, social workers will not be able to move freely across the continent in 1992, since the Professional Register of the European Community excludes the British professional social work qualification. British social work training courses are one year shorter than those in other European countries where there is a three year minimum.

Reasons for optimism

Amid the upheaval and uncertainties of the late 1980s and early 1990s, there *are* reasons for optimism. Social care training is soon to be available via NVQ to a wider range of workers whilst professional training is undergoing a radicalization and the new Dip. SW is expected to produce social workers better able to work more effectively within our multicultural society. Residential work is distancing itself from its institutional past and practice is being informed by the positive recommendations of the Wagner Report and the Social Care Association's Code of Practice which followed in 1988.

With regard to gender, there are signs of a heightened awareness of women's marginalization and the need to create and enforce non-discriminatory practices. Awareness alone is insufficient and needs to be accompanied by improved social provision for women. It is true to say that more women have made inroads into professional and management spheres and into new areas of work traditionally dominated by men, but their numbers are not substantial. So many are still held back by domestic and childcare responsibilities. Looking back over the last decade, Tessa Blackstone, Master of Birkbeck College, commented: 'The 80s have divided women in Britain. Professional women have advanced whilst many others have suffered. Their well-being has been jeopardized by the government's neglect. Child benefit has gone down and there has been a decline in the standards of many services which support the family. European countries' child care services have dramatically expanded, in Britain they have stood still, and care in the community policies have placed an additional burden on women who have to look after relatives' (*Guardian*, 28 December 1989).

For women to be able to lead richer and fuller lives and to be able to participate more fully in the world of work outside the home, there needs to be better social provision. Childcare services remain varied and generally un-developed throughout the country requiring many women who do not choose to stay at home to do so. Similarly, there are many women who are unsupported in their role of informal carer.

Some private and statutory organizations have introduced initiatives aimed at facilitating women's return to paid employment. But if the government is seriously intent on 'wooing' women back to the workforce in the 1990s, then provision needs to be more widespread and standard as well as accessible to all women, regardless of their capacity to pay. Some of the initiatives include: job sharing, flexi-hours, term timing (a mother's working day and holidays corre-spond with the times her children are at school), paid sick leave and unpaid leave for time spent off with sick children. Many women also need some form of pre-employment training, particularly if they have been out of work for a long period, even if this is just to improve their confidence. Of course for real change to occur these facilities should be equally open to men, and manage-ment should be trained to view the opportunities as realistic options for their male staff and not just for females. In this way true equality of outcome could be achieved.

Despite the slow progress in the implementation of equal opportunities policies concerning 'race', there has undoubtedly been a raised awareness of black perspectives and anti-racism during recent years. This has yet to be reflected in practical terms. Black people are still under represented in managerial and professional positions and over represented in the lower paid, lower status, less secure jobs.

Within the field of social care, there is an improved understanding of the needs of black people, although once again this has not been fully translated into practice. There is a slightly greater representation of black people within social and health care, even in the more senior positions, but there still needs to be more progress made. Social and health care practice has now moved towards centralizing the black perspective and has moved away from the tokenistic policies of the past. For example the British Association of Social Workers' (BASW) report, *Action Project into Ethnically Sensitive Social Work* (1990) stated, 'Managers should be prepared to challenge all *racist* incidents and should insist on the same stance from their staff' (p. 12). At the same time the Race Equality Unit of NISW has produced a code of practice on anti-racist work.

Similarly the Social Care Association has outlined their own code of prac-tice. Para. 1.1. describes a carer's role as one who 'will cultivate an understand-ing and awareness in relation to race, gender, culture, religion, class and sexuality and will implement an equal opportunity approach with all aspects of social care with which he or she is involved' (SCA, 1988, p. 2). As we have already pointed out the black perspective is now integrated in social care training at the NVQ level and through to full professional training at the Dip. SW level.

Social care practice has incorporated other changes, many of which have been brought about by the consumers themselves. For example the impact of social work clients with the HIV virus has forced carers to consider a whole range of new issues and to examine their own attitudes more closely, in particular on subjects such as sexuality, lifestyle and death. Furthermore HIV clients have tended to be younger and more articulate than other social work clients and have been more assertive in pressing their needs. Similarly, many physically disabled clients have made clear their objections to patronizing and debilitating care and have rightly insisted that they should be treated with dignity and respect. Indeed there has been a growth in the development of self advocacy amongst all client groups. For example the National Association for Young People in Care (NAYPIC) represents the voice of those children and young adults in care and is taken seriously by social care organizations.

Advocacy on behalf of clients has been an area of growing activity, for example, amongst people with learning difficulties. In areas where someone may meet hardship (e.g. employment, legal and welfare rights, courts and the criminal justice system), if a person is unable to speak for herself or himself, or act as her or his own advocate, then a worker or other representative will perform this role for that person. This is considered to be part of the *empowerment* process.

Much of the legislation regarding recent social care and social work policy places the client in the central position enabling her or him to determine as far as possible the kind of service which is appropriate. The centrality of the consumer is embodied in the proposal that clients undertake to be their own care manager within the proposed community care arrangements. It has also been suggested that clients may contribute to the NVQ assessment of staff.

The 1990s will require a much improved co-operation between all the caring agencies and a breakdown of traditional rivalries. *Child Care, the Butler-Sloss Inquiry into Child Abuse in Cleveland* (1987), recommended collaboration between doctors, nurses, social workers, teachers, the police and the staff of voluntary organizations and the 1989 Children Act laid down a statutory framework for multi-disciplinary co-operation. Similarly, the effect of the NHS review *Working for Patients* and the 1989 White Paper *Caring for People* is expressed in the National Health Service and Community Care Act and urges health and social care workers to co-operate.

Given the advancing philosophy and progress made in social care practice, it is crucial that this is matched by the provision of adequate resources. The gradual erosion of the welfare state, combined with the ideological pressure to pursue individual materialistic gains, represents a severe threat to the spirit of altruism and public service. Gross inequality and the presence in our society of an 'underclass' and others who are structurally deprived, ultimately threatens our corporate life and availability of collective community provision. It is important that social care advances in step with and in support of the enhanced desires of social groups which have thus far been marginalized.

Having made encouraging progress over the last few years towards establishing positive anti-discriminatory practice, it is necessary that this impetus is maintained by social care organizations. The recent upsurge in client self determination, empowerment and the drive for greater choice should encourage us as social carers to work in partnership for more appropriate and democratic services.

Appendix

The group Black Perspectives in Care (1990) have produced a set of questions that address issues of anti-discriminatory practice in respect of NVQ:

1. Are the competencies presented in a way that does not discriminate against individuals or groups of candidates? e.g. literacy, sensory or physical impairment.
2. What positive steps are to be taken to prepare the candidates to undertake a set of competencies?
3. What steps are to be taken in order not to discriminate within the selection process?
4. How are the assessment processes to be demonstrated to be fair and just to all candidates?
5. How are the selection of assessors, mentors, verifiers etc. to be anti-discriminatory?
6. What positive steps are to be taken to ensure fair representation of black assessors, verifiers etc.?
7. What previous experience of assessing black candidates would be expected of white assessors and verifiers?
8. What systems are to be instituted to monitor the assessors' and verifiers' performance?
9. What procedures are there going to be to monitor the experiences of disadvantaged groups through the NVQ system?
10. How will you ensure that the black voluntary organizations and training agencies have access to and are involved in the training consortium?
11. What arrangements have been made to prepare the white candidates to work in a multicultural environment?
12. What steps will be taken when any candidate fails to demonstrate anti-discriminatory practices?
13. How are the positive/negative life experiences of the black individuals to be assessed in a way which does not further discriminate against them?
14. What recourse do candidates have when they are considered 'not yet competent'?

Exercises

1. The purpose of this exercise is to reveal the extremes of bad practice in order to emphasize the value of non discriminatory practice. In small groups design a 'racist', 'sexist' or 'disablist' day nursery that would discriminate against children either directly or indirectly. Consider all aspects of nursery provision including staffing, selection procedures, decor, materials, food, rules and regulations.

2. *Library exercise*
Undertake one of the following tasks.

i) Locate a copy of the Wagner report, *A Positive Choice* (NISW, 1988). Read through the personal evidence sections on 'good practice', 'bad practice' and 'mixed' practice which can be found in Appendix 1, 'A Guide to the Evidence – The Personal Evidence' (pp. 129–160). Read through the 45 recommendations of the report (which can be found on pp. 115–119) and discuss each in turn with other members of the group.

ii) Locate a copy of the White Paper – *Caring for People: Community Care in the Next Decade and Beyond*, HMSO, 1989. Read through the various definitions of community care which can be found in the following places: Para. 1:1 (p. 3); Para. 1:8 (p. 4); Para. 1:10 (p. 5); Para. 2:2 (p. 9). Devise a definition of community care which amalgamates the information of all four separate definitions as succinctly as possible.

3. Imagine you are a member of a staff team in an elderly people's home run by the local authority. In an attempt to try to improve the quality of care for your residents, you have agreed to try to formulate a policy document specifying the principles underlying the quality of care which you are aiming to provide. In your staff team draw up a policy document which would be used by staff members and would be given to residents and their family and friends. You may like to include headings such as: admission procedures, after admission, detailed and general principles.

4. *Core performance criteria and good practice*
The whole group should divide into groups of three. Of these:

i) One will act as a client/service user who is elderly or has a physical disability or learning difficulty
ii) One will act as a social carer
iii) One will act as a practice assessor

Each group of three should then choose one of the following 'simple' practical tasks:

i) Dressing – say, putting on shoes, or a jumper or overcoat
ii) Feeding – say jelly or yoghurt
iii) Washing face and brushing teeth

Now, each group of three should read the six NVQ 'Core Performance Criteria' reproduced below. These are the core of good, anti-discriminatory practice required of all social carers.
  The social carer:

– Discusses, confirms and respects as far as possible the clients choice, wishes and preferences at all times.
– Recognizes and takes account of the clients culture, political beliefs, race, religion, sexual identity, age, gender, physical and mental condition.
– Recognizes and responds to the emotional needs of the client using advice, assistance and guidance as necessary.
– Uses language and other forms of communication suitable to the needs of the client (where necessary, this will include the assistance of an interpreter).
– Respects the confidentiality of all information and sources and only discloses information to those who necessarily require it after discussion with client and, when appropriate, receiving his/her permission.
– Correctly applies all relevant health and safety requirements and precautions.

The social carer should then carry out the task, with the client being as unco-operative, co-operative or 'difficult' as they choose! The Practice Assessor should make her or his assessment. Allow 15 minutes for this task.

After the task, the Practice Assessor should relay her or his assessment to the other two members, who should also provide feedback on their experience of the exercise. A discussion among the whole group can follow.

5. *Assessment methods in social care*
Study this list of assessment methods:

i) Written evidence from care programmes, reports, records, diaries/incident books etc.
ii) Written or oral tests of a social carers' knowledge.
iii) Direct (or naturalistic) observation of a social carer at work carrying out their normal duties and tasks.
iv) Role play of a social care situation.
v) Other simulation, which might include demonstrating the use of equipment, aids or adaptations, but will not include people.
vi) Audiotapes of a social care situation e.g. a home carer (home help).
vii) Discussion between the social carer and her or his Practice Assessor, after the completion of a task.
viii) Written assignments on specific areas of practice e.g. Equal Opportunities Policies, Health and Safety Policies, the side effects of medication.
ix) Video tapes of a social care practice situation.

Now provide your own assessment of each method, of their reliability and usefulness. Can you *rank order* them in relation to their reliability and usefulness? Can you think of social care tasks which each might be best applied to?

Questions for essays or discussion

1. Politicians are not interested in community care as 'good practice' – for them it is merely a cheaper way of providing services.
2. Equal opportunity policies for women and black people have not achieved significant positive results. Rather they have created ill-feeling and resentment.
3. Social carers and social workers merely provide individual solutions to problems caused by economic, political and social policy changes.
4. Some elements of the social care task are immeasurable. Discuss this in relation to the proposals for competency testing under NVQ(SVQ).
5. David Marsland suggests that we should 'retrain social workers away from dependency-generating rights – demanding ideologies' (*Social Studies Review*, November 1989). What ideology does his statement contain?
6. Anthea Tinker, Professor of Social Gerontology, King's College, London, one of the author's of the Church of England report entitled *Ageing* (Church House, 1990), said that it was 'essential that basic services should be funded through general taxation'. How far do you agree with this statement?

Further reading

Academic sources

Centre for Policy on Ageing, *Home Life – A Code of Practice for Residential Care*, Centre for Policy on Ageing, 1986. The report of the working party sponsored by the Department of Health and Social Security and convened by the Centre for Policy on Ageing under the chair of Kina, Lady Avebury.

Centre for Policy on Ageing, *Community Life – A Code of Practice for Community Care*, Centre for Policy on Ageing, 1990. Devised by a panel convened by the Centre for Policy on Ageing and chaired by Lady Lloyd. A companion to *Home Life*, a short and very readable manual about good care practice in the community.

Griffiths Report. *Community Care: Agenda for Action.* A Report to the Secretary of State for Social Services. Chaired by Sir Roy Griffiths. HMSO, 1988. The terms of reference were 'to review the way in which public funds are used to support community care policy and to advise (the Secretary of State) on the options for action that would improve the use of these funds as a contribution to more effective community care' (p. iii, para. 2).

Jordan, B., *The Common Good – Citizenship, Morality and Self-Interest*, Basil Blackwell, 1989. A philosophical and political critique of a society based on 'individual choice' and the author's alternative, based on the 'common interests' of all.

McCarthy, M., (ed.), *The New Politics of Welfare – An Agenda for the 1990s*, Macmillan, 1989. A range of writers look back over the 1980s and study a number of pertinent issues such as the personal social services, health, housing, social security, community care and criminal justice. In so doing, they look forward to developments over the next 10 years.

Wagner, G., *Residential Care – A Positive Choice*, NISW/HMSO, 1988. This comprehensive report, in two parts, is very readable and informative. One part deals with the history of residential care and the current state of care provision for all client groups. The second part deals with the principles and recommendations of the report in detail.

Caring for People: Community Care in the Next Decade and Beyond, (The White Paper on Community Care), Command 849, HMSO, 1989. The government's proposals for legislation on community care, including a greater role for the private and independent sectors compared to the statutory sector.

Other literary sources

Armitage, S., *Zoom*. Bloodaxe Books, 1989.

Dickens, M., *The Listeners*. Penguin, 1970.

England, H., *Social Work As Art: Making Sense For Good Practice*. Allen and Unwin, 1986.

Konrad, G., *The Case Worker*. Hutchinson, 1975.

Laken, B., *More Than A Friend*. Lion, 1984.

Morris, C. (ed.), *Literature And The Social Worker: A Reading List For Practitioners, Teachers, Students and Voluntary Workers*. The Library Association, 1975.

9   Towards positive practice

In order to develop positive practice it is necessary for carers to identify with, and more fully understand, the needs of those people for whom they care. There is a requirement for carers to have a good working knowledge of the effects of social discrimination and the process of marginalization. Throughout this book we have seen how various groups of people are structurally disadvantaged within society and how prejudicial attitudes and discriminatory practices combine to impoverish their lives, so that they do not participate as fully in society as they otherwise might. An acknowledgement of the structural disadvantage experienced by the majority of our clients helps the social carer or social worker to resist the temptation to blame the person, or people, for whom they care. Seeing the client in her or his social setting rather than in isolation is one step towards obtaining a more rounded perspective of the client. In pursuing positive practice we should be aiming to reduce the gap which often exists between social carers and their clients. Indeed many of the recently produced social care and social work directives, with their focus on the client, may help facilitate this.

We have seen from our examination of social class and the 'underclass' that many members of our society are deprived of full citizenship and suffer a range of deprivations. The same is true for many women, black people and members of other minority groups such as elders, people with disabilities, gay men, lesbians and travellers. We must attack the marginalization which prevents all these groups from fully participating in our society and aim for *full citizenship* for all.

In order to achieve this, we need as far as possible to aim to see the world through the eyes of those for whom we care. We need, therefore, to develop an empathy for others regardless of any differences in social class, gender, racial origin, culture, sexual orientation, age or life-style. We should note that we are not capable of absolute empathy because our experience will never fully correspond with that of another person. We should, however, always aspire to be as sensitive to others as possible.

There are a number of essential qualities that are needed in an effective carer in addition to empathy. These include personal qualities such as sensitivity, assertiveness, love and compassion, and a predilection to demonstrate the basic courtesies of politeness and respect. Also needed are communication and interpersonal skills, including the ability to listen, and the ability to like people and show warmth, friendliness and cheerfulness.

It is also important that carers can demonstrate practical abilities in order to instil confidence in those they care for: the ability to lift and assist with mobility and to apply nursing skills, including emergency First Aid. Certain attitudes

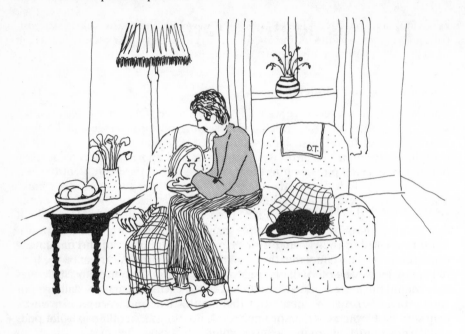

Knowledge and communication are an integral part of practical social care.

are also essential such as patience, tolerance and acceptance. Of course knowledge must precede all good practice. This might be academic knowledge in the social sciences; an awareness of the role and functioning of caring and other organizations; an insight into the needs of minority ethnic cultures; an ability to draw on personal life experience and a commitment to increased self knowledge; and a developed political awareness.

NB: These qualities are more fully explained in Chapter 8 of *Inside the Caring Services* (Tossell and Webb, 1986).

Change and the agencies in which we work

Some of us in social care and social work will be working in large, often bureaucratic organizations. It is very tempting to feel overwhelmed and to feel 'swamped' as an individual in such a large set-up. Frequently, this feeling is accompanied by a pessimism about our agency's ability to change or develop in a positive way. Large bureaucracies can seem to have a life of their own, one which is resistant to change. We need to acknowledge that many caring organizations, in common with other institutions and establishments, have a vested interest in maintaining the *status quo*. They are, in the main, dominated by white, middle-class, middle-aged males.

It is important not to become despondent about the inherent resistance of all bureaucracies because this can only be disabling. Instead, we need to be more positive and remember that we *can* control what we do – that is, our own behaviour and practice. These will often in small, immeasurable ways contribute to change around us and eventually to change in wider society, although we will not always be conscious of this process.

Self-awareness and self-development

The most important resource we bring to social care is ourselves. This is not a static entity, but a resource which is undergoing constant change and development. In order to retain a high standard of personal practice, we need to continually examine our attitudes, behaviour and approach, and to develop our own personal strategies for effective care.

Taking risks and being assertive

In addition to monitoring our own personal practice, we also have a responsibility to challenge the practice of others and the policies of the employing organization when we feel that these are having a detrimental effect on the lives of clients. However, this will often involve taking risks because our challenges may offend those we work with and may, in the extreme, actually damage our career advancement. We need to overcome this fear and in an assertive way confront bad practice. Compromise and, worse still, collusion with poor standards of practice are never acceptable.

For example, a carer may be tempted to tolerate racist comments made by an elderly white resident in an elderly person's home towards a black member of staff or a fellow resident. The carer may compromise by only making a tentative objection, or collude by ignoring its occurrence, in order not to offend the white resident. Neither option is satisfactory. It is all too easy to patronize and make excuses for someone's age or cultural background. Our behaviour and that of others should be consistent at all times and in all settings.

Empowerment

The principle of *empowerment* in social care has been around for some time in different guises, although the word itself has only recently come into common parlance. Even now the word is open to a range of varying interpretations, but it fundamentally concerns issues of power and control, and how these effect clients' lives.

It is more useful to consider empowerment as a continuum rather than in absolute terms. It would be extremely difficult to find situations of either complete empowerment or of its total absence. Most practice will lie somewhere in between.

Full empowerment	←——————— partial empowerment ———————→	Complete lack of empowerment

Some people object to the concept of empowerment because they do not believe that permanent power can ever be *given* to another person or group. If it were possible to give it, it could just as easily be possible for it to be taken away. Further they feel that power can only truly be seized. Others would see

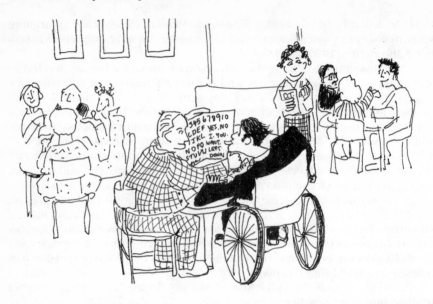

The use of an alphabet board enables a person with cerebral palsy to express exactly how he likes his food. By pointing to individual letters with his tongue, he indicates to his friend or carer his precise requirements. This is an example of empowerment.

this as representing a rather extreme philosophical objection that denies the power inherent in the caring role. Such people feel that any intervention which is aimed at enabling clients, by definition, automatically makes a contribution to their empowerment. For example, the creation of a safe environment in which a client is able to express her or himself freely, or the creation of structures where clients make more decisions for themselves, is part of the process.

Advocacy and self-advocacy

The idea of advocacy is an old one. We are familiar with someone acting on behalf of another who may not be able to speak for themselves. She or he speaks for that person and in so doing represents her or his best interests. A daily example can be found in the criminal courts where solicitors or barristers act as advocates for those they represent.

More recently the term has been introduced into social care and social work to describe such occasions when, for example, a social worker represents the interests of her or his client at a tribunal; a community psychiatric nurse attends her or his client's job interview, or when a probation officer supports her or his client at the housing department in an attempt to secure accommodation.

Advocacy however can be seen to be patronizing because the social carer or social worker in a position of authority mediates or negotiates on behalf of the client who is relatively powerless. It is of course very often this power differential which makes advocacy essential; it defends the weak against the strong. Malcolm Payne describes the essential nature of advocacy as 'arguing for change where power has created an existing decision or predisposition against the client' (1986, p. 118).

The negative implications of the patronizing nature of advocacy has led to the development of self-advocacy and a growing number of self-advocacy projects. It is seen that a social carer may actually 'disable' a client by acting 'for' them and may prevent them from acting assertively. Instead self-advocacy aims to enable clients to act on their own in their own best interests – to speak for themselves. It is therefore central to the concept of empowerment. It is about making decisions and choices for oneself and about being assertive.

Frequently, a self-advocacy project will develop from some collective or group activity in which common problems are shared, for example with a social welfare agency or housing department. Ways of tackling the problem may be explored and at a later stage rehearsals, simulations or role plays may take the participants further. All are designed to lead to a point where the client feels at least reasonably safe and confident to make contact or intervene on their own behalf. This does not of course rule out the possibility of the group remaining in existence as a background support.

Anti-discriminatory practice

As we have said earlier, our social care practice should be aimed at counteracting the marginalization of anybody in our society, whether on grounds of class, gender, race or culture, age, disability, sexual orientation or life-style. In this regard, we should be continually vigilant in examining ourselves and our attitudes. In order to help this process we can read, think, observe and discuss relevant issues with family, friends, colleagues and clients. One of the most important things to check out is our own *language* – how we speak or write is usually how we think and it reflects our attitudes and beliefs. The words we use will convey to others how we see them. Certain words and phrases will carry negative and possibly harmful connotations. Others will communicate dignity and respect: for example 'elderly' and 'elders' have increasingly replaced terms like 'old' and 'aged'; 'physically disabled' or even 'physically challenged', have replaced 'cripples'; 'people with learning difficulties' and 'people with special needs' are replacing the label of 'the mentally handicapped' and 'subnormal'. This is part of an ongoing process which has already seen the demise of such terms as 'lunatic', 'imbecile' and 'cretin'. Furthermore, certain terms such as 'the disabled' and 'these people' serve to distance the user from the client group. Words such as 'sufferer' or 'victims' are used to invoke pity or sympathy where it may not be welcome. Consider for example the more positive attitude conveyed by the use of 'people living with HIV' as opposed to 'AIDS sufferers' or the 'victims of AIDS'.

Anti-racism

There has been an increasing recognition of the central need for anti-racist practice. Social care organizations have provided their own Codes of Practice. In 1990, the Social Care Association produced a short *Action Checklist* for practitioners and managers in order to promote good practice. According to this booklet, anti-racist practice:

- is the responsibility of all practitioners;
- challenges racism in all practice settings;
- takes steps to remedy the shortcomings of provision for black people;
- is active in seeking out racism;
- consciously highlights the multi-racial nature of our society.

The Social Care Association's 'strategy' for putting this checklist into operation is also extremely useful:

- *Think* about your racism together with that of your colleagues.
- *Accept* that the problems exist.
- *Plan* for action.
- *Challenge* racism including the racism inside yourself.
- *Review* progress and decide on further action.

The checklist also provides more details and encourages us to aim for personal goals, which may include the ability:

'to actively seek awareness and understanding of our own racism and that of others; to examine how your attitudes and behaviour contribute to racism . . . to seek to avoid cultural and racial stereotyping; to openly disagree with any racist joke or action; and to promote a positive image of black people within social care settings.'

An important part of our anti-racist practice is to support our colleagues who work for changes in practice. We must oppose policies which collude with the marginalization of black people. It is important to be clear that anti-racism is not about preferential treatment; it is aimed at redressing inequality and establishing social justice. It is therefore something for us all to be involved in. Frequently a single black person can be made a scapegoat, or labelled as 'difficult' or a 'trouble-maker' by colleagues who simply disagree with her or him. We should also avoid a situation in which we contribute to one black person in a team being pressurized into being the so-called 'expert' on race issues or on racism. Instead we need to ask questions directly of policy makers, administrators and managers.

We need to continually update our practice in order to remain in touch with social change. One way in which we can do this is to attend anti-racist courses and encourage others to take part, in order to share what we have learned and to try to apply it to the work setting. It is important to discuss the issues involved in an open and honest way.

Other ways in which we can be anti-racist are to introduce positive images and experiences of black people: to share their history and life stories; to celebrate their customs and festivals; to have their food prepared in traditional ways; and enjoy culturally appropriate music, dance, games and pastimes. Decisions relating to any, or all of these, may depend upon management policies. However, we each have a responsibility to press for their introduction.

If we work with many people from different cultures, for example, Greek, Chinese, Punjabi or Polish, and a large number of that community do not speak English, we may need to learn the language in order to improve communication. The least we can do is to learn the most common 100–200 words and some regularly used phrases, and thus help to break down barriers.

Anti-sexism

Men must examine the sexism within themselves and not tolerate it or collude with it in other men, regardless of age. Often sexism will be subtle or unconscious, as when for example a man 'talks over' women in a team meeting. It may not be easy for a man to even realize he is doing this. However, men need to monitor their behaviour in this respect, perhaps by talking to others. It should be pointed out that it is not only women who are 'talked over'; the same thing happens to some men. Not everybody is comfortable expressing themselves in public, and we need to recognize that all of us have a valid contribution to make, whatever our style. What we can do to facilitate this is to make space and give encouragement to others so that everyone has a full opportunity to be heard.

All clients, but particularly women, should have the right to choose a carer of their own gender. This is important in situations of providing physical care as it is when intimate matters are under discussion, for example, in counselling. Similarly, all women should have the opportunity to be able to choose to be supervised by another woman whether they are paid social carers, volunteers, or students on training courses or placements. They may find this arrangement less threatening and more conducive to learning and self-disclosure.

Anti-disableism

People with disabilities are commonly patronized, pitied or ignored. All of these unhelpful responses contribute to the marginalization of people with disabilities or with learning difficulties. Treating them in this way prevents them from living as fully integrated and fulfilled people. The very word disability is in itself disparaging. This point is confirmed by the Wagner Report (1988) which states, 'The commonly applied label "disabled" emphasizes disability at the expense of ability and, without discussion, assumes dependency. Which one of us would wish to be characterized by what we are unable to do?'.

Not only do disabled people have to come to terms with their particular physical or mental limitation, they also have to cope with society's disablist attitudes when they want to be seen as ordinary people with ordinary human emotions who are capable of making a valuable contribution to society. How they are dealt with and depicted affects their self-image and self-belief. As Ann MacFarlane says 'It can be difficult, almost impossible, to have a good self-image and confidence if you are being "cared for" as a disabled person in a way which lends you to perceive yourself as a "burden" or "helpless" (*Arthritis News*, February 1990).

Equal opportunities

Many people feel their employers' equal opportunities policies are merely statements of good intent but are not translated into effective practice and there is some evidence of this being the case. One way of ensuring their relevance and application is for each of us to familiarize ourselves with what has been laid down by our employer. In order to keep the issues alive, we need to

share our understanding of equal opportunities with other people and continually monitor its application, and in order to reflect our changing society it
should be kept under review. A standardized equal opportunities statement is
likely to be taken for granted or ignored and will run the risk of being merely
'tokenistic'.

Positive practice today

Positive practice in social care should involve affirming some or all of the
following, both as policy and as practical action.

Rights

Insisting that clients' *citizen*, *legal* and *welfare* rights are upheld and respected
at all times. This is clearly a very important part of full social citizenship. It also
requires all carers to gain as much reliable, up-to-date information about any
rights which may improve the quality of life of those for whom they care.

User involvement

This is another term, currently very much in fashion, which needs to be
translated into practice in order to avoid becoming mere rhetoric. Clients can
be involved at all stages: in planning services, and how they are to be most
effectively delivered, and in running their own services as much as possible and
in budgeting for those services. Except in exceptional circumstances, all clients
should be present and involved in their own 'case conferences'.

The new proposals for community care offer exciting possibilities for user
involvement. They embody a client-centred approach, new procedures for
assessment, and the newly created role of care manager, and enable the client
to be more centrally involved in her or his own care. This can involve a real shift
in power in favour of the client, to the point where, as Terry Bamford, writing
in *Social Work Today*, has suggested, 'a client might become her or his own
care manager'. In fact some elderly people or people with disabilities are
already fulfilling this role.

Robert Taylor is paralysed from the neck down after a motorbike accident,
and is totally dependent. He runs his own self-care scheme and employs two
care assistants who 'live-in' at his home while on duty. They work a two week
rota system working about 11 hours per day. He funds the scheme from three
sources: the local authority, a DSS attendance allowance, and his own personal
income.

The care assistants perform very personal work including washing, dressing,
bladder and bowel care as well as general domestic duties. In addition, they
perform social duties which include entertaining and provide transport for
Robert as necessary. He writes, 'Independent living is not just living on your
own. It gives you the chance to live a normal life, make decisions, however
important or unimportant, to live in a normal house in a normal street with
normal people . . . With a fuller life you can put something more back into the
community' (*Community Care*, 27 April 1989, p. iii).

For many years Peter Beresford and Suzy Croft have been studying user
involvement in services which, in their own words, are 'more democratic and
appropriate'. But, as they point out, there are pitfalls; for example, when social

care agencies merely want user-involvement to help deliver a cheaper, more cost effective service. However, if it is done well, the clients involved can gain more confidence and learn new skills and abilities. At best, they say, 'where empowerment is the aim, people decide the agenda for themselves . . . This model comes closest to realizing the idea of self-advocacy in social services' (*Community Care Supplement*, 27 April 1989).

Access to records

Social care agencies hold a great deal of information about clients, much of it of an extremely personal nature. Apart from a small number of cases where the sharing of some of the information held would be unwise, we should strive to make the records and files we hold on others as open to them as possible; we should share the case records and even write them on a co-operative basis. This should increasingly become a natural part of regular practice because this is an essential constituent of empowerment.

Complaints and redress

When things go wrong, as they sometimes do, we must make it as easy as possible for those who are not happy with the service we deliver to make complaints and receive redress. If such procedures are built into normal daily practice they will also make it easier and less threatening for those of us who are on the receiving end of complaints. Readily admitting an error is one step towards developing good practice.

Get to know your community

In following our aim of seeing our clients in their social setting and not in isolation we need to acquaint ourselves with their immediate physical environment and local community. Getting to know the 'patch' where you work, whatever its setting, residential, day care, domiciliary or field, will involve a knowledge of all the resources in the neighbourhood including shops, clubs, pubs, community groups, and any specialist facility, for example, for those with disabilities or for a particular ethnic minority group.

A good up-to-date knowledge of the community in which we work can especially help to break down barriers in a residential setting which may seem rather cut off from the neighbourhood life around it. We always need to be aware that residential provision is an integral part of community care.

Find support

Whether we are paid social carers or volunteers, most of us need and benefit from the support of others. Where a form of support, possibly a group, already exists we should think of joining it to make our own unique contribution. If no form of support exists, we should think about starting one because there are usually others who feel isolated and who will benefit from contact. The same applies to carers of a dependent relative or relatives; they could find out whether or not a local group of the Carers' National Association exists in their area. If there is not, they could go about forming one.

The value of a support group for informal carers is the opportunity to express

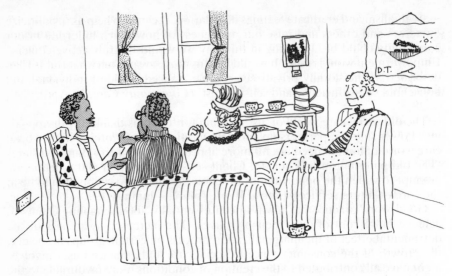

Informal carers can derive mutual benefit and support from regular meetings.

themselves, share their problems and learn from other carers. For some, the group can be a great source of confidence and support. In particular, Nick Fielding outlined the special value of an all black carers group, one of several black, Asian or Chinese carers groups which have been set up throughout the country.

'The group gives an opportunity for its members to discuss their problems and to share them – realizing that someone else has to deal with similar issues can often be uplifting. It also allows the members to socialize, share recipes and discuss issues relating to the black community or home background which they might feel constrained to mention in a predominantly white group.'
    'Sometimes it's just important to talk in our own "Patois"' added one of the members.

(*Community Care*, 11 January 1990)

Conclusion – the personal and the political

Political and social policy issues, such as poverty, poor housing, a lack of childcare provision or community facilities, cannot be separated from personal circumstances – each affects the other. As a reflection of this, individual positive practice in social care often needs to be accompanied by action for political change for a more humane, kinder, less unequal and unjust society. There are a number of ways which we, as social carers, can combine the personal and the political in a meaningful, life enhancing way.

If we join with either staff or clients to press for a new facility, for example, play space or the installation of a creche, or the provision of a regular meeting room in our local area, this *collective experience* can energize us, galvanize others into action and give us a valuable experience of shared assertiveness. Such an experience can help us, as carers and clients, to break out of our individualism and eradicate feelings of isolation. It can also help us to politicize ourselves and others and raise our awareness of how much fuller life in our community could be. In acting in this way we would be truly active citizens! Empowerment would result. It would help us move away from what Bill Jordan described as the 'totally privatized, commercialized world of individual and household self-sufficiency and self-interest' (*Community Care*, 19 April 1990, p. 28).

The old social care world of 'us' working for 'them' is thankfully disappearing. Power sharing, partnership and democratic ways of working in the social care world of human need are far more appropriate. As Terry Bamford states 'The old paternalism will not do. Client self-determination and a deliberate attempt to widen the opportunities for choice available to clients should be at the core of future services' (*Social Work Today*, 4 January 1990).

Good work practice has always been essentially about enabling clients to achieve more control over their own lives. The increased awareness of the detrimental effect of the marginalization process on certain groups in society, the growth of the consumer voice in social care and enhanced user involvement have all contributed to the creation of conditions more favourable to the enabling process. Any client-centred social care practice that fully acknowledges the importance of the clients' social setting will help to translate the theories and policies of Community Care and so move towards a more caring community.

Exercises

1. *Integration or special provision?*

You are a social worker working with a family of a 13-year-old child who has moderate learning difficulties; she is physically disabled and a wheelchair user. The girl, Marva James, has been offered the opportunity of attending a mainstream school full time, and whilst her father would support such a move her mother is against it, primarily because she feels Marva is too vulnerable and would 'only experience failure'.

To date Marva has been attending the same special school since she was four years old. The school was purpose built and is constructed on one level; it has wide corridors and hand rails throughout the building. Care within the school is of a very high standard and teaching takes place in small groups with a low staff/student ratio. The facilities are good and pupils can receive physiotherapy and hydrotherapy on the school premises. The academic emphasis is mainly on developing basic reading and writing skills. Marva likes school and has achieved a great deal.

Over the past 12 months Marva has also been attending a mainstream comprehensive; initially one day per week during the first term, and finally for three days of the week during the third term. The school is not fully adapted to wheelchair use but it is mainly on one level. Marva has been provided with her own word processor and is eligible for additional individual teacher support with lessons under the conditions of her educational special needs statement. In other words she is entitled to the exclusive support of an additional teacher in the classroom. However, this facility has not yet been arranged by the local education authority.

Marva likes her new school and no longer wants to go to the special school. She does not see herself as having the same problems of other children with learning difficulties and would regard a permanent move to a mainstream school as an achievement in itself. She wants to take up the chance of repeating the second year and to start full time in September.

Mrs James, Marva's mother, is concerned that Marva will now be exposed to the possibility of ridicule from other children and may even be at risk of physical injury in a large mainstream school. More significantly she worries that Marva will 'only experience failure'. Marva would have to study for GCSE's which both her mother and father fear she will not do well in. 'I want her to be able to read and write . . . but because of the National Curriculum she has to do French. What good will that do her?'

Despite the reservations of her mother Marva's father would like to see his daughter experience mainstream full time education in order that she may encounter some of the difficulties presented by the outside world as early as possible in her life. He argues that the younger she is when she is exposed to the reactions of 'able-bodied' people, the better adjusted she will be by the time she reaches adulthood. Mrs James is concerned that her daughter's already low self-image will be further damaged when she spends time away from the protective and supportive surroundings of the special school.

How would you go about helping the parents make a decision about Marva's full time education?

2. 'Empowerment'

The diagram on p. 219 shows a continuum ranging from *full empowerment* on the left to a *complete lack* of *empowerment* on the right. The area in between is regarded as partial empowerment. Consider each of the following five case studies. In particular, regard the clients' circumstances and the care regimes of the homes or establishments in which they are placed. Now place each case at a different point on the continuum. Compare your assessments with other members of the group.

Case 1

Ms Pillai is 85 years old and has been a resident of an elderly person's home for six months. She had some difficulty walking before she came into the home owing to her arthritis but now she rarely has to walk. The staff have provided her with a wheelchair which enables her to get around quicker and more easily. A retired teacher, she is happy with her own company and enjoys reading. She does not seem to like the activities provided by the home such as crochet, cards and bingo, although she participates from time to time usually following some persuasion from a member of staff. She is getting more used to the food now. Initially she refused to eat much of it and lost a little weight as a result. She still misses the food her daughter used to provide before she came into the home.

Her main interest is gardening. She has pictures of flowers in the room she shares in the home. The grounds of the home are not very well cared for but she likes to get outside when she can. Unfortunately, she is dependent upon a care officer making the time to take her out. The door to the garden remains locked in order to deter residents from wandering. Mrs Pillai has made a friend of the person she shares a room with. She doesn't mind sharing but would prefer a bed near the window. She is the only Asian person in the home. She misses her cat and looks forward to the monthly visits from her daughter who left the area with her young family recently.

Case 2

Derek Pendry is in his early thirties and now lives in a large communal home which has been adapted by a voluntary society that aims to provide housing and support for vulnerable people. Two former terraced houses have been converted to provide a 10-bedroomed house with separate w.c. and bathroom facilities on each of the three floors. In addition there is a lounge, an office and a large kitchen which everyone shares.

Derek has been ill for some time, although since he has been in the communal house he has improved. He is a university graduate who suffered the onset of 'atrophy of the brain' in his final year at Cambridge. He has not been able to find full-time work since, although he has recently had an interview with the rehabilitation officer with a view to exploring work possibilities once again. In the meantime he will continue his job two mornings per week of assisting a person who has multiple sclerosis, which involves preparing food and escorting her for appointments. He prefers this to the hospital day centre work he was formerly involved in.

The household functions rather like any ordinary large family, although there are a greater number of adults. The voluntary society insist that a minimum number of residents are 'dependent' and so the house provides places for two women with learning difficulties, an ex-prisoner suffering with psychiatric problems and another man who is recovering from longer term mental illness. The rest of the household are ordinary members of society; a student, a teacher, a caterer and two people who are unemployed. Their ages range from 24 to 63.

The voluntary society's philosophy is based on the principle that 'everyone has something to offer' and so household tasks are shared as far as possible. When work rotas are drawn up, attempts are made to match dependent people with those more able and that people are given tasks that they can manage. Certain members take responsibility to ensure that another's medication is taken and that any hospital or other appointments are kept.

Decisions regarding the home are taken at communal meetings which are rather informal and sometimes held during the evening meal. Derek is part-membership secretary for the whole housing co-op, a task he shares with another person. He enjoys the responsibility of being actively involved in the home and this experience of representing the house at wider co-op meetings has increased his confidence. He enjoys living in the house, which after three years he regards well and truly as his home. He spends more time than most in the house. He enjoys the variety offered by the different people in the house which is run very much along egalitarian principles which he supports. His medical condition has left him unable to concentrate for long periods on any task and he is obsessive about tidyness to a point where it may upset others, although tidyness is generally appreciated in a large, mixed household. He talks to himself and displays idiosyncratic behaviour such as walking away without explanation during conversations. Nevertheless, Derek is well liked and valued within the home and makes a contribution as full as that of anyone else.

Case 3
Mui Wingate is a 39-year-old Chinese woman who is married to an English
school teacher and has two teenage children. In her early thirties Mui
contracted multiple sclerosis (MS) and is now without any lower body limb
control. She can't bear weight and relies on a wheel chair to get around. Six
months ago she left her home and family to become a resident of the Young
Person's Disabled Unit (YDU) based in the general hospital. Mui recognizes
that she is dependent on others for physical care but no longer wants to be a
'burden' on her husband and children who found difficulty coping. She made an
active choice to be a full time resident at the YDU.

Although her right arm shakes perpetually, she has some steadiness in her
left arm. At the YDU the care staff have provided her with an arm support and
this device enables her to paint with watercolours by holding the brush with her
steadied right hand. After an initial period of settling in, she felt more sure that
she could now have a more fulfilled life than when she was at home. She
arranged for herself, via a local community group, the provision of regular
transport to take her to a local art class each week. Her husband and children
visit regularly and they all went on holiday as a family. Mui sometimes stays at
home over the weekend.

Mui now feels that she and her husband have a more equal relationship now
that he doesn't have to be her physical carer. She prefers to be 'in the hands of
professionals' whom she feels are competent and caring and 'unfussy' in their
attention to her needs.

Case 4
Arthur Denton is 60 years old and recently had a stroke, which paralysed him
down his left side, making it difficult for him to speak without slurring. He lives
at home with his wife, Margaret, who is 12 years younger and reasonably
healthy. The last of their five children has now left home. Mr Denton led a very
active life before his stroke. He was active in sports, was the captain of the
bowls team and a keen gardener. He used to commute to his professional job in
the city from which he had to retire prematurely. Mrs Denton has never
worked outside the home except as a student nurse before their marriage 30
years ago. She is very fit for her age and manages as well as possible to attend to
her husband's needs, although she finds lifting him very difficult in spite of her
earlier training as a nurse.

Financially the couple are well off and recently Mrs Denton has decided to
pay for a private nurse to bathe her husband three times a week. She does not
want any social services involvement partly because she is unaware of the range
of help they can provide and partly because she is reluctant to draw on 'welfare
provision'.

Mrs Denton is a voluntary worker for a national charity organization and an
active member of the branch of a political party. She is therefore out of the
house for some of the evenings in the week. She always ensures that her
husband has eaten, has been taken to the toilet and is comfortable before she
leaves. She ensures that the central heating is correctly set and that the TV
remote control switch is on the table within easy reach of her husband's right
hand.

Since his stroke Mr Denton has been depressed. He has lost interest in many of the issues that previously concerned him. He looks forward to the occasional visits from his son, Howard, who has promised to widen the back door entrance and construct a ramp alongside the step to enable his father to get out into the garden. He has also promised to construct a low level garden wall and patio but wants to wait for better weather. In the summer Howard will take him to a weekend bowling tournament which is held annually on the east coast. In the meantime Mr Denton tries to present a cheerful face, especially to his two grandsons who visit occasionally with their parents.

Case 5
Jane Biggs is 19 years old and has moderate learning difficulties. She has recently completed her full time education at a special school where she has been for all her school life. She is the only child of parents who have a tendency to over protect her. She has recently moved to a small group home situated in the local community. Her move follows the persistence and encouragement given to Jane by a Mencap social worker whom she knows through the local Gateway youth club. Both Jane and her parents were initially anxious about her living full time away from the family home, but after six months everyone is more resigned to Jane living in the small group home.

There are five other residents of the home including one full time live-in social worker. Other social workers are on duty during the day but don't usually sleep over. The residents are being trained in self-care and independent living skills including cooking, shopping, budgeting, personal hygiene and general household tasks. This programme is being reinforced by the local Social Education Centre (SEC) where all residents attend. Jane's aim is to eventually obtain some form of 'sheltered' employment. The local Mencap group are involved in providing a range of social activities in the evenings and at weekends.

Jane goes home to her parents most Saturdays and sometimes stays over-night. Occasionally she visits other relatives with her parents. Jane has her own room at the group home and shares the communal areas of the house with the other residents and support workers. She has recently become very friendly with a young man at the SEC. Her social worker is currently undertaking to arrange sexual counselling to ensure that she has appropriate advice and guidance regarding sexual and emotional matters.

In what ways can the subjects of the above cases be empowered?

3. *Carers' handbook*
You are employed by a voluntary organization working with people with disabilities and have been given responsibility for preparing a booklet for those who care for people in their own home. Include information on financial benefits, community resources, leisure facilities, statutory help, relevant organizations, local support networks and availability of aids and adaptations.

4. *Examining our behaviour in positive practice*
Most of the time we behave in one of the four ways described below:

   i) non-assertive or withdrawing – 'I will withdraw or retreat from the situation'.

ii) aggressive – 'I will win at all costs.'

iii) manipulative – 'I will use any method at my disposal.'

iv) assertive – 'I will speak my mind, but will also take into account how others feel or think.'

Most of the time in our work as carers, we might assume that being assertive is the most useful. However, at times the other three might be appropriate. Think of examples of situations when each of the four behaviours might be the most appropriate.

5. *Dealing with prejudice in practice*
Read the following three case studies. After each one consider the following questions:

i)   How would you deal with the situation?
ii) What issues does this case study raise?
iii) What are the attitudes underlying the person's prejudice?
iv) What might you say directly to this person?

Case 1.
You are the Deputy Principal of an Elderly Person's Home. A resident, Mrs Coles, aged 84, has complained on and off for the last couple of days about stomach pains. You noted this in the change-over book when you went off duty 24 hours ago. On your return, the Principal says during change-over

'Mrs Coles is still moaning about her stomach.'

She has taken no action. You see Mrs Coles who appears to be in pain and says, 'Will you get me the Doctor? The Principal wouldn't. Said I should expect it at my age.'

You ring the GP. He refuses to attend with any urgency saying,

'They're all the same at that age, moaning about every ache and pain. They ought to expect it. It'll only be wind. I waste too much of my time dealing with old women when I should be seeing those who really need me . . .'

Case 2.
You are a care assistant in a hostel for mentally handicapped adults. You have heard that the council is putting on courses for care staff dealing with race awareness. Staff in other units have been sent, but you have heard nothing. A number of staff would like to attend the courses. On their behalf, you go to talk to the Principal. When asked why she has not informed you, she says,

'I binned them. They're not relevant to us. We've only white residents and staff here. Anyway, we're so short staffed, I couldn't have afforded to let anyone go. I have to decide priorities you know. Now, if they had been about gender I'd have sent someone, because that's relevant to us. Anyway, the memo from the Director said they were advisable not compulsory.'

Case 3.
You are the Principal of a family group home. One of your residents, Sally aged 15, has applied without your knowledge for a place on an engineering YTS course at a local college. She comes into your office very distressed having had a letter of rejection. Sally is an intelligent girl who attends the local comprehen-

sive but is only expected to get GCSE grade D's. She missed a lot of schooling due to her epilepsy which is now successfully stabilized. Sally is black.

'They just turned me down. Didn't even see me. Didn't even say why.'

You ring the scheme co-ordinator to get more information.

'Sally? . . . Oh yes, I've got her school record here. The black girl . . . Crazy idea wanting to be an engineer when you're epileptic. I mean, workshops are dangerous places. We couldn't take the risk with someone like that. I mean she could get caught up in a machine or something, and then what would it look like? . . . And she'd get teased by all the lads on the course. Not many normal girls even do engineering you know . . . You know I couldn't have people having fits all over the place, especially in workshop three . . . Anyway we all know that kids in care never finish courses.'

Questions for essays or discussion

1. Discrimination awareness training introduces new terms and language but drives prejudice and discrimination underground.
2. Normalization is not a concept generated by minorities themselves, rather it has been devised and imposed by middle class professionals.
3. The idea of 'full citizenship' is not attainable in an unequal society like our own.
4. Empowerment and its application with regard to user involvement is flawed because the power involved is granted rather than taken.
5. All advocacy is disabling and patronizing. People have to do things for themselves.
6. Individual positive social care practice is divorced from wider social change.

Further reading

Academic sources

Ahmed, A., *Practice with Care*. Racial Equality Unit, 1990. A very detailed code of practice aimed at those working with black communities within the social services context. It highlights the relevance of the Race Relations Act to other aspects of social work legislation and provides examples of good practice.

Hicks, C., *Who Cares? Looking After People at Home*. Virago, 1988. Based on a study of 80 individuals who are caring for disabled people in their own homes, this book focuses on the practical and emotional conflicts experienced by carers. Comprehensive and very readable.

Kohner, N., *Caring at Home*. Third edition, NEC, 1989. A reliable mine of information for anyone caring for someone at home, including services available, financial and legal advice, and how to take 'time out'.

Langan, M., Lee, P. (eds), *Radical Social Work Today*. Unwin Hyman, 1989. With contributions from a number of practitioners as well as academics, this book assesses the progress made (or otherwise) in radical practice since the mid 1970s.

Tossell, D., Webb, R., *Inside the Caring Services*. Edward Arnold, 1986. An accessible, simple and comprehensive overview of the caring services, including both statutory and voluntary sectors. The book also highlights ways of performing social care and social work and the basic qualities of a carer.

Worsley, J., *Taking Good Care – A Handbook for Care Assistants*. Age Concern (England), 1989. A very accessible basic guide to caring, whether in a residential home or in the community.

Other literary sources

Alain-Fournier. *Le Grand Meaulnes*. Penguin, 1966.
Axline, V. M., *Dibs – In Search Of Self*. Penguin, 1990.
Bach, R., *Jonathan Livingston Seagull*. Pan, 1973.
Fynn, *Mister God this Is Anna*. Fount/Collins, 1977.
Jefferies, R., *The Story Of My Heart*. Macmillan, 1968.
Salinger, J. D., *The Catcher In The Rye*. Penguin, 1958.

Appendix

Useful addresses*

General

Campaign for Press and Broadcasting Freedom
9 Poland Street
London W1V 3DG

Carers' National Association
29 Chilworth Mews
London W2 3RG
Telephone: (071) 724 7776

Equal Opportunities Commission (EOC)
Overseas House
Quay Street
Manchester M3 3HN
Telephone: (061) 833 9244

National Citizen Advocacy (NCA)
2 St Paul's Road
London N1 2QR
Telephone: (071) 359 8289

Black people

Commission for Racial Equality (CRE)
Elliot House
10–12 Allington Street
London SW1E 5EH
Telephone: (071) 828 7022

Institute for Race Relations
2–6 Leeke Street
Kings Cross Road
London WC1X 9HS
Telephone: (071) 837 0041

Joint Council for the Welfare of Immigrants
115 Old Street
London EC1V 9VR
Telephone: (071) 251 8706

* (correct in January 1991)

Elders

Age Concern (England)
Bernard Sunley House
60 Pitcairn Road
Mitcham
Surrey CR4 3LL
Telephone: (081) 640 5431

Age Concern (Ireland)
6 Lower Crescent
Belfast BT7 1NR
Telephone: (0232) 245729

Age Concern (Scotland)
54a Fountain Bridge
Edinburgh EH3 9PT
Telephone: (031) 228 5656

Gays and lesbians

Campaign for Homosexual Equality
PO Box 342
London WC1N 0DU
Telephone: (071) 833 3912

Lesbian Line
BM Box 1514
London WC1X 3XX
Telephone: (071) 251 6911

HIV and AIDS

Body Positive
51B Philbeach Gardens
London SW5 9EB
Telephone: (071) 835 1045

The Terrence Higgins Trust
52–54 Grays Inn Road
London WC1X 8JU
Telephone: (071) 242 1010

Learning difficulties

Learning Difficulties – Values into Action
Oxford House
Derbyshire Street
London E2 6HG
Telephone: (071) 729 5436

Royal Society for Mentally Handicapped Children and Adults (MENCAP)
123 Golden Lane
London EC1Y 0RT
Telephone: (071) 253 9433

Mental health

National Association for Mental Health (MIND)
22 Harley Street
London W1N 2ED
Telephone: (071) 637 0741

National Schizophrenia Fellowship
78 Victoria Road
Surbiton
Surrey KT6 4NS
Telephone: (081) 390 3651/2

Physically disabled people

Physically Handicapped and Able Bodied (PHAB)
12–14 London Road
Croydon
Surrey CR0 2TA
Telephone: (081) 667 9443

Poverty

Child Poverty Action Group
1–5 Bath Street
London EC1V 9PY
Telephone: (071) 253 3406

Low Pay Unit
9 Upper Berkeley Street
London W1H 8BY
Telephone: (071) 262 7278

Prisoners, ex-prisoners and their families

National Association for the Care and Resettlement of Offenders (NACRO)
169 Clapham Road
London SW9 0PU
Telephone: (071) 582 6500

Prison Reform Trust
59 Caledonian Road
London N1 9BU
Telephone: (071) 278 9815

Single parents

Gingerbread
35 Wellington Street
London WC2E 7BN
Telephone: (071) 240 0953

National Council for One Parent Families
255 Kentish Town Road
London NW5 2LX
Telephone: (071) 267 1361

Women

Northern Ireland Women's Aid
143a University Street
Belfast BT7 1HP
Telephone: (0232) 662385

Scottish Women's Aid
Ainslie House
11 St. Colne Street
Edinburgh EH3 6AG
Telephone: (031) 225 8011

Welsh Women's Aid
38–48 Crwys Road
Cardiff CF2 4NN
Telephone: (0222) 390874

Women's Aid Federation (England) Ltd.
PO Box 391
Bristol BS99 7WS
Telephone: (0272) 633542

References

Acton, T., *Gypsy Politics and Social Change*, Routledge and Kegan Paul, 1974.

Age Concern, *Older People in the UK. Some Basic Facts*, Age Concern, 1990.

Archbishops' Commission on Rural Areas, *Faith in the Countryside*, Churchman, 1990.

Archbishop of Canterbury's Commission on Urban Priority Areas, *Faith in the City*, Church House, 1986.

Audit Commission, *Making a Reality of Community Care*, HMSO, 1986.

Bayley, D., in Punch, M. (ed.), *Control in the Police Organisation*, MIT Press, 1983.

Blackstone, T., *Prisons and Penal Reform*, Chatto and Windus, 1990.

Box, S., *Recession, Crime and Punishment*, Macmillan, 1987.

Boyson, R., *The Defence of the Family. The Battle Against Permissiveness*, The Church Society, 1987.

British Association of Social Workers, *The Obstacle Race. Report of the Action Project into Ethnically Sensitive Social Work*, BASW, 1990.

Brown, G. W., Brolchan, M. N., Harris, T., Social class and psychiatric disturbance among women in an urban population. *Sociology*, 1975, **9**, 225–54.

Bulmer, M., *The Goals of Social Policy*, Unwin Hyman, 1989.

Campling, J. (ed.), *Learning the Hard Way. A Feminist List*, Macmillan, 1989.

Central Council for Nursing, Midwifery and Health Visiting, *Project 2000 – A New Preparation for Practice*, CCNMHV, 1986.

Child Poverty Action Group, *Poverty – The Facts*, CPAG, 1988.

Church Action on Poverty, *Declaration – Hearing the Cry of the Poor*, CAP, 1989.

Church of England Report, *Ageing*, Church House, 1990.

Cochrane, R., Stopes-Roe, M., Women, marriage, employment and mental health. *British Journal of Psychiatry*, 1981, **139**, 137–45.

Cohen, B., *Caring for Children. Service Policies for Childcare and Equal Opportunities in the UK*. Report for the European Commission Child Care Network. Commission of the European Communities, 1988.

Commission for Racial Equality, *From Cradle to School – A Practical Guide to Race, Equality and Childcare*, CRE, 1989.

CRE, *Living in Terror – A Report on Racial Violence and Harassment in Housing*, Chairman Sir Peter Newman, CRE, 1987.

CRE, *Annual Report*, CRE, 1983.

CRE/ADSS, *Multi Racial Britain – The Social Services Response*, CRE, 1978.

Connor, S., Kingman, S., *The Search for the Virus*, Penguin, 1989.

Department of Health. Statistics and Management Division. HMSO, 1990.

Department of Health, Social Security, Wales and Scotland White Paper on Community Care, *Caring for People. Community Care in the Next Decade and Beyond*, HMSO, 1989.

Department of Health White Paper, *Working for Patients*, HMSO, 1989.

DHSS, *Better Services for the Mentally Handicapped*, HMSO, 1971.

DHSS, *Inequalities in Health*, Chairman Sir Douglas Black, HMSO, 1980.

Disability Alliance, *The Financial Circumstances of Disabled Adults Living in Private Households. Briefing paper No. 2*, Disability Alliance, 1988.

Esam, P., Oppenheim, C., *A Charge on the Community*, CPAG/LGIU, 1989.

Equal Opportunities Commission, *Information Pack Part II. Education and Training*, EOC, 1989.

Fitzgerald, M., *Key Facts on Minorities of Afro-Caribbean and Asian Origin. Based on Labour Force Survey Data 1985-7*, HMSO, 1989.

Formiani, H., *Men – The Darker Continent*, Mandarin, 1990.

Fryer, P., *Staying Power – The History of Black People*, Pluto Press, 1984.

Giddens, A., *The Class Structures of the Advanced Societies*, Hutchinson, 1973.

Giddens, A., *Sociology – A Brief but Critical Introduction*, Macmillan, 1982.

Goldsmith College Media Research Group, *Media Coverage of Local Government in London*, Methuen, 1987.

Goldthorpe, J., *Social Mobility and Class Structure in Modern Britain*, Oxford University Press, 1980.

Gordon, P., *Racial Violence and Harassment*, Runnymede Trust, 1986.

Gorz, A., *Farewell to the Working Class*, Pluto Press, 1982.

Griffith, J.A.C., *The Politics of the Judiciary*, Longman, 1985.

Griffiths report, *Community Care: Agenda for Action*, Report to the Secretary of State for Social Services. Chairman Sir Roy Griffiths, HMSO, 1988.

Hanmer, J., Statham, D., *Women and Social Work – Towards a Woman Centred Practice*, Macmillan, 1988.

Health Education Council (HEC), *The Health Divide: Inequalities in Health in the 1980s*, HEC, 1987.

Hennessy, P., *What the Papers Never Said*, Portcullis Press, 1985.

Heidensohn, F., *Gender and Crime*, Macmillan, 1985.

HMSO, *Gypsies and Other Travellers*, HMSO, 1967.

Hite, S., *Women and Love*, Penguin, 1988.

Holdaway, S., *Inside the British Police*, Blackwell, 1983.

Home Affairs Committee, *Report on Racial Attacks and Harassment*, HMSO, 1986.

Hough, M., Mayhew, P., *Taking Account of Crime. Key Findings from the 1984 British Crime Survey*, Home Office Research Study no. 85, HMSO, 1985.

House of Lords Select Committee on the European Commission, *Income Taxation and Equal Treatment for Men and Women*, HMSO, 1985.

Hyman, M., *Sites for Travellers – A Study in Five London Boroughs*, London Race and Housing Research Unit, 1989.

Inner London Education Authority, *Race, Sex and Class. 6. A Policy for Equality*, ILEA, 1985.

Jefferson, J., Smith, I., Watching the Police, in *Critical Social Policy, no. 13*, pp. 124–33, 1985.

Joint Council for the Welfare of Immigrants, *Target Caribbean – The Rise in Visitor Refusals from the Caribbean*, JCWI, 1990.

Jones, C., *State Social Work and the Working Class*, Macmillan, 1983.

Jones, T., Maclean, B., Young, J., *The Islington Crime Survey*, Gower Press, 1986.

Jordan, B., *The Common Good – Citizenship, Morality and Self-Interest*, Basil Blackwell, 1989.

Lea, J., Mathews, R., Young, J., *Law and Order – 5 Years On*, Middlesex Polytechnic Centre for Criminology, 1987.

Letts, P., *Double Struggle–Sex, Discrimination and One Parent Families*, NCFOPF, 1983.

Lister, R., *The Exclusive Society. Citizenship and the Poor*, CPAG, 1990.

Littlewood, R., Lipsedge, M., *Aliens and Alienists*, Pelican, 1982.

London Borough of Newham, *Report of a Survey of Crime and Racial Harassment in Newham*, London Borough of Newham, 1987.

Mack, J., Lansley, S., *Poor Britain*, Allen and Unwin, 1985.

Mallinson, I., *The Social Care Task*, SCA, 1988.

Mama, A., *The Hidden Struggle – Statutory and Voluntary Sector Responses to Violence Against Black Women in the Home*, Race and Housing Research Initiative, 1989.

Marshall, G., Newby, H., Rose, D., *Social Class in Modern Britain*, Hutchinson, 1988.

Marx, K., Engels, F., *Manifesto of the Communist Party*, Foreign Languages Press, 1975.

Matthews, R., from Justice of the Peace, quoted in Alcock, P., Lee, P. (eds), *Into the Third Term: Thatcherism and the Future of Welfare*, Sheffield City Polytechnic, 1988.

McNeil-Taylor, E., *Bringing up Children On Your Own*, Fontana, 1985.

Morgan Thomas, R., AIDS risks, alcohol, Drugs and the sex industry – a Scottish study, in Plany, M. (ed.), *AIDS, Drugs and Prostitution*, Routledge, 1990.

Morley, D., Whitaker, B., *The Press, Radio and Television – An Introduction to the Media*, Comedia, 1986.

Murphy, A., *The Heavy Stuff no. 1*, London Class War, 1987.

National Association for the Care and Resettlement of Offenders, *Imprisonment in England and Wales: Some Facts and Figures*, NACRO, 1990.

NACRO, *British Crime Survey. The Fear of Crime: Some Facts and Figures*, NACRO, 1982.

NACRO, *Black People and the Criminal Justice System*, NACRO, 1986.

NACRO briefing, *Understanding Criminal Statistics*, NACRO, 1988.

NACRO, *Courts and Sentencing*, NACRO, 1989a.

NACRO, *Crime and Sentencing*, NACRO, 1989b.

National Council for One Parent Families, *Key Facts*, NCFOPF, 1990.

NISW/SCA, *Making National Vocational Qualifications Work for Social Care*, NISW/SCA, 1990.

Norman, A., *Triple Jeopardy: Growing Old in a Second Homeland*, Centre for Policy on Ageing, 1985.

OPCS, *Classification of Occupation*, HMSO, 1988a.

OPCS, *Surveys of Disability in Great Britain. The Prevalence of Disabilities Among Adults in Great Britain*, Report no. 1, HMSO, 1988b.

OPCS, *Surveys of Disability in Great Britain. The Financial Circumstances of Disabled Adults Living in Private Households*, Report no. 2, HMSO, 1988c.

Office for Population, Censuses and Surveys, Population estimates limit, *OPCS Monitor*, HMSO, 1990.

Orbach, S., *Fat is a Feminist Issue*, Hamlyn, 1978.

Payne, M., *Social Care in the Community*, BASW, 1986.

Prison Reform Trust, *Prison Report*, 1989, **8**, 2.

Race Equality Unit, *Community Care: Race Dimension*, Duff, R. (ed), REU/NISW, 1989.

Reid, I., *Social Class Differences in Britain*, Grant McIntyre, 1981.

Rex, J., Tomlinson, S., *Colonial Immigrants in a British City*, Routledge, 1979.

Reiner, R., *The Politics of the Police*, Wheatsheaf, 1985.

Rutherford, A., *Growing Out of Crime*, Penguin, 1986.

Ryan, W., *Blaming the Victim*, Vintage Books, 1976.

Sandford, J., *Gypsies*, Abacus/Sphere Books, 1975.

Saunders, P., *Social Class and Stratification*, Routledge, 1990.

Savage, S., *Law and Order*, Hyperion Press, 1986.

Scottish Drugs Forum Bulletin, 1990, **34**, 7.

Scull, A., *Decarceration*, Prentice Hall, 1984.

Sickle Cell Society, *Sickle Cell Anaemia (HbSS) and Sickle Cell Trait (HbAS)*, SCS, 1987.

Smith, D., Gray, L., *Police and People in London*, Policy Studies Institute, 1983.

Smith, M., *Gypsies: Where Now?* Young Fabian Pamphlet, no. 42, 1975.

Smith, P., *Language, the Sexes and Society*, Blackwells, 1985.

Smith, D., Fowles, A. J., *Crime and Penal Policy*, Longman, 1986.

Social Care Association, *Social Care in the Community*, BASW, 1986.

Stevens, P., Willis, C., *Race, Crime and Arrests*, Home Office Research Unit, HMSO, 1979.

Swann Report, *Education for All – The Report of the Committee of Enquiry into the Education of Children from Ethnic Minority Groups*, HMSO, Cmnd 9453, 1985.

Tossell, D., Webb, R., *Inside The Caring Services*, Edward Arnold, 1986.

Town, P., in Walker, A., Walker, C. (eds), *The Growing Divide*, CPAG, 1987.

Twitchin, J., *The Black and White Media Book. Handbook for the Study of Racism and Television*, Trentham Books, 1988.

Ward, S., Power, Politics and Poverty, in Golding, P., (ed.), *Excluding the Poor*, CPAG, 1986.

Wagner Report, *Residential Care – A Positive Choice*, Chairman Lady Wagner, NISW, 1988a.

Wagner Report, *Residential Care – The Research Reviewed*, Chairman Lady Wagner, NISW, 1988b.

Women In Mind, *Finding Our Own Solutions – Women's Experiences of Mental Health Care*, WIM, 1990.

Index

Access *see* Physical Disabilities and
    Access
Accreditation of Prior Learning
    (APL) 207
Active Citizen (The) 203–4
Adult Training Centres (ATCs) 103
Advocacy 212   *see also* Self-advocacy
Afro-Caribbean Mental Health
    Association 89
Age Concern 111, 112
Ageism (institutional) 112
AIDS *see* HIV
Alzheimer's disease 53
Anorexia nervosa 133
Anti-disablism 223
Anti-discriminatory language 221
Anti-discriminatory practice 221–4
Anti-racism 221–2
Anti-sexism 223
Anxiety 136
Apartheid 14
Asian people
    definition of 66–7
Assimilation
    of black people 85
Association for Social Care Training 208
Association to Aid the Sexual and
    Personal Relationships of the
    Disabled (SPOD) 143, 246
Asylum 137

BBC 174, 176, 183, 185–7
Benefits
    welfare 7–8, 116–7, 194
Black people 1–3, 64–94, 181, 211
    and crime 164
    definition of 66–7
    and the media 87, 181
    and mental illness 137
    and the penal system 165
    and the police 155
    and social care 87, 211
Black Report *see Inequalities in Health*

Bourgeoisie 15
British Association of Social Workers
    (BASW) 211
British Council of Organizations of
    Disabled People 143

Campaign Against Pornography and
    Censorship (CAPC) 58
Campaign for People with Mental
    Handicap (CMH) 100
Campaign for Press and Broadcasting
    Freedom 185–6
Caravan Sites Act (1968) 122
Carers
    informal x–xi, 5, 53–4, 95–6
    social xi, 7, 130, 191–2
Carers' National Association 209, 225
Care Sector Consortium (NVQ) xv, 206
Caste system 14
Census (national) 17
Certificate in Social Work (CSS) xii
Certificate of Qualification in Social
    Work (CQSW) xii
Charity 203
Child care 50–3, 211
Child minders 52
Child Poverty Action Group
    (CPAG) 26, 111, 193
Children 118–9
Children Act (1989) 212
Chronically Sick and Disabled Persons'
    Act (1970) 144
Church Action on Poverty (CAP) 28,
    193–4
Citizenship 25, 29, 74–5, 217, 224
City and Guilds of London Institute
    (CGLI) xv
Civil Service 3, 15, 42
Class *see* Social class
Clause 28 126, 128, 185, 209
Colonialism 70–2, 93
Commission for Racial Equality
    (CRE) 81–4, 87, 121, 204

Community Care 91, 137–9, 196, 197–200, 224, 227
Community Charge (Poll Tax) 200–2
Council of Europe 50, 167
Crime 151–73
  dark figure of 151–2
  media images of 169
  social class 159
  victims of 153–4, 162
Cutteslow Walls (Oxford) 12

Department of Health 139
Department of Social Security (DSS) 7, 15, 53, 89
Depression 37–8, 132–3, 136
Deviance 151
Diploma in Social Work (Dip. SW) 2
Disability 30   *see also* Physical disability
  models of (individual and social) 140
Disability Alliance 28, 140, 141
Disabled Persons Act (1986) 103, 143
Discrimination 3
  positive 86–7
Down's syndrome 100
Drugs 4, 8
  therapy 135, 137
Dyslexia 99

Education 21, 40
Education Act (1944) (Butler) 21
Education Act (1981) 102
Elders 109–114
Electro-convulsive therapy (ECT) 135, 137
Empowerment 31, 212, 219–20, 227–8
Engels, Friedrich 15
Equality 1–2
  formal 1
  of opportunity 1
  of outcomes 1–2
Equal Opportunities Commission (Manchester) 39, 46, 61, 197, 204
Equal Opportunities Policies 2, 10, 86–7, 128, 204, 211, 223–4
Equal Pay Act (1970) 45–6, 48–50
Ethnic minority
  definition of 66
European Economic Community (EEC) 51, 75, 210

Family Welfare Association (FWA) 193–4, 203
Feminism 45

Gammon (Travellers' language) 119
Gay Liberation Movement 128
Gay men 39, 124–32, 209
Gender 3, 8, 10, 12, 14, 16, 19, 30, 34–63
  and crime 162–4
  processing 36–7
  stereotyping 35
Gingerbread 118
Goldthorpe, John 17–18, 21, 31
Griffiths Report 97, 196–8
Gypsies *see* Travellers

Health and Community Care Act (1990) 199, 212
The Health Care Divide – Inequalities in Health in the 1980s 20–2
Health care workers xiii
Health Education Authority 19, 108
Health Education Council 20
Health Service (NHS) 7, 15, 19, 20, 22, 72, 87–8, 96, 112, 114, 134, 136–9, 199, 212
Help the Aged 112
Heterosexism 125–6
Heterosexuality 125–6
HIV (AIDS) 105–9, 127, 211–2, 221
  definition of 106
Homelessness 139, 195
Home Office 153, 157–8, 163–4
Homophobia 125
Homosexuality *see* Gay men and Lesbians
  definition 125
House of Commons 2, 42, 58
House of Lords 42, 50, 53
Housing 117
Housing Act (1980) 117
Housing Department 15

Ideology 15
Immigration 74–5
Inequality 1–3
  individual 2–4
  structural 2–4, 15, 31
Inequalities in Health (Black Report) 20, 22, 114
Institute for Race Relations 65
Institutionalization 41
Integration
  principle of 99, 227
Ius soli (right of) 75

Joint Council for the Welfare of Immigrants (JCWI) 74–5, 157

Labelling 4, 8
Learning difficulties (people
  with) 97–105, 133, 143, 212
  definition of 100
Lesbians 118, 124–32
Local Government Act (1988) 126, 209
London Charter for Gay and Lesbian
  Rights (1985) 131
Lumpenproletariat 25–6

Manchester Gay Centre 130
Marginalization 3–7, 95–7, 121, 163,
  221
  and gays 127
  and mental illness 134–5
  multiple 95, 121
Marx, Karl 14–16, 25–6, 31
Matriarchy 14
Means of production 15
Media 3, 4, 32, 43, 72, 110, 121, 127,
  144, 146, 148, 164, 169–71, 174–90
Mental handicap *see* Learning difficulties
Mental Health Act (1959) 196
Mental Health Act (1983) 81, 137
Mental illness 100, 131–39, 147–48
  causes of 133–34
  definition of 132

National Association for the Care and
  Resettlement of Offenders
  (NACRO) 164–5, 167
National Association of Local
  Government Officers (NALGO) 54
National Association of Prison Officers
  (NAPO) 126, 165
National Association of Young People in
  Care (NAYPIC) 212
National Council for One Parent
  Families (NCFOPF) 61, 115–8
National Council for Vocational
  Qualifications (NCQV) xv
National Gypsy Council 119
National Health Service Training
  Agency (NHSTA) xv, 206
National Institute for Social Work
  (NISW) 66–7, 197, 206, 211
Nationality Act (1948) 72, 74
Nationality Act (1981) 74–5
National Society for the Prevention of
  Cruelty to Children (NSPCC) 37
National Union of Miners (NUM) 178
National Vocational Qualifications
  (NVQ) xiv–xv, 91, 205–7, 210–14
Neighbourhood watch schemes 153

Normalization
  principle of 99, 104–5, 141
Nursery nurses 39

Official Secrets Act (1911) 185
Outrage 127

Patriarchy 14, 17, 42
Peace convoy 5, 180
Peace Movement 5
Penal system 162–9
Pensioners Link 112
Percy Commission 196
Physical disabilities 139–46
  and access 141–3, 146
  and the media 182
  and mobility 141, 146
  and sex 143–4
'Piss on Pity' 203
Police 42, 54, 57, 75, 79, 154–9, 200
  accountability 159
  culture 155
Police and Criminal Evidence Act
  (1984) 159
Police Complaints Authority 159
Police (Community) Liaison
  Committees 159
Policy Studies Institute (PSI) 155–7
Pornography 57–9, 61
Positive discrimination *see*
  Discrimination
Poverty 5, 10, 22, 28–9, 116, 119, 135,
  160
Prejudice 3, 4, 8, 115
Prevention of Terrorism Act (1984) 185
Prison 139, 154, 165, 166–70
Prison Reform Trust 165
Probation Service 60, 154, 163, 165,
  170, 200
Project 2000 91, 207–8
Proletariat 15
Psychiatric services 134–9
Psychoanalysis 136
Psychotherapy 136

Race 3, 10, 14, 19, 30
  definition of 64
Race Equality Unit (NISW) 197
Racialism
  definition of 65
Racism 64–94, 157, 165, 182
  camouflaged 80–1
  definition of 65
  institutional 80–1, 205

Race Relations Acts (1965, 1968, 1976) 74, 121, 164
Registrar General's Classification of Occupations 16–8, 31, 162
Residential care 197, 210
Right to Buy Legislation (Housing) 24
Rights (Citizen, Legal, Welfare) 224
Romany (language) 119
Royal College of Psychiatrists 138
Rule 43 (prison rules) 169

Schizophrenia 133, 136, 139
Scottish Vocational Qualifications (SVQ) xiv–xv, 206
Section 28 *see* Clause 28
Seebohm Report 22
Self-advocacy 220–1
Sex 34
Sex Discrimination Act (1975) 39, 46, 48–50
Sexism 34–63, 156, 182
Sexual harassment 54–7
Sexual Offences Act (1967) 125–6
Sexual orientation 30, 125–6, 128
Sheffield Men's Awareness Project (SMAP) 59
Shelta (Traveller's language) 119
Sickle cell disease 88
Single parents 4, 113–9
Slavery 14, 68–70, 93
Social care xi–xiv, 2, 7
  and disability 145
  and gay people 130–2
  and HIV (AIDS) 108
  and the media 186
  and travellers 124
Social Care Association (SCA) xiii, 206, 210, 211, 221, 222
Social class 3, 8, 12–33, 159–62, 177
  see also Underclass
Social Education Centres (SECs) 100, 103
Social fund *see also* Benefits 193–4
Socialization 38, 65
Social policy 194–7, 226–7
Social Security Act (1986) 112
Social Services Departments (SSDs) (England and Wales) xi, 15, 53, 59, 87, 91, 96, 103, 112, 138, 186, 199, 201–2, 209
Social work xi–xiv, 2, 7
  and HIV (AIDS) 108

Social Work Departments (SWDs) (Scotland) xi, 15, 59, 60, 103, 112, 163
Social Work (Scotland) Act (1968) xi
SPOD (Association to Aid the Sexual and Personal Relationships of the Disabled) 143
Status 14, 16
Stereotypes 3–5, 35, 37, 97, 140, 170
  and language 4
Stigma/stigmatization 4, 100, 117, 124, 135
'Sus' Law 157
Swann Report (1985) 80, 122

Tagging
  electronic (of offenders) 171
Time Poverty 5–6
Tokenism
  and black people 67–8, 224
Tracking
  of offenders 171
Travellers 119–24, 180

Underclass 13–33, 135–6, 141, 161–2, 192–3, 212, 217
  and the Criminal Justice System 159
Unemployment/Unemployed 7
User-involvement 224–5

Vagrancy Act (1824) 157, 195
Values into Action (VIA) *see* Campaign for People with Mental Handicap (CMH)
Victim Support Schemes 153
Volunteers xi, 153

Wagner Report 89–91, 97–8, 102, 117, 206, 210, 213, 223
Women 16, 18, 34–63
  and depression 136
  and discrimination 47–8
  and elders 112
  and media 180–1
  and the penal system 163–4
  and social care 59–60
  and violence 54–7
Women Against Violence Against Women 45
Women's Aid 45, 57
Women's Movement 45–6
World Health Organization (WHO) 108

Yuppies 23